SD

D1195778

HYPNOSIS AND BEHAVIOR THERAPY

Hypnosis and

Behavior Therapy

Edited by

EDWARD DENGROVE, M.D.

Diplomate, American Board of Psychiatry and Neurology
Former Secretary, The Society for Clinical and Experimental Hypnosis
Representative at Large, Association for
Advancement of Behavior Therapy

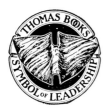

CHARLES C THOMAS • PUBLISHER

Springfield · Illinois · U.S.A.

Published and Distributed Throughout the World by
CHARLES C THOMAS · PUBLISHER
Bannerstone House
301-327 East Lawrence Avenue, Springfield, Illinois, U.S.A.

© *1976, by* CHARLES C THOMAS · PUBLISHER
ISBN 0-398-03336-0
Library of Congress Catalog Card Number: 74–20785

*With THOMAS BOOKS careful attention is given to all details of
manufacturing and design. It is the Publisher's desire to present books
that are satisfactory as to their physical qualities and artistic possibilities
and appropriate for their particular use. THOMAS BOOKS will be true
to those laws of quality that assure a good name and good will.*

Library of Congress Cataloging in Publication Data

Dengrove, Edward.
    Hypnosis and behavior therapy.

    1. Hypnotism—Addresses, essays, lectures.
2. Behavior therapy—Addresses, essays, lectures.
I. Title. [DNLM: 1. Behavior therapy. 2. Hypnosis.
WM415 D392h]
RC497.D44   616.8′916′2   74–20785
ISBN 0–398–03336–6

Printed in the United States of America
Q-1

To Ida,
my lovely and talented wife

CONTRIBUTORS

LEO ALEXANDER, M.D.
Lecturer in Psychiatry, Tufts University Medical School
President, New England Society of Clinical Hypnosis

THEODORE X. BARBER, Ph.D.
Medfield Foundation (Medfield, MA)

ALFRED A. BARRIOS, Ph.D.
Director of the Self-Programmed Control Center (P.O. Box 49939, West Los Angeles, CA)

GUS K. BELL, Ph.D.
Consulting Psychologist to Dede Wallace Mental Health Center and Cumberland House Re-Ed School (Nashville, TN)

JOHN E. BROWN, M.D.
Former Staff Psychiatrist, Veterans Administration Center (Biloxi, MS)

M. LYNN CARROLL, B.A.
Allied Psychological-Psychiatric Services (Philadelphia, PA)

JOSEPH R. CAUTELA, Ph.D.
Professor of Psychology, Boston College, Chestnut Hill (Boston, MA)

WILFRIED DEMOOR, Ph.D.
University of Tilburg (The Netherlands)

EDWARD DENGROVE, M.D.
Former Secretary of the Society for Clinical and Experimental Hypnosis
Representative at Large for Association for Advancement of Behavior Therapy

WILLIAM E. EDMONSTON, JR., Ph.D.
Department of Psychology, Colgate University
President of the American Society of Clinical Hypnosis
Editor, The American Journal of Clinical Hypnosis

J. HARRY FEAMSTER, Ph.D.
Staff Psychologist, Veterans Administration Center, (Biloxi, MS)

PETER B. FIELD, Ph.D.
Director of Research, The Morton Prince Center for Hypnotherapy (New York, NY)

CYRIL M. FRANKS, Ph.D.
Professor of Psychology and Director, Ph.D. Program in Behavioral Clinical Psychology, Graduate School of Applied and Professional Psychology
Rutgers University
Editor, Behavior Therapy
Former President, Association for Advancement of Behavior Therapy

ERIKA FROMM, Ph.D.
Professor, Department of Behavioral Sciences, University of Chicago (Chicago, IL)

BURTON S. GLICK, M.D.
Medical Director, Glen Cove Day Center (Glen Cove, NY)

JOHN HARTLAND, B.Sc., M.B., Ch.B., M.R.S.C., L.R.C.P.
Former President of the British Society of Medical and Dental Hypnosis
Editor, The British Journal of Clinical Hypnosis

SUZANNE L. HOROWITZ, Ph.D.
Psychiatry Clinic, Department of Psychiatry, Stanford University Medical Center (Stanford, CA)

MILTON JABUSH, M.D.
Late Associate Director, Institute for Research in Hypnosis (New York, NY)

ROBERT J. KELLEY, Ph.D.
Behavior Therapy Institute of Colorado (Denver, CO)

MILTON V. KLINE, Ed.D.
Director, Institute for Research in Hypnosis (New York, NY)

SAMUEL H. KRAINES, M.D.
Formerly Assistant Professor of Psychiatry, University of Illinois Medical School (Chicago, IL)

STANLEY KRIPPNER, Ph.D.

Senior Research Associate, Department of Psychiatry, Maimonides Medical Center (Brooklyn, NY)

WILLIAM S. KROGER, M.D.

Executive Director, Institute for Comprehensive Medicine (Beverly Hills, CA)

Consulting Neuropsychiatrist City of Hope Medical Center (Los Angeles, CA)

ARNOLD A. LAZARUS, Ph.D.

Professor of Psychology and Director, Doctor of Psychology Program in Clinical Psychology, Graduate School of Applied and Professional Psychology, Rutgers University (New Brunswick, NJ)

GARY MARSHALL, M.A.

Psychology Department, Stanford University (Stanford, CA)

CHRISTINA MASLACH, Ph.D.

Psychology Department, University of California (Berkeley, CA)

ROBERT G. MEYER, Ph.D.

Associate Professor of Psychology and Director of Psychology Clinic, University of Louisville (Louisville, KY)

A. S. PATERSON, M.D.

Late Physician-In-Charge and Lecturer in the Medical School, Department of Psychiatry, West London Hospital (London, England)

JOHN M. PLAPP, Ph.D.

Hincks Treatment Center (Toronto, Canada)

FRANCES D. ROTHMAN, Ed.D.

Allied Psychological-Psychiatric Services (Philadelphia, PA)

Department of Psychology, St. Joseph's College (Philadelphia, PA)

IRWIN ROTHMAN, V.M.D., D.O.

Psychiatric Director, Allied Psychological-Psychiatric Services (Philadelphia, PA)

Department of Psychiatry, University of Pennsylvania, and Philadelphia College of Osteopathic Medicine (Philadelphia, PA)

MORTON RUBIN, D.O.
Charter Clinical Fellow of the Behavior Therapy and Research Society

JEROME M. SCHNECK, M.D.
Attending Psychiatrist, Division of Psychiatric Training and Education, St. Vincent's Hospital and Medical Center of New York

DAVID L. SCOTT, M.R.C.S., L.R.C.P., D.A., F.F.A.R.C.S.I.
Founder Fellow, British Society of Medical and Dental Hypnosis

NICHOLAS P. SPANOS, Ph.D.
Medfield State Hospital (Medfield, MA)

DOROTHY J. SUSSKIND, Ph.D.
Professor of Educational Psychology, Hunter College (New York, NY)
Former Secretary, Association for Advancement of Behavior Therapy

HARVEY A. TILKER, Ph.D.
Associate Publisher, CRM Books (Del Mar, CA)

FREDERICK J. TODD, Ph.D.
Behavior Therapy Institute of Colorado (Denver, CO)

ANDRE M. WEITZENHOFFER, Ph.D.
Chief Research Psychologist, Psychology Service, Veterans Administration Hospital (Oklahoma City, OK)
Associate Professor of Medical Psychology, University of Oklahoma Health Sciences Center (Oklahoma City, OK)

GREG WHITE, M.A.
Psychology Department, Stanford University (Stanford, CA)

IAN WICKRAMASEKERA, Ph.D.
Assistant Professor of Psychiatry, University of Illinois (Peoria, IL)

PHILIP G. ZIMBARDO, Ph.D.
Department of Psychology, Stanford University (Stanford, CA)

FOREWORD

To TEACH Johnny Latin, it is necessary to know Johnny and Latin: to appreciate the use of hypnosis in behavior therapy, it is necessary to know something about both hypnosis and behavior therapy. Hypnosis is an effective clinical tool; it is not an end in itself. How it is used and to what end will depend upon the orientation of the therapist. For example, a psychoanalyst might use hypnosis to evoke regression to an earlier developmental level, whereas the behavior therapist might employ hypnosis to facilitate relaxation prior to desensitization. And the dentist might use hypnosis as a therapeutically unrelated device for the reduction of sensitivity to pain during treatment.

By contrast, behavior therapy is an established, conceptually independent approach to treatment with an identity of its own and a framework applicable—at least in principle—to any type of disorder falling within the domain of the psychiatrist or clinical psychologist. Behavior therapists—be they psychiatrists or psychologists, practicing clinicians or clinical researchers, working with the seriously disturbed hospitalized patient or the relatively intact outpatient, the individual unit or a complex social structure —all share a common allegiance. This allegiance is to no guru or school, it is to the methodology of the behavioral scientist with its dispassionate and constant evaluation of all theory in the cold light of emerging new data. At present, the emphasis is upon social learning theory, it may not always be so: increasingly, information derived from cognitive and affective sources is being incorporated into the behavioral model.

Modern day behavior therapy, in all its ramifications, is a comprehensive and self-sufficient means of coping with problems in mental health. It is *not* a series of techniques, a grab bag of gimmicks—no matter how effective—which any therapist, regardless of his primary orientation or intent, can more or less readily learn to apply, or have applied by a trained technician, in the limited treatment of certain specific symptoms. Behavior therapy is *not* a salve to be applied topically while the internist gets on with the more basic and lasting job of treating the disease process.

In its early stages—as with many meaningful new points of departure in man's thinking and technology—behavior therapy was inevitably simplistic, focusing upon the direct application of a few principles of classical and operant conditioning to the modification of specific deviant behaviors. From these somewhat naive beginnings, behavior therapy gradually evolved into the multimodal, sophisticated approach to virtually every facet of human functioning that it is today. And as behavior therapy becomes more complex, so do behavior therapists make increasing use of a variety of carefully planned adjunctive techniques and community resources. These include pharmacological agents, environmental intervention and numerous physical devices. Hypnosis falls into this adjunctive category; it is a tool to be used at the appropriate time to facilitate a particular goal.

Hypnosis and Behavior Therapy is ostensibly geared towards, on the one hand, hypnotherapists seeking to know more about behavioral techniques in order to apply them in their practices, and, on the other hand, behavior therapists who utilize hypnosis to facilitate specific goals as part of the overall process of behavior therapy. But, as I have tried to indicate, these two situations are by no means equivalent. To my way of thinking—and I may be wrong—an appreciable majority of hypnotherapists with professional training are primarily dynamically oriented clinicians who make greater or lesser use of hypnosis to facilitate the therapeutic process. They, themselves, would probably not regard the hypnotic process as an end in itself even though—and more about this shortly—they may view the various hypnotic phenomena as manifestations of some form of state or entity.

Unlike hypnosis, behavior therapy constitutes a well studied basis of knowledge with a conceptual framework which can legitimately lay claim to an independent identity. Thus, it makes considerable sense to think in terms of the behavior therapist seeking to know about hypnosis with a view to application in clinical practice or research; it makes less sense to think of somebody called a hypnotherapist seeking to acquire a behavior therapy package to tack on to his therapeutic armamentarium. He may try to do so, of course, in the mistaken belief that behavior therapy is a series of techniques to be readily acquired at a weekend workshop. Were he to acquire these techniques, and even to learn to use some of them with limited success, he would not be practicing behavior therapy in any meaningful sense of the word. It is neither desirable nor possible to be a theoretically eclectic, peripatetic advocate of the occasional use of behavior therapy if one wishes to be known as a "behavior therapist." It is perfectly possible, and even acceptable, for a therapist of any persuasion to use selected behavioral techniques in his or her practice, but it should not then be believed that he or she is practicing behavior therapy. Those who think otherwise do not really understand what behavior therapy is about. Hopefully this book—particularly Edward Dengrove's informative introductory sections—will go a long way towards the correction of this totally false impression of behavior therapy.

This book, then, is not primarily for the hypnotherapist who seeks to acquire a few techniques of behavior therapy. As my worthy friend, Edward Dengrove, has pointed out in the Preface, the behavior therapy literature has continued to neglect both the clinical role of hypnosis in behavior therapy and the contributions it can make to behavioral research. The behavior therapist would do well to consider adding a knowledge of hypnosis to his other skills, and it is primarily to this individual that the present book is directed.

Hypnosis has had its share of charlatans—perhaps more than its share—since its dramatic and potentially flamboyant image first made it a fertile source of exploitation for those seeking to exhibit its "wonders" to a gullible public. For untold eons, magnets had been used for the treatment of disease, with the magnet being regarded as possessing almost magical healing powers. Gradually, the intriguing notion arose that the body possesses magnetic properties of its own. According to the sixteenth century writer, Paracelsus, the human organism possesses two kinds of magnetism: the first attracts the planets and provides us with wisdom, judgment and other psychological attributes; the second attracts more earthly and material elements, producing the somatic aspects of body function. This notion, that there exists a pervasive magnetic principle which controls and accounts for all the interactions between people and natural phenomena, was further developed by leading thinkers, philosophers and scientists of the sixteenth and seventeenth centuries. It provided the fertile climate for the Viennese physician, Franz Mesmer, to write his 1776 doctoral dissertation on "The Influence of the Planets in the Cure of Diseases:" the heavenly bodies acted upon organic matter through the medium of a mysterious life fluid called "animal magnetism." Not long afterwards, Mesmer "discovered" that this animal magnetism, in sharp contrast with mineral magnetism, did not depend upon the use of metallic magnets to achieve its curative powers—the supernatural magnetic properties were within the body and could be transmitted to others by the use of appropriate induction techniques.

In 1774, Mesmer moved to Paris and published a paper announcing the epoch-making discovery of a principle which was capable of curing all diseases. Unfortunately for Mesmer, these claims failed to stand up to the professional scrutiny of his peers, and animal magnetism as a valid scientific principle was justifiably rejected. What was perhaps more unfortunate in the long run was that the data of animal magnetism—the observations which Mesmer documented—were thrown out along with his preposterous theory. It was not until 1841, when James Braid, a British surgeon and scientist of undisputed skill and integrity, came upon the scene, that the phenomena observed by Mesmer achieved scientific respectability. Influenced by Alexandre Bertrand, Braid applied the Greek term for sleep, *hypnos,* to the phenomena documented by Mesmer to denote their artificial, somnambulistic qualities. It was thus that hypnotism very soon achieved both scientific respectability—which was a good thing —and popular acclaim as a kind of eighth wonder of the world— which was probably not such a good thing.

Braid established the first potentially viable theory of hypnosis, explaining the various phenomena not in terms of magical liquids or currents but solely in terms of the physiological impressions made upon the central nervous system by the hypnotist. Out of such beginnings arose the interest in hypnosis as a legitimate field of scientific inquiry and clinical endeavor by neurologists, psychiatrists, psychologists, and others.

At this time, two things are certain: hypnotic phenomena do exist, and hypnosis can work. Its efficacy with selected problems may be undisputable. What does seem to be in dispute is the nature of hypnosis itself: What is hypnosis and why does it work? Traditional explanations attribute hypnosis to some little understood state of consciousness which is fundamentally different from being either asleep or awake. This hypnotic or trance state can be long lasting, with various levels or depths and characteristics which seem to be quite different from those to be found in either the waking or normally sleeping individual. But while such notions are certainly tenable—and many highly respected professionals take them very seriously indeed—the evidence remains equivocal. For example, to the best of my knowledge, no one has successfully demonstrated that the hypnotic trance possesses unique, or even distinctive, physiological concomitants (such as the rapid eye movements associated with dreaming). To recognize the marvels of hypnosis—and quite extraordinary physiological as well as psychological events have been reliably documented to occur while the individual is in the hypnotized condition—is one thing; to assume that this inevitably implies the existence of some underlying hypnotic core state is quite another.

More attractive, at least to the behavior therapist, are explanations in terms of what T. X. Barber calls a *cognitive behavioral viewpoint*. This posits no unique state of hypnosis and regards such terms as *trance induction, hypnotised* and *depth of hypnosis* as superfluous and even misleading. Subject to wide individual differences, the parameters of which are neither fully delineated nor agreed upon, people carry out so-called "hypnotic behaviors" when they have attitudes, motivations, and expectations towards the test situation which lead to a willingness to think and imagine with the theories or instructions that are being suggested.

From this stance, hypnotic phenomena can be understood and manipulated in terms of similar antecedent and mediating variables to those used to explain many other psychological phenomena. While not necessarily implying a facile identity, this point of view would enable us to ferret out elements of congruence between basic procedures in behavior therapy, such as systematic desensitization, and what occurs during "hypnosis." There may well be one or more orthogonal dimensions along which the various phenomena of such seemingly somewhat disparate areas as hypnosis, biofeedback, Yoga, psychedelic drug effects, transcendental meditation and such behavior therapy procedures as systematic densensitization and the Idealized Self Image can be placed. A judicious combination of factor analysis and psychophysiological investigation may well prove fruitful in this respect. Again, I should caution that this does not necessarily imply either identity or downgrading of the significance of any one of these processes.

This cognitive-behavioral point of view is surely of appeal, both intellectually and by inclination, to behavior therapists. The present book should contribute in no small measure to the ordered integration of the various hypnotic phenomena into the cognitive social learning system of the contemporary behavior therapist. Each of the papers in this innovative compendium has been selected by Dengrove with this goal in mind even when the use of hypnosis as presented by the author concerned is essentially nonbehavioral. Skillfully, the reader is led from an overview and discussion of basic concepts in behavior therapy and hypnosis in the first section of this book to the clinical and research application of both strategies in a variety of diverse situations.

While I do not share all Dengrove's views about either hypnosis or behavior therapy—what a sorry world it would be if we all thought alike or if Foreword writers were not permitted to be forward looking!—I can not but be impressed with the consummate skill and experience with which he has gathered together this comprehensive array of papers, and the acumen with which he has welded these diverse offerings into a meaningful and valuable whole. It fills a definite gap in the professional literature, and both he and the publisher are to be congratulated for their foresight in embarking upon this long overdue venture.

Cyril M. Franks, Ph.D.
Graduate School of Applied and
    Professional Psychology
Rutgers University
New Brunswick, New Jersey 08903

PREFACE

WHEN Payne Thomas asked me to edit a book on hypnosis and behavior therapy, I thought: (1) Why me? (2) With so many books on the market, is such a book needed? (3) With so much literature scattered in the field should this book be written from scratch, or edited from the existing literature?

Why Me? I have straddled both fields for a good many years. For two years I was Secretary of The Society for Clinical and Experimental Hypnosis, and an interest in hypnotherapy, together with its use, has been present ever since I began to practice psychiatry. My affinity toward behavior therapy extends back to the days of my psychiatric residency when behavioral techniques were used without awareness of the behavior therapy or modification fields. In time, this interest led me to become a co-founder of the *Association for Advancement of Behavior Therapy* (in those days it was called "Behavioral Therapies") and subsequently to becoming News and Notes Editor of *Behavior Therapy* from its inception in 1970. So why not me?

Why publish this book at all? At first, hypnosis was seriously considered to be a worthy preliminary to desensitization, then the experimenters determined that it was not a necessary component of this type of therapy. Thereafter, the behavior therapy literature de-emphasized the role of hypnosis, probably because so few persons took the time to be properly trained and/or did not have either the expertise or the confidence to use hypnotic techniques as an adjunctive therapy. It now seems to be dropped from the armamentarium of the behavior therapist, except for its use by an occasional enthusiast, such as myself.

This de-emphasis of hypnosis misses the point, for hypnosis has an important, though not indispensable, role in the practice of behavior therapy. Properly used, it adds leverage to treatment and shortens treatment time. Hypnosis accelerates the production of relaxation, and the patient can practice self-hypnosis at home; hypnotic vivification can be used to intensify visual images; time distortion techniques reassure him; hypnotic dream induction has proven of value; post-hypnotic suggestions reduce subsequent fears and motivate him to continue making contact with the feared object, situation or feeling, on a regular basis.

In contrast to this neglect of hypnosis by many behavior therapists, hypnotherapists have been flocking to the use of behavior therapy techniques. This is natural, since hypnotherapists have been using them for ages, although not in such a well-organized form nor as intensely researched as in behavior therapy. The hypnotherapist has much to gain by systematically learning behavior therapy techniques.

To answer the third question, whether this book should have been written from scratch or edited from the existing literature, it is clear that, collectively, the experts in both fields have said far more than I could possibly say and have said it much better. It thus became a matter of primarily searching out the literature, which I had already been doing for years. In addition, I decided to invite other experts to write articles on aspects of the subject that did not seem to have been properly covered in the existing literature.

The articles contained herein have something for everyone. The experimentalist has proof that hypnosis adds something extra to the process of conditionability, the behavior therapist is given a better understanding of the hypnotic techniques he can use to accelerate therapy and shorten treatment time, the hypnotherapist is shown a more ordered approach to the use of behavioral techniques, which he has already been using for some time.

I acknowledge with gratitude the help I received from Cyril M. Franks, editor of *Behavior Therapy*. Without his aid my job would have been much more difficult. His interest and encouragement have immeasurably eased the path. My whole-hearted thanks to my contributors without whom there would have been no book, and particularly to those workers who have written original articles to make *Hypnosis and Behavior Therapy* more complete. Lastly, I wish to thank my son and editorial assistant, Robert Dengrove—now a physician in his own right—whose comments and criticisms sharpened my own thinking.

E. D.

CONTENTS

USES OF BEHAVIOR THERAPY IN HYPNOSIS

HYPNOSIS AND BEHAVIOR THERAPY

SECTION 1

BASIC CONCEPTS

SECTION 1

INTRODUCTION

THIS INTRODUCTORY SECTION is written, on the one hand, for those hypnotherapists less well-acquainted with the principles of behavior therapy, and on the other, for those behavior therapists with an insufficient grasp of hypnosis. The intent is not to provide an exhaustive treatise on these subjects, the subject matter being limited primarily to information relevant to the purposes of this book.

For the hypnotherapist, there is a brief survey of the principal approaches and uses of behavioral techniques, emphasizing those problems most likely to be encountered in the practice of behavior therapy. For the behavior therapist, there is a chapter delineating the basic elements of hypnosis, a survey of the literature on hypnosis (suggestion) and behavior therapy, and a short review of the uses of hypnosis in behavior therapy.

CHAPTER 1

BEHAVIOR THERAPY

Edward Dengrove, M.D.

THIS CHAPTER IS DIRECTED toward the therapist with little experience of the principles and techniques of behavior therapy.

Behavior therapy consists of a number of treatment methods derived from research in experimental and social psychology, stressing the application of learning and conditioning principles, both classical and operant, and the methodological rigor of the behavioral scientist. These techniques constitute a break with traditional insight therapy, emphasizing behavior rather than personality review and change. They do not handle so-called unconscious dynamic factors; the symptoms, or behavior as a whole, are considered the disease, but cognizance is taken of the person behind the symptom, and consideration is given to values, attitudes, and beliefs. Neurosis is defined (Wolpe, 1958) as learned behavior that is persistent and unadaptive, and which is acquired in anxiety-generating situations. Historically, symptoms arise by training or trauma, by purpose or accident, during the life span of the individual who is more or less predisposed toward them.

Among the treatment methods are listed systematic desensitization; active, graded therapy; assertive techniques; sexual responses; and numerous others. These are preceded by a proper behavioral diagnosis (Dengrove, 1972b) in order to "target in" upon the symptom.

BEHAVIORAL DIAGNOSIS

Taking a patient's history is essential to a behavioral diagnosis. The patient's complaints are sought and found in the manner usually accomplished by a competent psychotherapist, and his past and personal history are recorded so that a better idea of the patient may be formed. A list of fears is then requested. Some behavior therapists utilize a Fear Survey (Wolpe and Lazarus,

1966) or other questionnaire. I often ask for an autobiography of undetermined length, to help fill in the gaps.

A behavioral diagnosis is unique in that it "targets in" upon the source of the presenting symptom and its reinforcing elements.

> An executive who stuttered excessively while dictating to his stenographer changed his stenographer, but to no avail. When asked to close his eyes and reconstruct the scene, he concluded that it was not the stenographer who caused him to become tense, but the fact that what he was saying was being made a matter of public record and he would be held accountable for it. Desensitization was directed thereafter to his concern for his stated words.

A useful technique for identifying source and reinforcement of a symptom or behavior is letter association (Dengrove, 1962).

> The patient is asked to sit back in the chair and relax, to close his eyes and think of a particular symptom, to relate it to the last setting or event (or the first, or any) in which it was felt, and to attempt to relive or reconstruct—to whatever extent is possible—the feeling tone of the complaint. He is then asked to give the very first letter that comes to mind, then the next one. When five letters are noted —the number is arbitrary—they are listed vertically in order. At this point the patient is allowed to open his eyes if he wishes; he is requested to give the first word—again only the first one—that comes to mind and which begins with each of the letters previously chosen. He is to make up sentences using each word or freely to associate the words. In the majority of instances one is able to pinpoint the immediate cause of the symptom or to trace it back to its source.

SYSTEMATIC DESENSITIZATION

Systematic desensitization (Wolpe, 1968a) is a process of relearning whereby, in the presence of an anxiety-evoking stimulus, a nonanxiety-producing response is continually repeated until it extinguishes the old, undesirable response. The various treatment methods based upon this principal usually have four components:

1. Contact with the feared object, situation or feeling.
2. A graduated approach to this contact.
3. Motivation of the patient to make this contact on a regular basis.
4. Fear reduction—induced by reassurance, relaxation training, medication, distraction, hypnosis, or other technical means.

Systematic desensitization is achieved through visual imagery in the doctor's office; in this process the patient lives through his fears and anxieties while in a relaxed state. Active, graded therapy requires contact with the feared object, situation, or feeling in a realistic manner.

A complete list of fears is secured from the patient and anxiety hierarchies are set up for each one. A hierarchy is a list of stimuli to which the patient reacts with anxiety, from the least disturbing to the most frightening.

> For instance, to the woman who is afraid to leave the house, the least disturbing stimulus would be just looking out of the widow or opening the door and putting out one foot. The most frightening would be walking about town freely. Relaxational methods are then taught, using hypnosis, a modified Jacobson technique (Wolpe, 1958; Wolpe, 1961; Wolpe and Lazarus, 1966) of differential relaxation of various muscle groups, medication, or other means. Only when she is completely at ease will treatment be effective. As she lies on the couch or sits in the chair with her eyes closed and at peace with herself, the least anxiety provoking stimulus from the hierarchy is presented to her visual imagination. For instance, she is asked to visualize herself looking out the window of her home. If she retains her composure and continues at ease while viewing the scene, she informs us by a signal that it is not disturbing to her. She may have been asked to raise her hand slightly or to move her head a bit, up and down for yes, side to side for no; not enough to disturb her equanimity. The next stimulus on the list is then presented. She is asked to view herself putting a foot out of the door; then to walking a few steps; to view herself walking to the street in front of her house; to walking on the street as far as the house next door; and so on. If there is anxiety at any one presentation, she is asked to view the preceding scene, which she can do again with greater ease. At this point the session is terminated, although a number of fears may be so handled in one session. At the next session, the desensitization process starts with the last item that did not evoke anxiety at the previous meeting, and treatment moves ahead from there. In the interim, the general level of anxiety has apparently diminished so that she can cope with further elements in the hierarchy. Transfer of the relief from anxiety in these fixed situations to real life situations occurs.

Psychological desensitization is much like chemical desensitization for an allergic disorder, wherein the patient is injected with minute quantities of the allergen and gradually exposed to larger and larger doses until he or she is able to cope with the natural environment. As a rule, there is an acceleration of progress as one moves along.

In active, graded therapy, real-life approaches are made to the feared feeling, object, or situation.

> Consider the child who is afraid of dogs. The child is held by a trusted person who allows him to suck on a lollipop (food is used as a counter to anxiety also) and points to a dog on a leash in the distance. A little later, the child, still held, is encouraged to view a dog through a pet-shop window. Still later, he is brought closer to a dog; and later, closer still. With the pleasure of the food and the security of being held by a trusted person, the child gradually experiences a reduction of his fear. One may use pictures of dogs or toy dogs at first, gradually progressing to small, friendly dogs and then to medium-sized dogs. In the end, the child is able to reach out and touch a dog.

One must do the very things that one fears. A fear cannot be overcome by avoiding it, nor by trying to drown it out with continued medication. Medicine, while useful, is to be reduced gradually and finally discarded. Avoiding the phobic situation or object only perpetuates the fear by reinforcement of the escape response. So, while giving the patient the tranquilizer or sedative, insist that he or she make attempts toward overcoming the fears, in a graduated fashion and with reassurance, persuasion, or the security of your presence.

The patient is not expected to attempt any activity that produces overwhelming anxiety. But he is encouraged to try tasks that are mildly upsetting, at the same time attempting to quiet himself. If the anxiety persists, he is to stop what he is doing, for this will only set him back. Instead, he is to return to doing those things that he can do without getting upset. The patient is exposed at first only to those fears he can cope with, gradually increasing contact with those productive of more and more anxiety. One can get accustomed to almost any new situation that is approached gradually.

Interestingly, as the milder fears are overcome, the more disturbing ones concurrently lose their intensity. However, the patient must proceed at his own pace; he is assured that there is no reason to feel guilt or shame if progress is slow. At times, under pressure of need or anger, large strides are made, but this is the exception. Sometimes it is only after the patient has completed an activity that he realizes what he has accomplished without apprehension or anxiety.

ASSERTIVE RESPONSES

Some patients fear to raise their voices to the therapist, or to swear even mildly, or to express anger in any form. Such patients are encouraged to shout or scream; to swear, first without looking at the therapist and then looking at him; to smash his fist into the couch or on the arm of the chair. In effect, the patient is taught to express his anger toward the authoritative figure of the therapist. Of course there are limits to how much can be expressed outwardly, but at least the patient can allow himself to feel the anger and not repress or suppress it. The learned freedom is carried over to real life. The patient is made happier and more capable by this character change.

Wolpe and Lazarus (1966) emphasize that, although the most common class of assertive responses involved in therapeutic action is the expression of anger and resentment, the term "assertive behavior" is used broadly to cover all socially acceptable expression of personal rights and feelings. A polite refusal to accede to an unreasonable request; a genuine expression of praise, endearment, appreciation, or respect; an exclamation of joy, irritation, adulation, or disgust—all may be considered examples of assertive behavior. Diminishing the object of fear by poking fun at it also makes it easier to overcome. Making fun of one's emotional responses will do the same. The "paradoxical intention" of Frankl (1960) is based upon this type of approach.

SEXUAL RESPONSES

Learning to relax during coitus is another shortcut to overcoming impotence and, often, frigidity. Wolpe's method (1958), which has been particularly effective in many cases of impotence, consists of teaching the patient to relax in the act and not become anxious over inability to produce an erection. The wife is told not to expect performance on her husband's part for a while; partners are just to caress and enjoy each other, whatever the outcome. When the man no longer feels that he is *obliged* to perform, he discovers that he is able to do so once again. No effort is made to work through long periods of life history. Of course there are some situations in which impotence is due to lack of love and the lack of real interest in the spouse, but in the absence of this, many patients will respond successfully to this simple Wolpeian approach within two to six sessions.

AVERSIVE TECHNIQUES

Aversive stimuli (e.g. electrical, chemical, noise) have been used to modify behavior for many years, in real life situations, imaginary ones, and under hypnosis. They may be used to decrease the probability of a response, as in punishment; or to increase the probability of a response by removing the aversive stimulus, as in negative reinforcement (e.g. aversion relief).

The use of punishment to modify behavior sometimes is self-defeating. When punishment is not closely related to its cause, the corrective value is lost altogether. If too mild, the inhibiting punishing stimulus is not effective. If it is too severe, a nonspecific anxiety or fear state may occur so that all behavior leading to reward is inhibited.

Aversion relief (Dengrove, 1972a) may function as a distraction, as in thought block, to teach the patient ways of overcoming obsessive thoughts. The patient at first is taught to escape from the effect of an aversive stimulus, i.e. electrical shock, by changing a "bad thought" to a "good" one; then allowed to avoid the aversive stimulus altogether by changing to a "good thought" before a shock is applied. In this way he learns how to dispense with unwanted and unnecessary ideas, which is highly useful in treating obsessive-compulsive behavior and sexually deviant disorders.

Some thought must be given to matching the appropriate aversive stimulus to the particular sensory modality under treatment (Lazarus, 1968b). For instance, electric shocks are usually less effective in reducing addiction to alcohol and food, than unpleasant olfactory and gustatory stimuli; the reverse is often true in treating trichotillomania (i.e. an uncontrollable impulse to pull out one's hair).

Another aversive technique is time-out, usually employed with children suffering from conduct disorders. When the child is obstreperous and out-of-hand, swift removal from the group for a short period of time may be very effective in altering his behavior.

The ball and pad technique (Mowrer and Mowrer, 1938; Lovibond, 1964) has been moderately successful in conditioning against enuresis. When a few drops of urine strike a specially prepared electrical pad a noisy signal and/or bright light suddenly awakens the child so that he can go to the bathroom on his own volition.

Cautela (see article later) employs a similar but imaginary technique, "covert sensitization," which is used to produce aversion to certain foods, alcohol, tobacco, or sexual deviation. The scenes and responses may be vivified through hypnosis.

When aversive conditioning is employed, some basic principles must be strictly adhered to (Franks, 1966b):

1. The unconditional stimulus (the inherently aversive stimulus) and the conditional stimulus (a previously neutral stimulus which is intended to become aversive) must be amenable to exact control with respect to their intensity, duration, and precise time for onset and cessation. It is important that exposure to the stimulus have a rapid onset.

2. The conditional stimulus (CS) must precede the unconditional stimulus (UCS) and the interval between them must be precisely determinable and amenable to control.

3. Trials (pairings between the CS and the UCS) should be distributed over a longer period of time rather than massed. Therapeutically, the same number of pairings are more effective spaced out over time rather than carried out during short periods.

4. It is unnecessary for the UCS to have an excessively high level of intensity; a moderately aversive stimulus may be as, or more, effective.

5. The effect of conditioning tends to persist longer if a partial or random reinforcement schedule is followed. Instead of having the UCS follow every presentation of the CS, it is best to have it follow most but not all trials. It also helps to vary the time interval between trials.

6. The situation in which training is undertaken should be both realistic and as variable as possible, with the CS being easily discerned from other stimuli in the situation.

OTHER TECHNIQUES OF BEHAVIOR THERAPY

There are many other techniques that are available to the behavior therapist, the number limited only by the ingenuity of the therapist.

Flooding is the continued exposure of the patient to the phobic situation until anxiety and avoidance responses are extinguished. This exposure is greatly facilitated when carried out in real life situations rather than in fantasy (Marks, 1973); prolonged flooding in practice significantly reduces phobias (Marks, 1972; Stern and Marks, 1973). However, it may be that patients improve rapidly during *in vivo* treatment only after previous exposure in fantasy (Matthews and Gelder, 1974).

Behavior modification, involving operant techniques (Agras, 1972; Leitenberg, 1972) derived from Skinnerian research, embodies the psychology of positive and negative reinforcement with schedules of reinforcement. Emphasis is placed upon responses rather than stimuli; the consequences of an act determine the behavior, and by altering the response, behavioral change occurs. By applying selective positive reinforcement until the desired response is obtained, behavior is shaped; by removal of reinforcement, extinction occurs; by using aversive procedures, the subject is punished, or learns to escape or avoid certain behaviors. Token economies (Ayllon and Roberts, 1972) are special applications of reinforcement and extinction procedures applied to a group in a controlled environment, as in a hospital, ward, or classroom.

Self-reinforcement (Bandura, 1969), a crucial element of homework, frequently outweighs the influence of externally imposed systems of reinforcement in governing social behavior, particularly in the case of older children and adults. Modeling processes play a highly influential role in the transmission of self-monitored reinforcement patterns, together with imitation and role playing, and can, in fact, maintain behavior.

Massed or negative practice (Lehner, 1960), derived from the work of Dunlap (1932), has been used in the treatment of tics, stuttering, and other personal habits. The subject is required to repeat the action or word over and over again with no or very little time interval between repetitions. Dunlap found that practicing certain previously "wrong" responses led to the dropping out of these responses.

MULTIMODAL BEHAVIOR THERAPY

Lazarus (1973), who considers himself a "technical eclectic," insists that an effective therapist must have an armamentarium of scientifically derived skills and techniques to supplement his effective interpersonal relations. He states that lasting change is at the very least a function of combined techniques, strategies and modalities. He describes seven interdependent and interactive modalities (his BASIC ID) to which attention must be directed for proper treatment of the patient: Every patient-therapist interaction involves *behavior* (be it lying down on a couch and free associating, or actively role playing a significant encounter), *affect* (be it the silent joy of nonjudgmental acceptance, or the sobbing release of pent-up anger), *sensation* (which covers a wide range of sensory stimuli from the spontaneous awareness of bodily discomfort to the deliberate cultivation of specific sensual delights), *imagery* (be it the fleeting glimpse of a childhood memory, or the contrived perception of a calm-producing scene), and *cognition* (the insights, philosophies, ideas, and judgments that constitute our fundamental values, attitudes and beliefs). All of these take place within the context of an *interpersonal* relationship, or various interpersonal relationships. An added dimension with many patients is their need for medication or *drugs* (e.g. phenothiazine derivatives and various antidepressants and mood regulators).

SYMPTOM SUBSTITUTION

It has been my experience in the years during which I have used these techniques that symptom substitution or replacement does not occur if the underlying base for the symptom is no longer operative. Spiegel (1967) states that symptom removal is not dangerous if the therapist is not inept and does not convey expectations of harm to a sensitive, pliant patient. Lazarus (1971) found only the most tenuous indications of "symptom substitution" in a detailed and systematic follow-up inquiry of 112 cases. Yates (1970), Ullmann and Krasner (1967), and Rachman (1968) find symptom substitution a relatively rare event. Franks (1969) points out that, even within a Pavlovian framework, treating the "symptom" alone without also attempting to remedy the central pathology could result in response substitution. Bandura (1969), however, declares that the problem of deviant response substitution can be easily forestalled by including in the original treatment program procedures that effectively remove the reinforcing conditions which sustain deviant behavior and concurrently foster desirable alternative modes of behavior. These not only produce enduring changes in the selected direction, but may also set in motion beneficial changes in related areas of psychological functioning.

THE USES OF BEHAVIOR THERAPY

Initially, behavioral techniques were successfully used to treat phobic disorders. A review of the now voluminous literature, however, reveals extensive applications to many other disorders, together with a variety of treatment methods derived from experimental psychology. Behavior therapy is being used to treat anxiety reactions, depressive reactions and grief states, jealousy, obsessive-compulsive disorders, psychosomatic illnesses, sexual difficulties, study blocks, and numerous other psychological disorders from simple habit disorders to behavior problems in psychotic states. Often, one defines the basic phobic unit, which is the lowest common denominator, and desensitizes to it; the phobic concept is not limited to fear of objects, situations or feelings, but includes social fears, i.e. fear of inadequacy, criticism, or rejection.

CLINICAL PROBLEMS

No therapeutic approach is without difficulties that challenge the alert and inventive therapist. The following problems are illustrative.

Improper Behavioral Diagnosis

Without correct identification of the relevant stimulus elements, one may expend a great deal of time and effort without result.

Stevenson and Hain (1967) insist that one does not consider merely a specific phobia; for example, fear of barber shop. There may be a dread of scrutiny by others, a rebelliousness against social customs, impatience with delays, aversion to confinement, fear of mutilation, anxiety-arousing experiences with chairs resembling barber chairs; sexual arousal; issues of seniority; and other explanations for the phobia—a multiplicity of stimuli that touch off the central response.

The presence of historically earlier sources of anxiety, according to Meyer and Crisp (1966), may complicate recovery until ferreted out. Clarke (1968) has shown that relearning, too, will fade if it is not reinforced. Lazarus and Serber (1968) concede that maladaptive behavior may not be due to anxiety, but to naiveté or poor verbal skills; therapy therefore aims not at desensitization but at re-education, modeling, and practice. Other instances they cite include complaints secondary to psychotic processes that respond to antipsychotic medication, and phobic disorders in patients suffering with depression who are better treated with antidepressant medication or by advice to secure employment, invitation to join a supportive therapeutic group, and training to develop assertive response.

Difficulties in Relaxation

Relaxation is probably indispensable to success in most cases using systematic desensitization, but the method used to relax the patient is not so important as the depth of relaxation it produces. An effective criterion of adequacy of depth for purposes of desensitization is the patient's subjective estimation. The patient must feel not partially or nearly relaxed, but completely so. Wolpe (personal communication) asks a patient to imagine a situation in which he has felt panic and to label this "100." Then he is asked to imagine a situation in which he has felt most calm and at ease, and to label this "0." The percentage of relaxation must be over 85 percent to be effective for desensitization.

> It is my custom to ask a patient to nod his head up and down or side to side in answer to the question, "Do you feel relaxed. Are you at ease?" Often, if I am not sure of the answer, I will add, "Are you completely relaxed, completely at ease?" Interestingly, these may differ, the patient nodding yes to the former and no to the latter. I have found, too, that when a patient indicates he is still not at ease, it is most helpful to ask him to put himself at ease, without further suggestions from myself, over the next few minutes. Often this is effective.

> Sometimes progress is slowed because the patient indicates that he is relaxed when he is really only resting, i.e. merely lying still but with continuing muscular tension. A greater difficulty lies with patients whose bodies are relaxed but who remain obsessed with trying to retain control.

Difficulties in Application of the Hierarchies

Lazarus (1968a) comments: "The patient may not be picturing the scenes described; he may fail to signal anxiety only because the time interval is too short to permit vivid imagery; he may introduce extraneous variables without the therapist's knowledge; he may experience immediate associations of which the therapist ought to be aware; and so forth . . ."

I have found an occasional patient whose facile mind races ahead, and although he is not anxious about the scene being presented, he is disturbed by the scene he is associating on his own; he anticipates me. A minority of patients do not experience anxiety at all when they imagine situations that in reality are disturbing (Wolpe, 1958, Wolpe, 1961). In some of these patients, anxiety can be evoked when they are asked to describe the scene they imagine (Jaspers, 1963). Others may have to resort to active, graded desensitization.

Differences in Individual Conditionability

Phobic conditions are seen in three separate groups of patients: obsessive-compulsives, schizoid, and post-traumatic. The obsessive-compulsive perfectionistic pattern is the most common and the most intensively affected. These people are neat, systematic, conscientious, orderly, concerned that everything should be in its right place and that there is a right place for everything. They want to please everyone excepting their spouse. Feelings of inadequacy are always present. Assertive techniques and role playing are utilized in order to develop an increased self-confidence, less perfectionism, ability to cope with dominant people, and an "I don't really care" attitude.

The schizoid personality develops phobic complaints within a pansymptomatic picture, the central issue being an inner helplessness and difficulty in coping with hostile feelings. Desensitization to both are necessary, assisted by therapeutic group techniques.

Other Means of Systematic Desensitization

When a patient cannot be sufficiently relaxed for systematic desensitization to take place, other means of countering the phobic anxiety must be employed. Sexual and assertive feelings are often used together with a variety of techniques limited only by the ingenuity of the therapist.

> Lazarus (1965; 1966) used anger as a counterdevice in systematic desensitization. In place of relaxation, his patients overcame each item in the hierarchy by an angry response. He also reported the use of directed muscular activity, such as pounding one's hands against a padded stool. With children, he and Abramovitz (1962) employed a process of visual imagery, with the child incorporating his phobic symptoms into a fantasy situation, using the hero to overcome the feared object. Similar techniques (Lazarus, 1968a), using emotive or assertive imagery and cognitive variables, have been employed with adults. I have found it of value, where relaxation is insufficient, to ask the patient to signal me when he is taking his fearful situation "in stride," rather than being completely without anxiety; or to visualize himself helping others in similar situations and being constructively useful. Some situations (e.g. sexual ones) do not call for relaxed responses, but for pleasurable ones.

The literature of behavior therapy is filled with the inventiveness of therapists who have devised ways to get around the relaxational barrier. Whatever method is used, however, must reduce fear from one session to the next one.

Faith, Trust, and Expectation: The Placebo Effect

The patient comes to the therapist expecting help and motivated toward getting better. Beacher (1959) has pointed out that 35.2 ($\pm$ 2.2) percent of patients are placebo reactors and that placebo reactivity is directly related to experienced distress or suffering. Wolf (1962) considers this the effect of meaningful situations, whereas Gantt, Newton, Royer, and Stephens (1966) credit a positive expectancy reaction. Truax (1966) points out that therapists who are low in communicated empathy, nonpossessive warmth, and genuineness are ineffective. Lazarus (1968c) enhances therapeutic potency by adding structure to the usual behavior therapy framework. Leitenberg, Agras, Thompson and Wright (1968) maintain improvement by feeding back information as to the patient's progress in treatment.

Anticipation or the Fear-of-Fear Itself Phenomenon

There is a difference between the fear of an object or situation and fearful anticipation of them. It is the difference between the armed bandit actually pointing the gun at you, and your expectation that you might be held up. In the former, one is actually faced with the threat; in the latter, it may never happen.

> Often a patient will say that it is not the actual happening of an event that bothers her but the worry about it ahead of time. As one woman related, "I worried and worried about it, but when I finally forced myself to go there, it wasn't at all what I thought. I got along fine." Many of us have undergone similar experiences when taking examinations; yet once we were engaged in writing the examination, we quieted down. We had somewhere to go with our aroused state, and provided we had done our work beforehand, we could concentrate on the task at hand with a certain amount of equanimity. Frequently the task is to convince the patient to make the try.

MacLean (1967) relates expectation to the brain's electrical activity. A slow, negative shift in potential builds up in the frontal cortex and does not collapse until the subject has made a decision. Goldstein (1964) characterizes individuals by their mode of response, some responding chiefly by means of the autonomic nervous system, some by muscle tension, and others with overt muscle activity. Autonomic components are often the only discernible symptoms in neurotics.

> One needs to desensitize not only to the act, but to anticipation of the act, as a separate hierarchy. I attempt to decondition the patient to anxiety by having him feel fright; open his eyes widely, suck in air, and hold his breath in an inspiratory position, urging him to re-experience the feeling of dread as much as possible. Imitation of anxiety responses must be actually felt. Additionally, the patient is made aware of the heart beat, and assisted in becoming used to the visceral sensations, to accept the inevitable and say "to Hell with it!" Operant techniques (Gavalas, 1967) may be used to reinforce autonomic responses. Sometimes the anticipation takes on an obsessive quality, at which time we must revert to thought-blocking procedures (Dengrove, 1972a) or aversion relief methods (Solyom, Kenny, and Ledwidge, 1969).

Delay or Inability to Transfer Improvement from Office to Real Life

The difficulty carrying over improvement to everyday real life results from problems involving behavioral diagnosis and motivation.

> A twenty-year-old woman was doing well in the office with systematic desensitization to her fears of walking and driving from her home, whereas elsewhere she had made no progress at all. Asking her to make attempts in real life produced only excuse after excuse during each session as to why it had been impossible for her to do anything that week. She had an anticipatory fear response, of such degree that she would not make the slightest attempt, even with help. Further diagnostic exploration revealed her fear that if she were free to come and go as she pleased, she would simply go and not return. She had no respect for her immature husband, yet feared to give up her kind of life.

There are cases in which there is no solution to a conflict of conscience, in which secondary gain outweighs the pain of the neurotic solution and inhibits the danger of psychotic breakdown. When patients are making out reasonably well with monies received from insurance schemes, treatment may become well nigh impossible. The passive-dependent personality is only too happy to retire from the stresses and strains of competition and responsibility. When pressed, even lightly, the symptoms simply return or are aggravated.

Stevenson (1962) instructs a patient not to come for her next appointment unless she drives alone, or insists that a timid woman not call for her next appointment until she has discussed a feared operation with a surgeon, or offers a fee reduction to another patient if she will discuss her annoyance directly with her mother-in-law. He, himself, began riding elevators with a woman who feared doing so. The latter active, graded therapy, or *in vivo* training, is an important addition to systematic desensitization, and often the patient can be led to make attempts outside the office in a gradual manner.

Avoidance of Setbacks During Treatment

Relapses occur when the patient is pushed too fast, the phobic situation is reinforced, or a general overall increase in anxiety occurs. In a study of speed of generalization in systematic desensitization, Rachman (1966) showed that reductions in fear from imaginal to real-life situations occur almost immediately. Relapses, however, occurred in slightly less than 50 percent of the occasions tested during the succeeding hours and days. Though his experiments were conducted under limited test conditions, the need for reinforcement was indicated.

Gelder and Marks (1966) note that single panic attacks, whatever the reason, may undo the effects of weeks of treatment, and if less severe attacks of anxiety are repeated, the fear may also be relearned. Much of the skill of behavior therapy, they add, lies in tracing environmental causes for these unexplained attacks of panic.

> A male patient had a recurrence of fear in church. After four Sundays without difficulty, he again began to sweat and shake. It was quite hot in church, and he had started to sweat, which temporarily reinstituted his phobia.

According to Franks (1966a) two possible ways to cope with relapses are either to develop new counter conditioning techniques that minimize regression or to provide "booster" follow-up conditioning sessions.

Recurrence of Symptoms after a Lapse of Time

The return of symptoms is probably due to new situations rather than to reinforcement of old fears.

One of the first patients whom I treated with systematic desensitization was a woman in her early forties. She had suffered a phobic state for about twelve years. When treated with systematic desensitization, she progressed to a point where she could travel, not only from her home, but also to great distances. After a lapse of several years, she phoned for an appointment. She was frightened; her symptoms had returned. Examination, however, proved her alarm to be unfounded. She was suffering from some of the symptoms of menopause, had mistaken them for the return of her previous illness, and had panicked. Reassurance and estrogens limited her visits to one. She phoned to say that she was her renewed self again.

Another young woman who returned after a lapse of time had developed symptoms due to a fear that had not shown itself previously because she had had no occasion to encounter it. Treatment with systematic desensitization rapidly returned her to a symptom-free state.

The Importance of Concurrent Physical and Interpersonal Problems

Any circumstances that increase the general level of anxiety may delay progress (Rachman, 1968). Concern over physical disorders, justified or not, inhibits systematic desensitization. A doctor does not wish to overlook an undiagnosed physical disorder because of a mistaken notion that the basic trouble is a psychological disease.

When a patient complains of attacks of panic, with feelings of faintness, numbness, dread, perhaps chest and head tightness, and the like, one must give immediate thought to the hyperventilation syndrome. Having the patient breathe rapidly, with forceful expiration for one minute in the office quickly reproduces the same effects and reassures the patient. She is advised that all she needs to do to control these symptoms is to slow down her breathing, breathe into a paper bag, or take a sedative. Many symptoms of gas (eructations, borborygmi, abdominal pains, and spasms) are explained on the basis of throat tension, muscle spasm, or air swallowing. For patients who panic when their bodies tremble or shake without control, reassurance to allow the shaking to take place is often sufficient.

As to interpersonal obstacles in treatment, I advise patients that an understanding and cooperative spouse is not only helpful but also an essential part of treatment. Marital problems tend to retard progress and should be resolved.

Timidity and depression have an adverse effect on prognosis (Marks, 1967) by diminishing initiative. "Triers" do better because they encounter more opportunities to relearn and to adapt than patients who passively sit back and wait for things to happen to them. Paranoid irritability does not appear to affect prognosis. The presence of high anxiety (Rachman, 1968) impedes or entirely prevents the progress of systematic desensitization.

> Lazarus (1966) emphasizes the part played by others in the persistence of a symptom. In one instance he had to call in the patient's husband and mother and inform them that they were reinforcing the patient's dependency by displaying concern and expressing reassurance whenever she complained of minor somatic discomfort. They were requested not to pay attention to these negative statements, but to reward by attention, encouragement, and approval all positive self-reference and independent responses. He states that it is presumably impossible to become an agoraphobic without the aid of others who will submit to the inevitable demands imposed upon them by the patient. They play a vital role thereby in sustaining and maintaining the agoraphobic behavior, and make lasting therapeutic change unlikely unless they are treated concurrently.

The Effect of Antianxiety Medication

None of the present-day sedatives and tranquilizers quiet the patient without also producing a certain amount of drowsiness. This is a hindrance or danger to the patient who must work, think, drive, or use machinery. Many therapists do not prescribe medication, but treatment is made much easier and carried out more effectively in a shorter period of time when the patient has the reassurance that the pill in her hand will effectively terminate an anxious spell. Placebos have no place here, for even those responding to placebos will not do so on every occasion; once a patient is fooled, it becomes a difficult matter to get him to try to face the feared object, situation, or feeling once again. I have found it most useful to diminish the anxiety, on occasion, with medication. As the patient continues to expose herself to the noxious stimulus, I gradually cut down the dosage so that he or she is exposed to smaller amounts of anxiety and thereby to effective desensitization. This approach is helpful when a patient must work in the presence of the phobic stimulus.

One further problem with medication is the development of

dependency upon the drug. A few patients use the pill as a crutch, taking it in anticipation of an attack, rather than during one. These, too, must gradually be weaned from medication.

Although some therapists use behavior therapy techniques exclusively (Wolpe, 1968b), it seems best to employ them as an added tool in a broad armamentarium of therapeutic modalities (Abramovitz, 1970; Lazarus, 1967). In doing so, however, it is important to keep in mind Bandura's (1969) caution, "Psychodynamic and social-learning (behavioral) approaches to psychotherapy are equally concerned with modifying the 'underlying' determinants of deviant response patterns; however, these theories differ, often radically, in what they regard these 'causes' to be, a crucial difference which in turn influences the types of stimulus conditions favored in the respective treatments." In order to utilize the behavioral techniques successfully, it is essential to keep these differences in mind and to orient one's thinking to this different, i.e. behavioral, approach.

REFERENCES

Abramovitz, C. M.: Personalistic psychotherapy and the role of technical eclecticism. *Psychol Rep, 26:*255, 1970.

Agras, W. S.: The behavioral therapies underlying principles and procedures. In Agras, W. S. (Ed.): *Behavior Modification: Principles and Clinical Applications.* Boston, Little, Brown and Company, 1972.

Ayllon, T., and Roberts, M. D.: The token economy: now. In Agras, W. S. (Ed.): *Behavior Modification: Principles and Clinical Applications.* Boston, Little, Brown and Company, 1972.

Bandura, A.: *Principles of Behavior Modification.* New York, Rinehart and Winston, 1969.

Beecher, H. K.: *Measurement of Subjective Responses.* New York, Oxford University Press, 1959.

Clarke, A. D. B.: Learning and human development. *Brit J Psychiat, 114:*1061, 1968.

Dengrove, E.: A new letter-association technique. *Dis Nerv Syst, 23:*25, 1962.

Dengrove, E.: Thought-block in behavior therapy. In Letters to the Editor, *Behav Ther, 3:*344, 1972a.

Dengrove, E.: Practical behavioral diagnosis. In Lazarus, A. A. (Ed.): *Clinical Behavior Therapy.* New York, Brunner/Mazel, 1972b.

Dunlap, K.: *Habits: Their Making and Unmaking.* New York, Liveright, 1932.

Frankl, V. E.: Paradoxical intention. A Logotherapeutic Technique. *Am J Psychother, 14:*520, 1960.

Franks, C. M.: Clinical application of conditioning and other behavioral techniques. *Cond Reflex, 1*:36, 1966a.

Franks, C. M.: Conditioning and conditioned aversion therapies in the treatment of the alcoholic. *Int J Addict, 1*:61, 1966b.

Franks, C. M.: *Behavior Therapy: Appraisal and Status.* New York, McGraw-Hill, 1969.

Gantt, W. H., Newton, Joseph E. O., Royer, Fred L., and Stephens, Joseph H.: Effect of person. *Cond Reflex 1*:18, 1966.

Gavalas, R. J.: Operant reinforcement of an autonomic response: two studies. *J Exp Anal Behav, 10*:119, 1967.

Gelder, M. G., and Marks, I. M.: Severe agoraphobia: a controlled prospective trial of behavior therapy. *Brit J Psychiatry, 112*:209, 1966.

Goldstein, I. B.: Study in psychophysiology of muscular tension. I. Response specificity. *Arch Gen Psychiatry, 11*:322, 1964.

Jaspers, K.: *General Psychopathology.* Chicago, University of Chicago Press, 1963.

Lazarus, A. A.: A preliminary report on the use of directed muscular activity in counter-conditioning. *Behav Res Ther, 2*:301, 1965.

Lazarus, A. A.: Broad spectrum behavior therapy and the treatment of agoraphobia. *Behav Res Ther, 4*:95, 1966.

Lazarus, A. A.: In support of technical eclecticism. *Psychol Rep, 21*:415, 1967.

Lazarus, A. A.: Variations in desensitization therapy. *Psychotherapy: Theory, Research and Practice, 5*:50, 1968a.

Lazarus, A. A.: Aversive therapy and sensory modalities: clinical impressions. *Percept and Motor Skills, 27*:178, 1968b.

Lazarus, A. A.: Behavior therapy and graded structure. In Porter, R. (Ed.): *Ciba Foundation Symposium on the Role of Learning in Psychotherapy.* London, J. and A. Churchill, 1968c.

Lazarus, A. A.: *Behavior Therapy and Beyond.* New York, McGraw-Hill, 1971.

Lazarus, A. A.: Multimodal behavior therapy: treating the "Basic Id." *J Nerv Ment Dis, 156*:404, 1973.

Lazarus, A. A., and Abramovitz, A.: The use of "emotive imagery" in the treatment of children's phobias. *J Ment Sci, 108*:191, 1962.

Lazarus, A. A., and Serber, M.: Is systematic desensitization being misapplied? *Psychol Rep, 23*:215, 1968.

Lehner, G. F. J.: Negative practice as a psychotherapeutic technique. In Eysenck, H. J. (Ed.): *Behavior Therapy and the Neuroses.* New York, Pergamon Press, 1960.

Leitenberg, H.: Positive reinforcement and extinction procedures. In Agras, W. (Ed.): *Behavior Modification: Principles and Clinical Applications.* Boston, Little, Brown and Company, 1972.

Leitenberg, H., Agras, W. S., Thompson, L. E., and Wright, D. C.: Feedback in behavior modification: an experimental analysis in two phobic cases. *J Appl Behav Analysis, 1*:131, 1968.

Lovibond, S. H.: *Conditioning and Enuresis.* New York, MacMillan, 1964.

MacLean, P. D.: The brain in relation to empathy and medical education. *J Nerv Ment Dis, 155:*355, 1967.

Matthews, A., and Gelder, M.: Letter in *Brit J Psychiatry, 124:*104, 1974.

Marks, I. M.: Components and correlates of psychiatric questionnaires. *Brit J Med Psychol, 44:*270, 1967.

Marks, I. M.: Flooding (implosion) and allied treatments. In Agras, W. S. (Ed.): *Behavior Modification: Principles and Clinical Applications.* Boston, Little, Brown and Company, 1972.

Marks, I. M.: Reduction of fear: towards a unifying theory. *Can Psychiatry Assoc J, 18:*9, 1973.

Meyer, V., and Crisp, A. H.: Some problems in behavior therapy. *Brit J Psychiatry, 112:*367, 1966.

Mowrer, O. H., and Mowrer, W. M.: Enuresis: a method for its study and treatment. *Am J Psychiatry, 8:*436, 1938.

Rachman, S.: Studies in desensitization, III: Speed of generalization. *Behav Res Ther, 4:*7, 1966.

Rachman, S.: *Phobias: Their Nature and Control.* Springfield, Thomas, 1968.

Solyom, L., Kenny, F., and Ledwidge, B.: Evaluation of a new treatment paradigm by phobias. *Can Psychiatry Assoc J, 14:*3, 1969.

Spiegel, H.: Is symptom removal dangerous? *Am J Psychiatry, 123:*10, 1967.

Stern, R., and Marks, I.: Brief and prolonged flooding. *Arch Gen Psychiatry, 28:*270, 1973.

Stevenson, I.: The use of rewards and punishments in psychotherapy. *Comp Psychiatry, 3:*20, 1962.

Stevenson, I., and Hain, J. B.: On the different meanings of apparently similar symptoms, illustrated by varieties of barber shop phobia. *Amer J Psychiatry, 124:*3, 1967.

Truax, C. B.: Some implications of behavior therapy for psychotherapy. *J Consult Psychol, 13:*160, 1966.

Ullmann, L., and Krasner, L.: *A Psychological Approach to Abnormal Behavior.* Englewood Cliffs, Prentice-Hall, 1969.

Wolf, S.: Placebos: problems and pitfalls. *Clin Pharmacol Ther, 3:*254, 1962.

Wolpe, J.: *Psychotherapy by Reciprocal Inhibition.* Stanford, Stanford University Press, 1958.

Wolpe, J.: The systematic desensitization treatment of neuroses. *J Nerv Ment Dis, 132:*189, 1961.

Wolpe, J.: Psychotherapy by reciprocal inhibition. *Cond Reflex, 3:*234, 1968a.

Wolpe, J.: Editorial. In *Newsletter, Assoc Adv Behav Ther, 3:*1, 1968b.

Wolpe, J., and Lazarus, A. A.: *Behavior Therapy.* New York, Pergamon, 1966.

Yates, A. J.: *Behavior Therapy.* New York, Wiley, 1970.

CHAPTER 2

HYPNOSIS

Edward Dengrove, M.D.

DESPITE ITS LONG HISTORY, it is hard to specify just what hypnosis is. Hilgard (1965) describes the hypnotic state as an altered state of awareness with certain characteristics: (1) subsidence of the planning function, in which the hypnotized subject loses initiative and lacks the desire to make and carry out plans on his own; (2) redistribution of attention, which is a loose way of saying that attention is selective, that we do not attend equally to all aspects of the environment, and that under hypnosis selective attention and selective inattention (generally diffuse) go beyond the usual range; (3) availability of visual memories from the past, and heightened (made vivid) ability for fantasy production so that the hypnotist can suggest the reality of memories for events that did not happen; (4) reduction in reality testing (lack of criticality) and a tolerance for persistent reality distortion, with a trance logic (Orne, 1959) denoting the peculiar acceptance of what would normally be found incompatible; (5) increased suggestibility that is but one of the features of hypnosis, arising at least in part as a consequence of the foregoing changes in the state of the person, with the trance itself a product of suggestion; (6) role behavior, in which the subject will adopt a suggested role and carry on complex activities corresponding to that role; (7) amnesia for what transpired within the hypnotic state, a common but not essential aspect of hypnosis, which can be furthered through suggestion.

There are numerous degrees of hypnotic suggestibility (Hilgard, 1965) depending upon the demand characteristics of the hypnotic situation (Orne, 1959), the expectations of the subject, task motivation, imagination instructions, hypnotist-subject interaction, and other factors. Simulation may take place, perhaps to please the therapist, or to resist losing control of one's self, but this is often detectable, and may still be useful. The subject may say afterwards that he really was not hypnotized, which may or may not be true and may not even be of much consequence as long as the desired outcome is obtained.

Wolberg (1972) states that 10 percent of subjects resist entering into a trance for one reason or another, while 10 percent are capable of entering into the deepest (somnambulistic) stage of hypnosis; others can be hypnotized to some degree. The level of depth achieved with successive inductions is relatively stable. Unless an individual goes into a fairly deep trance at the beginning, he will not make gains with practice. Though not necessarily more deeply hypnotized, the evidence suggests that, with practice, a person tends to become more quickly hypnotizable. Generally, there is no correlation between depth of trance and effectiveness of therapeutic suggestion.

Available data (Hilgard, 1965) suggests that all normal infants are born with the potential to develop the ability for profound hypnotic experiences; some people lose it because involvement in fantasy or adventure is not encouraged by example, or tolerated or rewarded in preadolescence. It is evident that much learning is involved, whether that learning be a result of associative repetition, the influences of rewards and reinforcement or some subtle process of imitation and contagion little represented in contemporary learning theories.

Some kinds of behavior outside hypnosis have been found to have low positive correlations with later hypnotic behavior (Hilgard, 1965): the ability to become deeply involved in reading novels, adventure, mystery stories; to become deeply involved in viewing or acting in the dramatic arts; to derive keen pleasure from sights and sounds, such as nature lovers or music lovers; to have a sense of religious devotion and discipleship; to reveal a spirit of adventure, and have a rich curiosity about the ranges of human experience. The hypnotizable person is one who has rich subjective experiences in which he can become deeply involved; one who reaches out for new experiences and is thus friendly to hypnosis; one who is interested in the life of the mind, and not a competitive activist; one who accepts impulses from within and is not afraid to relinquish reality testing for a time. Or, as Meares

(1961) points out, an individual who is willing to accept a "lack of criticality" for a time.

One of the most puzzling aspects of hypnosis has been the immediate readiness of the susceptible subject to be hypnotized within a few minutes, regardless of many variations in the hypnotist's qualifications or practices (Hilgard, 1965). In hypnosis, the subject responds to the power of words, uses "trance logic," and shows a more or less active receptivity, entering into varying degrees of role-enactment, role-involvement, and partial dissociation. Normal subjects are more hypnotizable than those who border on the neurotic or are frankly neurotic. The hypnotic interaction goes on most smoothly in conflict-free areas; if a conflict area is tapped in the hypnotic interaction defenses are aroused that may interfere with the hypnosis.

Many techniques of induction are available to the hypnotist. But techniques of induction, consideration of levels of hypnotic responses, and theories of hypnosis, are outside the purview of this chapter. Reference is made to some of the extensive literature in these subjects (Meares, 1961; Weitzenhoffer, 1957; Hartland, 1971; Kroger, 1963; Teitelbaum, 1965).

THE BEHAVIOR THERAPIST AND HYPNOSIS

One of the comments made by observers of systematic desensitization is that it bears some similarity to hypnosis. Ullmann and Krasner (1969) state that if hypnosis is defined as a role enactment, then there is much overlap between hypnosis and systematic desensitization; both are potential forms of social influence and, if used to alter behavior directly, of behavior therapy. Horowitz (1970) found a positive relationship between improvement and the subject's self-report of hypnotic depth. On the other hand, Cautela (1966a, 1966b) analyzed the relationship between the hypnotic induction procedure or suggestibility and the desensitization process and concluded that these variables are not significant aspects of the desensitization process.

Many studies evaluating the role of suggestion (both suggestion under hypnosis and instruction for therapeutic change without hypnosis) have come up with contradictory findings. Litvak (1970) emphasized the possible role of hypnotic suggestion and autosuggestion in the desensitization therapies utilizing mental operations (in contrast to desensitization techniques carried out *in vivo*). McGlynn, Mealiea, and Nawas (1969), Borkovic (1973), Oliveau, Agras, Leitenberg, Moore, and Wright (1969), Kazdin (1973), Woody (1973), and Woody and Schauble (1969) also found evidence supporting the positive effects of suggestion. Woody and Schauble further pointed to the possibility that either consciously or unconsciously, the behavior therapist employs subtle suggestions of improvement. The suggestion is made that a more appropriate approach would be to determine what kind of suggestions should be given and to give these consistently, much in the same manner as reinforcers are predetermined and administered in verbal conditioning. Kohn (1955) demonstrated that a hypnotic group showed somewhat higher suggestibility than a relaxation group.

On the other hand, Paul (1966), Lang (1969), and Lang, Lazovik, and Reynolds (1965) found no correlation between suggestion and therapeutic outcome in behavior therapy. Lang stated that the addition of limited hypnotic procedures did not contribute to the efficacy of desensitization, and eliminated hypnosis from his procedure, with no apparent change in rate of success. He added, however, that direct suggestion appeared to be as efficient as scene visualization in producing short-term reduction in fear behavior, and that hypnotic experience in the context of therapy may produce fear change, in part related to individual hypnotic susceptibility, but indicated that hypnotic susceptibility is not related to the specific desensitization effect.

In evaluating these contradictory findings, one must keep in mind that suggestibility is not hypnosis, but only one of the features of hypnosis, arising at least in part as a consequence of the changes in the state of the hypnotized person (Hilgard, 1965). Nevertheless, it is convenient to study hypnosis in terms of alterations in suggestibility, regardless of how these changes come about.

Marks, Gelder, and Edwards (1968) compared hypnosis with desensitization in the treatment of the phobias and concluded that both treatments produced significant improvement, with desensitization producing slightly more improvement in phobias than did hypnosis-relaxation. Hypnosis was induced with suggestions of relaxation and arm levitation and forceful suggestions made to the patients that their phobias would gradually disappear; only a general suggestion was given, without imagery or suggestions that the patient should enter particular situations. Patients were asked to relax at home but no graduated task was given, unlike the instructions given to patients who received desensitization.

THE USES OF HYPNOSIS IN BEHAVIOR THERAPY

Though not indispensable, hypnosis does have an important role in the practice of behavior therapy. When properly used, it adds leverage to treatment and shortens treatment time.

Hypnosis makes treatment easier in three ways: (a) in relaxing the patient, (b) in easing the path to visual imagery, and (c) in providing techniques which aid in the management of the more difficult patient.

In my experience, and if not too time-consuming, relaxation induced by hypnosis can be quite deep and satisfactory.

Barber and Hahn (1963) insist that hypnosis (a 20-minute "hypnotic induction procedure" consisting of suggestions of relaxation, drowsiness, and sleep) is no more effective in the production of relaxation than mere instruction to sit quietly, as indicated by physiological criteria. Paul (1969b) compared relaxation training and hypnosis (induction patterned after Kline's visual imagery technique, with an eye fixation induction emphasizing suggestions of heaviness, drowsiness, sleep and relaxation, directed to the subject's image of herself, and followed by a test challenge for arm immobilization). The conclusion was that, in general, while both methods were effective in reducing subjective reports of tension-distress, even within a single session, progressive relaxation training was more effective than hypnotic suggestion in producing desired physiological changes. One must keep in mind other features that form part of the hypnotic state and which are useful to systematic desensitization, chiefly the altered suggestibility of the subject, or, as Meares (1961) terms it, the "lack of criticality," which provides an added bonus to therapy.

Besides the usual suggestions to relax, there are numerous "tricks of the trade" available through hypnosis. Lazarus (1963) has the patient simulate a state of sensory deprivation and finds it highly useful in treating pervasive "free-floating" anxiety. Weitzenhoffer (1957) and Lazarus (1958) also use autohypnosis to reduce a feeling of panic to one of calmness. Patients are taught relaxation at home by autosuggestion. Weitzenhoffer details another "sensorimotor" method, in which the individual is hypnotized without his awareness (The postural sway can be considered a form of sensorimotor induction).

Under hypnosis, suggestions are made to the effect that, in response to a signal from the therapist, in the next session the patient will enter into a more deeply relaxed state, and in a much shorter time, thereby reducing the time taken by the patient in adopting the relaxed posture. In no way is the patient pressured.

When there is difficulty in visualizing the next step in a hierarchy (a list of stimuli to which the patient reacts with anxiety, arranged from the least disturbing to the most frightening), hypnotic vivification can intensify the visual image. A statement given in the hypnotic trance, such as "When I touch your shoulder, you will visualize it with ease and comfort," will often gently nudge the patient along. Schubot (1967) found that hypnotic susceptibility and vividness of hynotic imagery were positively related to reduction of fear in highly anxious subjects. In another study, Paul (1969a) found evidence clearly supporting the theoretical assumption that relaxation induced through brief relaxation training or hypnotic suggestion does inhibit the physiological response to stressful imagery, and that hypnotic treatment resulted in significant reduction in systems not under direct voluntary control.

Time distortion techniques may be used for desensitization. One can project a patient into the future and have him live through an anxious situation as if it were happening in the present, but in a relaxed manner. On awakening, he can be left with the feeling that he has been through all of this before and has progressed adequately.

The induction of dreams by hypnosis, particularly if they are repetitive, is a useful desensitization device with graduated responses. Patients are given tasks to perform in the "dream state" and suggestions are paced to the progress of the patient, or the patient may be told to set the pace himself.

Tart (1965, 1966) casts doubt on the notion that most hypnotic dreams are dream-like. However, experiments reveal that posthypnotic suggestions may affect the content of dreams at night, often quite markedly. The patient may be instructed under hypnosis to dream of doing those very things he fears most, but with ease and pleasure. Barber, Walker, and Hahn (1973) gave presleep suggestions to hypnotic and nonhypnotic subjects and found that these suggestions were equally effective in altering the contents of nocturnal dreams when they were given with or without an hypnotic induction procedure. However, they had the greatest effect on dreams when they were given authoritatively to the hypnotic subjects and permissively to the nonhypnotic subjects.

By associating new and pleasant stimuli with old responses, it is possible to diminish general anxiety. At the conclusion of a session, posthypnotic suggestions to the effect that the patient will continue to feel relaxed and will carry out that which he performed in the session can be most helpful. For example, Mrs. O. feared she might hurt her infant son with a knife. She was told to visualize herself cutting bread in front of her child, but to see the baby happy and laughing, and to visualize herself quite pleased with her son posthypnotically. This proved most helpful to her.

Erickson (1966) employs posthypnotic suggestions to the effect that the patient will experience panic episodes but that they will be brief and last only seconds and that the patient will be amazed at how shortlived the feeling is.

Aversive responses produced through hypnosis have been used to extinguish unwanted behavior for years. Typical, perhaps, is the posthypnotic suggestion used to modify a patient's smoking habit. Under hypnosis it is suggested to the subject that he view rat dung rubbed into the tobacco used to prepare the cigarette which he then puts into his mouth, lights up, and inhales deeply, producing intense nausea. Cautela (see Chapter 13) employs a similar technique which he calls covert sensitization and which is used to produce aversion to certain foods, alcohol, tobacco, or sexual deviation. The scenes and responses may be vivified with hypnosis.

Feamster and Brown (see Chapter 27) successfully used aversive treatment through hypnosis to control excessive drinking. A somnambulistic trance was achieved and the patient was instructed to relive his worst hangover whenever he smelled, tasted, looked at, or even thought of alcoholic beverages. After recovery from the hangover, he was to feel hungry and eat a satisfying meal and achieve relaxation by pressing together his left index finger and thumb. Brief reinforcement was required. Other authors (Miller, 1959; Abrams, 1964) have used hypnotically induced conditioned aversion techniques successfully in the treatment of alcoholism.

When aversive conditioning is employed, basic principles must be strictly adhered to (Franks, 1966), as noted in Chapter 1.

The creative use of hypnosis makes it possible for the behavior therapist to satisfy the basic requirement for aversive conditioning in a manner not easily achieved by any other technique. Some of the examples cited above illustrate this point and suggest some of the ways appropriately chosen posthypnotic suggestions can be employed in the context of conditioning therapy. Behavior therapists are noted for their ingenuity, but hypnotherapists have long shown a more extensive inventiveness because of the extra leverage of hypnosis.

In recent years a wide range of behavior therapies have been developed. Only systematic desensitization and aversive conditioning have been discussed here. These and other methods are effective without employing any hypnotic techniques; however, many outstanding therapists report hypnosis to be an extremely useful adjunct in their practice. It would seem that there are many situations where some of the special characteristics of hypnosis can be employed to great advantage in a behavior therapy setting. The exciting possibilities inherent in the combination of hypnosis and behavior therapies have barely been tapped.

REFERENCES

Abrams, S.: An evaluation of hypnosis in the treatment of alcoholics. *Am J Psychiatry, 120*:1160, 1964.

Barber, T. X., and Hahn, K. W.: Hypnotic induction and "relaxation": an experimental study. *Arch Gen Psychiatry, 8:*295, 1963.

Barber, T. X., Walker, P. C., and Hahn, K. W.: Effects of hypnotic induction and suggestions on nocturnal dreaming and thinking. *J Abnorm Psychol, 82:*414, 1973.

Borkovec, T. D.: The effects of instructional suggestion and physiological cues on analogue fear. *Behav Ther, 4:*185, 1973.

Cautela, J. R.: Desensitization factors in the hypnotic treatment of phobias. *J Psychol, 64:*277, 1966a.

Cautela, J. R.: Hypnosis and behaviour therapy. *Behav Res Ther, 4:*219 1966b.

Erickson, M. H.: Experiential knowledge of hypnotic phenomena employed for hypnotherapy. *Am J Clin Hyp, 8:*299, 1966.

Franks, C. M.: Conditioning and conditioned aversion therapies in the treatment of the alcoholic. *Int J Addict, 1:*61, 1966.

Hartland, J.: *Medical and Dental Hypnosis and Its Clinical Application,* 2nd ed. Baltimore, Williams and Wilkins, 1971.

Hilgard, E. R.: *The Experience of Hypnosis.* New York, Harcourt, Brace and World, 1968.

Horowitz, S. L.: Strategies within hypnosis for reducing phobic behavior. *J Abnorm Psychol, 75:*104, 1970.

Kazdin, A. E.: The effect of suggestion and pretesting on avoidance reduction in fearful subjects. *J Behav Ther Exp Psychiatry, 4:*213, 1973.

Kohn, H. B.: Suggestion relaxation as a technique for inducing hypnosis. *J Psychol, 40:*203, 1955.

Kroger, W. S.: *Clinical and Experimental Hypnosis.* Philadelphia, Lippincott, 1963.

Lang, P. J.: The mechanics of desensitization and the laboratory study of human fear. In Franks, C. M. (Ed.): *Behavior Therapy: Appraisal and Status.* New York, McGraw-Hill, 1969.

Lang, P. J., Lazovik, A. D., and Reynolds, D. J.: Desensitization, suggestibility and pseudotherapy. *J Abnorm Soc Psychol, 70:*395, 1965.

Lazarus, A. A.: Some clinical applications of autohypnosis. *Med Proc, 14:*848, 1958.

Lazarus, A. A.: Sensory deprivation under hypnosis in the treatment of pervasive ("free floating") anxiety: a preliminary impression. *S Afr Med J, 27:*136, 1963.

Litvak, S. B.: Hypnosis and the desensitization behavior therapies. *Psychol Rep, 27:*787, 1970.

Marks, I. M., Gelder, M. G., and Edwards, G.: Hypnosis and desensitization for phobias: a controlled prospective trial. *Brit J Psychiatry, 114:*1263, 1968.

McGlynn, F. D., Mealiea, W. L., and Nawas, M. M.: Systematic desensitization of snake avoidance under two conditions of suggestion. *Psychol Rep, 25:*220, 1969.

Meares, A. A.: *A System of Medical Hypnosis.* Philadelphia, Saunders, 1960. Reissue 1972 by The Julian Press, New York.

Miller, M. M.: Treatment of chronic alcoholics by hypnotic aversion. *JAMA, 171*:1492, 1959.

Oliveau, D. C., Agras, W. S., Leitenberg, H., Moore, R. C., and Wright, D. E.: Systematic desensitization, therapeutically oriented instructions, and selective positive reinforcement. *Behav Res Therapy, 7*:27, 1969.

Orne, M. T.: The nature of hypnosis: artifact and essence. *J Abn Soc Psychol, 58*:277, 1959.

Paul, G. L.: *Insight vs Desensitization in Psychotherapy: an Experiment in Anxiety Reduction.* Stanford, Stanford University Press, 1966.

Paul, G. L.: Inhibition of physiological response to stressful imagery by relaxation training and hypnotically suggested relaxation. *Behav Res Ther, 7*:249, 1969a.

Paul, G. L.: Physiological effects of relaxation training and hypnotic suggestion. *J Abnorm Psychol, 74*:425, 1969b.

Schubot, E. O.: The influence of hypnotic and muscular relaxation in systematic desensitization of phobias. *Dissert Abst, 27*:3681, 1967.

Tart, C. T.: The hypnotic dream: methodological problems and a review of the literature. *Psychol Bull, 63*:87, 1965.

Tart, C. T.: Some effects of posthypnotic suggestion on the process of dreaming. *Int J Clin Exp Hypnosis, 14*:30, 1966.

Teitelbaum, M.: *Hypnotic Induction Technics.* Springfield, Thomas 1965.

Ullmann, L. P., and Krasner, L.: *A Psychological Approach to Abnormal Behavior.* Englewood Cliffs, Prentice-Hall, 1969.

Weitzenhoffer, A. M.: *General Techniques of Hypnotism.* New York, Grune and Stratton, 1957.

Wolberg, L. R.: *Hypnosis: Is It For You?* New York, Harcourt, Brace Jovanovich, 1972.

Woody, R. H.: Clinical suggestion and systematic desensitization. *Am J Clin Hypnosis, 15*:250, 1973.

Woody, R. H., and Schauble, P. G.: Desensitization of fear by video tapes. *J Clin Psychol, XXV*:102, 1969.

HYPNOSIS AND CONDITIONABILITY

THIS SECTION PRESENTS a number of experimental articles relating hypnosis and conditioning phenomena. Hypnosis can
influence conditioning in a number of ways and be used to modify
its effects.

Alexander and Kraines view hypnosis as a physiological phenomenon. Conceptualizing it in Pavlovian terms (though one
should keep in mind that hypnosis is not sleep), posthypnotic
suggestion is seen as an example of Pavlov's second (verbal)
signaling system. Plapp and Edmonston's experimental analysis
of Pavlov's cortical inhibition theory of hypnosis indicates that
the type of response conditioned may be an important determinant of the effect obtained. Barrios' point of departure is neurophysiological. Hypnosis facilitates higher order conditioning, and
the greater the effectiveness of the hypnotic induction the more
effective the conditioning produced by the posthypnotic suggestion.

In the laboratory, the hypnotic state has been used to facilitate
experimental procedures. Writing on the use of instrumental
learning to modify glandular and visceral responses, Miller (1969)
suggests the use of "hypnotic suggestion to achieve similar results
by enhancing the reward effect of the signal indicating a change
in the desired direction, by producing relaxation and regular

breathing, and by removing interference from skeletal responses and distraction by irrelevant cues."

Following these lines, Paterson uses hypnosis to inhibit and facilitate conditioned responses, to condition voluntary and involuntary autonomic responses, and to indicate that suggestion under hypnosis appears to be more potent than the conditioned reflex principle. The article by Zimbardo, Marshall, White and Maslach reports an operant conditioning methodology to validate the viability of hypnosis in the induction of altered time perception. Incidentally, these authors have expanded this theme more fully elsewhere (Zimbardo, Marshall and Maslach, 1971).

Horowitz's presentation moves into conditioning following hypnotic induction. It is shown that conditioning involving relaxation, fear arousal, and posthypnotic suggestion reduces phobic responses, and that the subject's depth of hypnosis is positively related to degree of improvement.

Finally, Kline defines the hypnotic experience, conditioning, and the resultant behavioral changes in neurophysiological terms. He is of the opinion that both voluntary and involuntary functions can be conditioned under hypnosis, with hypnosis facilitating conditioning.

REFERENCES

Miller, Neal A.: Learning of visceral and glandular responses. *Science*, 163:434, 1969.

Zimbardo, Philip G., Marshall, Gary, and Maslach, Christine: Liberating behavior from time-bound control: expanding the present through hypnosis. *J Appl Soc Psychol*, 1:305, 1971.

CHAPTER 3

CONDITIONAL REFLEXES AS RELATED TO HYPNOSIS AND HYPNOTIC TECHNIQUES*

Leo Alexander, M.D.

THE CONCEPTIONAL FRAMEWORK of current theories of psycho-therapy does not explain the three most important aspects of hypnosis.

THE INDUCTION OF THE TRANCE

The traditional idea that trance induction comes about by sub-mission and surrender of important ego functions to the therapist is contradicted by the experience that trance states in resistant subjects can be induced by encouraging the patient to resist as much as he can, and in anxious or suspicious patients by a mere explanation of the trance state and the subjective experiences the patient may achieve (Alexander, 1965; Erickson, 1954; Haley, 1963).

By contrast to the traditional excessively simply psychothera-peutic model, Pavlovian physiology (Pavlov, 1932) explains most of the variegated phenomena of the trance and of the particular psychological set which hypnotic psychotherapy provides. Pavlov (1941) concluded from his studies in the dog that "hypnosis can be produced by the continuation of one and the same stimulus, finally resulting in an inhibitory state" (p. 75) irrespective of the nature of this stimulus. In man it is quite obvious that it is the monotony and repetiveness of the hypnotist's discourse and the

* Originally published in *The American Journal of Clinical Hypnosis*, Volume X, Number 3, January 1968, pages 157–159. Copyright 1968 by the American Society of Clinical Hypnosis.

unchanging sameness of the setting and of the position of the patient which is the most convenient way to induce trance. Also, Helge Lundholm's method (1942) of deepening hypnosis by counting is explainable by this important and simple finding of Pavlov.

THE FACILITATION OF PSYCHOTHERAPY
DURING THE TRANCE

One of the outstanding characteristics of the trance is the remarkable, almost instantaneous enrichment of the creative imagination of the patient which brings long forgotten or repressed memories and emotional material into clear insightful awareness. This phenomenon is the key to effective hypnotic psychotherapy; I regard it as the most clinically useful aspect of hypnosis (Alexander, 1942). It is this remarkable and hitherto inexplicable stimulation of the creative imagination of the person under hypnosis which had so impressed the members of the Philadelphia Philosophical Society as early as 1784 (Alexander, 1965).

The most cogent explanation of this phenomenon is Pavlov's recognition of the fact that the human mind encompasses two almost mutually exclusive aspects (p. 79): 1) "The magnificent representation of the external world through the afferent fibers" (named by Spitzer (1924) the oikotropic system), and 2) "An extensive representation of the inner world of the organism" (Spitzer's idiotropic system). "These two projections are very different. While the projection of the skeletal muscular apparatus can be finely adjusted to the representative of the external energies, such as the auditory and visual, the projection of the other internal process remains sharply separated. Perhaps this depends upon the slight practical use made of this agency. In every case it is a constant physiological fact. On this basis the voluntary and involuntary functions of the organism are separated, the activity of the skeletal musculature being counted as voluntary." "On account of the state of hypnosis the motor analyzer is inhibited but all the remaining part of the cortex is free" (p. 79). Pavlov believes that the inhibition of the part of the cortical apparatus which deals with the outside world is of the paradoxical type (p. 80); therefore its stimulation at this point no longer leads to its excitation but to a further deepening inhibition. Its inhibition, according to the law of reciprocal induction (p. 81), then induces excitation of the other part of the cortical apparatus, namely, the one dealing with the inner world of the organism.

This most ingenious analysis of Pavlov's observations in the dog explains most beautifully the most perplexing, mystifying and fascinating part of the hypnotic state in man, namely, the remarkable enrichment of the inner world when the person's capacity of dealing with the outer world is inhibited by closure of the eyes and immobility which separate the person from distracting details of the outside world. The resulting reciprocal stimulation of the awareness of the inner world, skillfully enhanced by the suggestions of the therapist, then brings about those surprising, remarkable and astute insights which are possible in the hypnotic state (Alexander, 1942).

THE POST-HYPNOTIC SUGGESTION

The compelling nature of an effective post-hypnotic suggestion which becomes fully incorporated into the mental life of the patient, who accepts it as an idea of his own rather than something he learned from the therapist, is inexplicable by traditional psychodynamic concepts. It is characterized by what is best described as the compulsive triad (Spiegel, 1959), namely: compelling power of the suggested idea, amnesia of the source of the idea, and confabulatory rationalization of the amnesia if challenged.

These characteristics are remarkably analogous to those of a conditional response. It is well known that a person may show a consistent, i.e. "compelling" conditional response to a conditional signal while no longer consciously remembering the stimulus by which it had been conditioned. But it is not generally appreciated that the third item of the triad, namely confabulatory rationalization of the otherwise inexplicable response, may also occur. In 1957 I made a pertinent observation while studying polygraphic measurement techniques of conditioning sequences (Alexander, 1959). After having been conditioned to respond with cessation of eye movements to a high tone, I retired to my study two doors down from the experimental laboratory to do some reading, while

my collaborator continued to condition other normal control subjects. As I was reading, I noted that ever so often the smooth
progress of my reading would come to a stop at a certain word.
My first thought was that some obstruction on my eye glasses was
interfering with my vision at a certain angle. So I took off my
glasses and cleaned them, but this did not remedy the situation.
I then noticed that whenever the interruption of my visual progress along the lines occurred, the faint sound of the high tone to
which I had been conditioned was audible through two closed
doors, every two minutes for five seconds. My earlier rationalization of the obviously conditioned effect upon my eye muscles
reminded me of my patients' rationalizations of post-hypnotic
suggestions and alerted me to the relevance of conditioning theory
to hypnotic phenomena. The most satisfactory explanation of the
post-hypnotic suggestion is conditioning by means of the second
(verbal) signaling system in accordance with Pavlov's concept
of establishment of new connections between functions by this
means. This explanation adequately explains all three crucial
characteristics of the post-hypnotic suggestion, namely: its consistent compulsivity, its unconscious incorporation into the higher
nervous activity, and its rationalization when some or all of its
effects are brought into awareness. Viewed in this light, the hypnotic state, by means of the post-hypnotic suggestion, offers the
psychotherapist the opportunity to establish a new connection
between a new conditional stimulus and a basic unconditional
drive.

This technique of associating a new conditional signal to an
unconditional need or to extinguish an old and noxious conditional need to new, more desirable associations, is particularly
important and feasible in the treatment of sexual deviations, such
as homosexuality (Alexander, 1967) because in sexual behavior
a sharper distinction between its conditional and unconditional
determinants is possible than in other aspects of human behavior.
The effectiveness of a post-hypnotic suggestion can be explained
only by the fact that true conditioning by means of the second
signaling system employed by the hypnotherapist has been established.

SUMMARY

Conditional reflex physiology is of importance in explaining the production and some of the crucial features of the hypnotic state. Understanding of these basic physiologic aspects is helpful in rendering hypnotic psychotherapy more effective.

The hypnotic state is produced in the dog as well as in man by repetitive monotonous stimuli which set up a state of inhibition of those nervous functions which deal with the mastery of the environment (the oikotropic system). The inhibition of these functions effects a reciprocal release of those nervous functions which deal with the autonomic functions and emotions as well as the self and the inner life of the person (the idiotropic system). This explains the remarkable upsurge of creative thinking and spontaneous insight so characteristic of the trance state.

Conditionability during the hypnotic state is increased to the point of ready demonstrability of paradoxical and ultraparadoxical phases. It is therefore possible to extinguish conditioned associations, as well as to form and establish new ones. This is most strikingly demonstrable in the treatment of sexual deviations, because in sexual behavior a sharper distinction between its conditional and unconditional determinants is possible than in other aspects of human behavior.

The "compulsive triad," characteristic of an effective posthypnotic suggestion, is best explained as a conditional response established by means of the second signaling system.

REFERENCES

Alexander, L.: Clinical experiences with hypnosis in psychiatric therapy. *Am J Clin Hypn,* 7:190–206, 1965.

Erickson, M. H.: Special techniques of brief hypnotherapy. *J Clin Exper Hypn,* 2:109–129, 1954.

Haley, J.: *Strategies of Psychotherapy.* New York, Grune and Stratton, 1963, Vol I–X, pp. 1–204.

Pavlov, I. P.: *Lectures on Conditioned Reflexes.* Transl. and ed. W. Horsley Gantt. Volume II: Conditioned reflexes and psychiatry. Chapter 47: Contributions to the physiology of the hypnotic state in the dog. From: Reports of the physiological laboratory of Pavlov, Volume 4, 1932 (with M. K. Petrova), London, Lawrence and Wishart, 1941, pp. 75–82.

Lundholm, H. and Lowenbach, H.: Hypnosis and the Alpha activity of the electroencephalogram. *Charact Personal,* 11:145–149, 1942.

Alexander, L.: Hypnosis. *North Carolina Med J,* 3:562, 1942.

Spitzer, A.: Anatomie und Physiologie der Centralen Bahnen des Vestibularis. Arb. a.d. Wiener Neurologischen Institut., 1924, Vol. 25, p. 423.

Spiegel, H.: Hypnosis and transference: a theoretical formulation. *Arch Gen Psychiat,* 1:634–639, 1959.

Alexander, L., and Kris, C.: Polygraphic measurement technique of conditioning sequences in mentally disturbed and normal control subjects. (Abstract). *EEG Clin Neurophysiol,* 10:363–364, 1958.

Alexander, L.: Psychotherapy of sexual deviation with the aid of hypnosis. *Am J Clin Hypn,* 9:181–183, 1967.

CHAPTER 4

HYPNOSIS: PHYSIOLOGIC INHIBITION AND EXCITATION *

S. H. KRAINES, M.D.

DEFINITION AND THEORY

HYPNOSIS IS A HIGHLY LABILE STATE of physiologic inhibition and excitation of the cerebral cortex. Though induced by psychologic techniques, hypnosis alters cerebral physiology. There are two sets of theories as to the fundamental nature of hypnosis: *Psychologic* theories advance the concept that it is: (1) a form of hysteria (Eysenck, 1963); (2) a dissociative phenomenon (Janet, 1920); (3) a form of suggestion (Hull, 1933, Weitzenhoffer, 1948); and (4) that it reflects psychoanalytic concepts such as an unconscious desire for libidinal gratification (Ferenczi, 1916), a relationship to love (Freud, 1922), an erotic gratification (Schilder, 1956). *Physiologic* theories are based on (1) hypnotic phenomena in animals (Hull, 1933); (2) an "ideomotor" hypothesis (Eysenck, 1963; McDougall, 1926; Wolberg, 1948); and (3) a Pavlovian concept (Pavlov, 1928) that hypnosis and sleep are identical and that both are the result of inhibition of the cerebral cortex.

It is the thesis of this paper that the Pavlovian concepts can explain the phenomena of the hypnotic state. It is further postulated that utilization of these concepts can deepen the level of hypnosis and enhance the therapeutic benefits.

THE PAVLOVIAN CONCEPT

Working primarily in the vast field of conditioned reflexes, Pavlov found that certain conditioning techniques would put

* Originally published in *Psychosomatics*, Volume X, January–February, 1969, pages 36–41.

dogs to sleep. He advanced the thesis that sleep and hypnosis result from an inhibition of cerebral activity. He further postulated that conditioned responses were ultimately based on areas of cerebral excitation and inhibition.

Two of the many experiments reported by Pavlov will illustrate the principles he advanced.

1. A lively animal is placed in a light harness on a stand. He struggles—his paws are bound, the head straps tightened— he becomes quiet, drowsy, and falls asleep.

2. "Suppose that in a certain dog we always give the conditioned stimulus ten seconds before reinforcing it, i.e. adding the food or acid. In the course of ten seconds, we have an extreme degree of both motor and secretory (salivary) reaction. . . . If the unconditioned stimulus is applied not ten seconds but thirty or sixty seconds after the beginning of the conditioned stimulus, drowsiness sets in and the animal falls asleep."

In the first experiment, Pavlov postulates that the dog, finding that struggle is futile, inhibits his motor restlessness. This inhibition which initially involves the motor cortex irradiates over the entire brain thus producing sleep.

In the second experiment, the conditioned stimulus initially produced a state of excitation in the cerebral cortex, reflected in increased motor and salivary activity. When the unconditioned stimulus was not given at the expected time, the excitation was reversed; inhibition appeared; and the irradiation of this inhibition resulted in rapid sleep. During this so-called sleep, the dog stood as if he was carved of wood.

In innumerable experiments, Pavlov, with varied and refined techniques, illustrated this mechanism of cortical excitation and inhibition. Several of his conclusions are applicable to the concepts advanced in this paper.

1. Hypnosis and sleep result from inhibition of the cerebral cortex.

2. Both the inhibitory and the excitatory processes are physiologic phenomena.

3. When one area of the cortex is stimulated (stimulation of one spot on the skin will stimulate the corresponding area in the cerebral cortex) the excited cortical area irradiates

its excitability over the entire brain; inhibitory phenomena similarly irradiate from one locus of cortical inhibition.

4. The inhibitory and the excitatory phenomena can become concentrated in certain areas; areas of intensified cortical stimulation can be surrounded by areas of inhibition.

5. An isolated and continuous stimulation of a definite point in the cerebral hemispheres leads infallibly to drowsiness and sleep.

6. Marked individual differences exist (from dog to dog) as to the degree of irradiation and/or concentration of inhibition and/or excitation.

Hypnosis in animals is induced primarily by forced immobilization. This hypnosis is manifested as catalepsy in many animals. The thesis is advanced that the fear induced by this forced immobilization—with no opportunity for flight or fight—results in a generalized cerebral inhibition of activity. Preyer (1958)—as quoted by Moss and Forel—noted in these hypnotized animals such signs of fear as trembling, rapid respiration, and rapid heart beat. Birds hypnotized by the slowly undulating snake are "frozen with fear" with the escape mechanism negated by the fixation of attention. In animals hypnotized by fear—no matter how induced —there is a general cerebral inhibition * of all muscles—a cerea flexibilitas.

Clinical Evidence of Inhibition/Excitation in the Cerebral Cortex

In the human subject, the following occur:

1. Inhibition of independent evaluative thinking.

2. Inhibition, (e.g. paresis) or excitation (e.g. rigidity) of muscle groups.

3. Inhibition (anesthesia) or excitation (parasthesia, hyperesthesia) of sensation.

4. Inhibition or excitation of functions controlled by the autonomic nervous system (e.g. in viscera).

5. Inhibition (e.g. amnesia) or excitation (enhanced recall) of memories.

---

* R. Heidenhain in 1880 suggested that hypnosis resulted from inhibition of cortical ganglion cells.

It is significant that these manifestations are all functions of the cerebral cortex.

Clues from Induction Techniques

There are three basic types of induction techniques which demonstrate the role of cortical inhibition: (1) sensory fixation, (2) monotonous repetition of the word "sleep," and (3) mutually contradictory commands.

1. Sensory fixation is best exemplified by eye fixation. It matters little on what the eye is fixed, be it a bright light, a spot on the wall, or a swinging pendulum; the end result of prolonged gaze will be an "exhaustion" or inhibition of the cortical representation of vision. With adequate technique, this area of inhibition is then made to irradiate over the rest of the cortex and produce a hypnotic state. Remember Pavlov's conclusions: "An isolated and continuous stimulation of a definite point of the cerebral hemispheres leads infallibly to sleep."

2. Monotonous repetition of auditory or other stimuli induces sleep and hypnosis. Not only does the monotonous repetition of a single stimulus fixate the attention on this stimulus, but it also simultaneously inhibits attention (via cortical inhibition) to other stimuli. Moreover, it is probable that the monotonous, rhythmic, regularly recurring sounds act to synchronize the input from the reticular system to the cerebral cortex—E.E.G. studies show that the cortical synchrony is associated with sleep whereas asynchronic activity is associated with alertness (Gellhorn and Loofbourrow, 1963).

When in the overall setting of pleasant quietness the therapist rhythmically and monotonously repeats the word "sleep," all the connotations of this word facilitate those physiologic processes which induce sleep. The consequent cortical inhibition is the prologue to hypnosis.

3. By far the most common technique is that of "mutually contradictory commands." In these commands, one of the pair is subordinate and the other dominant; the words used by the hypnotist, his tone of voice, his persuasiveness, all determine the dominant one of the pair. For example, the hypnotist may say, "Close your eyes and relax them to the point where they will not

work. When you are sure they will not open, test them. Try to open them, but make sure that you can't. Try, try hard; the harder you try the more tightly they are glued together."

The cerebral cortex receiving the contradictory commands must inhibit one of them. In the proper setting, this inhibition is accomplished smoothly, easily, and the patient apparently is unaware of the illogicality of the commands. The inhibitory process, once initiated, becomes the locus from which inhibition can radiate over the entire cortex.

Many of these mutually antagonistic commands are given directly—"Clasp your hands together so tightly that you cannot pull them apart; try to pull them and make sure that you can't." "Your finger is so rigid that it will not bend no matter how hard you try; try to bend it and make sure you can't." However, there are many indirect suggestions which imply mutually antagonistic actions. The subject is directed to perform actions which are contradictory to natural patterns. "Naturally," one lifts his hand only for a purpose; one stands still without marked swaying or falling. However, in hand levitation, the hypnotist suggests that the hand will gradually rise and remain suspended without any effort by the subject; in the postural sway test, the patient is told that he will sway back and forth like a pendulum, or that standing, he will fall rigidly backward. A hand floating in air, a standing body swaying like a pendulum or falling backwards all imply an inhibition of "natural," habitual patterns.

In both the direct and indirect suggestions of mutually contradictory commands, there is an excitation of the cortical areas carrying out the act accompanied by an inhibition of the opposing action. It is the inhibiting force which then—on the command, "Go to sleep"—irradiates over the cortex.

ADJUNCTIVE PROCEDURES

There are several adjunctive techniques which facilitate the induction of the cortical inhibition and/or excitation. The primary one is that which "sets the stage" for acceptance of the suggestions. These procedures include preparing the patient, enhancing his desire, utilizing both authority and rapport.

Any technique which decreases cortical resistance such as

drugs will facilitate the acceptance of suggestions. Intravenous sodium amytal is particularly useful as an inducing procedure, (Kraines, 1967) but sedatives given orally are also effective. It is even possible by producing a temporary cerebral ischemia (the carotid sinus compression technique) (Weitzenhoffer, 1948) to bring about a rapid cortical inhibition.

Although the fear technique is rarely recommended, it can be used to frighten patients so that they are in a state of "functional decortication" (cortical inhibition) and thus amenable to suggestion. It is possible to hypnotize a sleeping person. In sleep, the asynchronous activity of the reticular system is inhibited and the synchronous activity results in secondary, "passive" inhibition of the cortex. In hypnosis, the cortex is actively inhibited. Proper induction techniques can quickly change the passive inhibition of sleep to the active inhibition of hypnosis. Children's behavior problems are particularly responsive to this procedure.

Suggestion is utilized in hypnosis both to induce trance and to obtain desired responses. Hypersuggestibility is merely a *function* of the hypnotic state and not its essence; hypnosis is a state of cortical inhibition.

Suggestions will not be effective in inducing hypnosis unless the subject is first prepared to accept them. There are many methods of such preparation, the most frequently used being the establishment of a pleasant cooperative feeling tone, providing persuasive "rationalizations," asserting the influence of authority, and even by inducing a state of confusion wherein the subject—transiently disoriented—accepts unquestionably the orientation of external origin.

Suggestions given to induce hypnosis have three purposes: (1) to orient and fix the subject's attention on an object, act or image (concentration of cerebral excitation), (2) to limit conscious awareness of other stimuli as a result of this fixation of attention, with concomitant general cortical inhibition of response to other stimuli, and (3) to command the performance of an act which, in turn, increases cortical inhibition.

Each suggestion (attention fixation, command) when executed adds to the cortical inhibitory state eventuating in a hypnotic trance. In the trance, a suggestion (command) is carried out automatically, evaluative thinking having been suspended.

CEREBRAL PHYSIODYNAMICS OF THE HYPNOTIC STATE

The exact mechanism of the inhibitory process—a process which is fundamental and inherent in the entire nervous system —is unclear. It is recognized that inhibition is an active and not a passive process—the inhibited neurones are not passively inactive but they have, in effect, "restrained activity." The cortical inhibition involved in hypnosis is an active restraint of activity.

The areas of cortical excitation (in the Pavlovian sense) are apparently (as judged by clinical results) areas of greater than usual, *supramaximal* activity. Not only is there increased activity of the "excited" cortical cells, but also all of the component fibers, association tracts, correlating subcortical nuclei, have a subsequent increase in their activity levels.

The consequent activity of the hypnotized patient—and the therapeutic benefits from the hypnotic procedure—do not result simply from the cortical areas of inhibition. Cortical inhibition is an essential preliminary state, but the areas of concentrated excitability produce the suggested actions and benefits.

When the hypnotist establishes areas of concentrated excitability—via appropriate suggestions—the effectiveness and completeness of the subject's response will be proportionate to the intensity of the concentration of excitability.

As a rule, the deeper the hypnotic state—that is, the more diffuse and the more intense the inhibition of the cerebral cortex —the easier it is to establish areas of excitability and to intensify their concentration.

From this general thesis, specific variations may be established. Thus, it becomes possible to establish localized areas of inhibition which surround areas of concentration. In his conditioned animals, Pavlov has achieved discrete areas of inhibition/excitation. The hypnotized subject may have several isolated areas of inhibition/excitation—the rigid finger in the totally relaxed hand, the localized area of hyperesthesia surrounded by an area of anesthesia, or the tubular vision. Although cortical inhibition tends to irradiate to other areas, it can be localized and concentrated.

Multiple areas of concentrated rings of inhibition surrounding areas of concentrated excitability can co-exist while other areas of the cortex remain relatively "normal" and unaffected. Accordingly, the subject who appears to be in a light trance can nevertheless obtain great therapeutic benefits from these localized and concentrated areas of inhibition/excitation.

It is again emphasised that the subject's execution of commands, whether it be for theatrical exhibition or as a therapeutic procedure, is effective in proportion to the intensity of concentration of excitement in the involved cortical area; the more intense and widespread the inhibition, the greater and more intense the evoked excitation. It is as if the potential energy of the entire cerebral cortex were channeled through the specific area of excitation.

In states of induced cortical inhibition, the human is not asleep. What appears to be sleep is suggested amnesia and though appearing to be deeply asleep one is aware of all activities in his environment and can recall when re-hypnotized even those stimuli which were presumably blocked out by selective amnesia. Even Pavlov's dogs were not truly asleep. He reports that they stood as statutes, as if carved from wood, whereas in true sleep, the dogs' muscles would be relaxed. In Pavlov's dogs there was an active cortical inhibition; they were truly hypnotized. Many studies have shown that the brain does not respond in hypnosis as it does in sleep (Bass, 1931; Jenness, 1937; Loomis, et al; 1936; Nygard, 1937).

The primary clinical result of hypnosis in man is the *suspension of evaluative judgment*. Independent thinking is "by-passed" in the hypnotic state; the person reacts on a stimulus-response basis. The grossest distortion of logic is accepted by the subject because he does not and *cannot* evaluate. Commands which arouse a specific fear mechanism (e.g. relating to rape or to murder) result in the disruption of the cortical inhibition and hence of the hypnotic state. The physiologic base for this loss of evaluative power lies in the inhibition of the cerebral cortical activity so that the free flow of associations is impaired. So that many experiences can be compared, a free flow of associations is essential for the normal evaluative process.

In consequence of this abdication of evaluative judgment, the cortex then responds on a "literal" basis and not to innuendos, connotations, and implications. Each request must therefore be

specifically designed to obtain a specific response. A surgical patient, under hypnosis, was told he would not feel the pain of
surgery. He did not, but he responded violently to the hot water
used. "Pain of surgery" meant to him only the pain of the scalpel.

The establishment of areas of excitation is done by orientation
and attention directing. The hypnotist orients the subject's attention by suggesting that he concentrate on a specific part of
the body, a particular memory, a definite concept. The cortical
area subserving the somatic area, the specific memory, or the
suggested concept, is thus alerted and becomes the area of excitation. By adequate techniques, this area of excitation becomes
concentrated.

The cerebral cortex functions in terms of *patterns of functional
activity* and not in terms of isolated anatomic units. Incoming
stimuli are integrated and synthesized by the cerebral cortex into
a pattern; the resultant response is in terms of a function which
includes different anatomic and physiologic entities. Thus the
cortex becomes aware not of the specific pricking of a particular
nerve fiber in a finger, but a painful sensation in that finger; it
responds not only by withdrawal of the involved finger but of
the entire hand. When, for example, suggestions are made during
hypnosis to bring on or postpone a menstrual flow, to curtail an
"emotionally induced" diarrhea, to relieve a "spastic colitis" con-
stipation, or to eliminate a headache, the response of the cortex is
not in terms of the musculature, the nervous or vascular supply,
but in terms of functional units. In a similar fashion, the hypnotic
fixation on a particular memory tends to arouse all of the tribu-
taries of that memory; the creation of a concept by suggestion
tends to activate—and be acted on—by all the subject's associations to that concept.

There are three primary areas which can be influenced therapeutically: somatic, mnemonic, and conceptual. Suggestions
made in the hypnotic state can influence any and all functions of
the soma—sensory, motor, visceral.

The inhibition (amnesia) or excitation of memories (recall of
those forgotten) operates on the same principles. Memory is
essentially a neurophysiologic function, the exact mechanism of
which is still unclear. Penfield (1951) has shown that mechanical

stimulation of temporal lobe areas activates memories. Apparently the electrical impulse from an external source activates a neural trunk which in turn results in the conscious evocation of certain memories. The as yet primitive techniques do not permit electric stimulation of specific memories but the principle is clear: memories radiate like the branches of a tree; the stimulation (via areas of cortical excitation) coursing down a given "branch" brings the memories involved into consciousness.

In the hypnotic state, the area of concentrated excitability, designated by the hypnotist, can be applied to a memory chain. There is a greater than usual flow of impulses down this memory trail; half-forgotten, distantly remembered, long-disused memories are now activated by this increased flow of impulses from the area of concentrated excitability. Hypnoanalysis finds this technique most useful.

The conceptual aspect involves pattern and image formation. The hypnotist suggests to the subject a concept, a pattern of thought or action; on the stage it may be the concept of being a monkey, a ballet dancer, Napoleon; in the therapist's office, the concept of being calm in situations that previously evoked anger, of being detached when criticized by a particular person, or of being interested in the meaning of an academic course. If adequately hypnotized, the subject accepts this suggestion without the usual independent evaluation. The more specific the concept delineated by the hypnotist, the more vivid it is, the more strongly will it be fixed. The more the appropriate emotional connotations (Kraines, 1963) of this concept the hypnotist can activate, the more deeply will the concept or image be fixed in the subject's mind.

The subject then draws on his own experiences which he feels are appropriate to the concept—each person has his own associations to the concept of a monkey, a ballet dancer, a Napoleon— and unless otherwise directed, he will act out the assigned role in terms of his own associations, his own functional patterns. The associations activated by the conceptual stimulus may be many, but they pertain only to the specific concept suggested and not to connotations or related concepts. Although it is infinitely easier to "act like a monkey" than to "be calm" (since emotionally-toned patterns are complex and require psychodynamic restructuring), nonetheless, the same principles apply.

Once such a concept is formed, it can then be associated with a stimulus (post-hypnotic suggestion); this stimulus occurring after the trance will arouse the suggested concept in the manner of a conditioned reflex. As a rule, conditioned reflexes in the human can be quickly implanted by the hypnotic procedure.

The greater the concentration of excitability in that portion of cortex involved in the formation of a given concept, the more firmly imprinted will it be. Concepts evoked during hypnosis have the quality of "reality." The persistence of the imprinted concept will depend upon the intensity of its fixation during the hypnotic state.

SUMMARY

The thesis is advanced that hypnosis is essentially a physiologic phenomenon involving both an active inhibitory process as well as areas of "concentrated excitation" in the cerebral cortex.

This thesis is supported by (1) application to human beings of Pavlovian concepts; (2) clinical responses of the hypnotized subjects; and (3) evidence from various trance-induction procedures.

Although induced by psychologic procedures, the cerebral physiodynamics of hypnosis result in the inhibition of the "normal" flow of intracortical associations. Since "evaluative thinking," is dependent on the free flow of associations which permits comparison of different memories and experiences, this cortical inhibition results in the suspension of evaluative thinking.

With the suspension of evaluative thinking, the subject becomes "hypersuggestible," reacting on a stimulus-response basis.

Desired somatic responses can be evoked by the activation of specific cortical areas via fixation of attention or command. Memory processes can similarly be enhanced, since the physiologic basis of memory resides in the cerebral cortex. Concepts and patterns of action, also dependent on cortical activity, can be created and activated by the inhibitory-excitatory mechanism. The concept that hypnosis is a state of cortical inhibition and excitation not only explains the various phenomena of hypnosis; it also can be used as a spring board by which the hypnotic trance can more easily be induced, intensified, and therapeutically enhanced.

REFERENCES

Bass, M. J.: Differentiation of the hypnotic trance from normal sleep. *J Exper Psychol*, *14:*382–399, 1931.

Brown, W.: *Psychology and Psychotherapy.* Baltimore, W. Wood, 1934.

Eysenck, H. J.: Suggestibility and hypnosis. *Proc Roy Soc Med*, *36:*349–354, 1963.

Ferenczi, S.: *Contributions to Psychoanalysis* (transl. by E. Jones). Boston, Badger, 1916.

Freud, S.: *Group Psychology and the Analysis of the Ego,* (transl. by J. Strachey). New York, Bone and Liveright, 1922.

Gellhorn, E., and Loofbourrow, G. N.: *Emotions and Emotional Disorders.* New York, Harper and Row, 1963.

Heidenhain, R.: *Hypnotism or Animal Magnetism* (transl. by L. C. Wooldridge). London, K. Paul, Trench, and Trubner, 1906.

Hull, C. L.: *Hypnosis and Suggestibility.* New York, Appleton-Century, 1933.

Janet, P.: *The Major Symptoms of Hysteria.* New York, Macmillan, 1920.

Jenness, A., and Wible, C. L.: Respiration and heart action in sleep and hypnosis. *J Gen Psychol*, *16:*197–222, 1937.

Kraines, S. H.: Emotions: A physiologic process. *Psychosomatics*, *4:*313–324, 1963.

Kraines, S. H.: Sodium amytal, hypnosis, and psychotherapy. *Am J Psychiat*, *122:*458–460, 1965, and *Int J Neuropsychiat* *3:*248–256, 1967.

Loomis, A. L., Harvey, E. N., and Hobart, G.: Brain potentials during hypnosis. *Science*, *83:*239–241, 1936.

Nygard, J. W.: Cerebral circulation prevailing during sleep and hypnosis. *Psychol Bull*, *34:*727, 1937.

McDougall, W.: *Outline of Abnormal Psychology.* New York, Scribner, 1926.

Pavlov, I. P.: *Lectures on Conditioned Reflexes* (transl. by W. H. Gantt). New York, International Publ., 1928.

Penfield, W.: Memory Mechanisms, *Trans Am Neurol Assoc*, *76:*15–31, 1951.

Preyer, W., quoted by Moll, A.: *Study of Hypnosis.* New York, Julian Press, 1958.

Schilder, P.: *The Nature of Hypnosis.* New York, Intern'l Univ. Press, 1956.

Weitzenhoffer, A. M.: *General Techniques of Hypnosis.* New York, Grune and Stratton, 1948.

Wolberg, L. R.: *Medical Hypnosis.* New York, Grune & Stratton, 1948.

Young, P. C.: Experimental hypnotism: a review. *Psychol Bull*, *38:*92–104, 1941.

CHAPTER 5

EXTINCTION OF A CONDITIONED MOTOR RESPONSE FOLLOWING HYPNOSIS*

John M. Plapp, Ph.D.
AND William E. Edmonston, Jr., Ph.D.

INTRODUCTION

The administration of a standard hypnosis induction procedure to 6 randomly assigned experimental Ss resulted in the disappearance of a recently acquired conditioned motor response. When hypnosis was terminated by another standard procedure the CR reappeared. On subsequent trials its appearance followed the usual extinction pattern. An equated control group (6 Ss) gave responses that followed the usual extinction pattern during both a "hypnosis-control" period and an identical 2nd block of extinction trials. Possible interpretations were considered and suggestions for further study made.

NOTICING that the repetition of a conditioned stimulus (CS), without any presentation of the unconditioned stimulus (UCS), caused a lethargic or drowsy state in his animals, Pavlov (1927) developed a theory which clearly linked the conditioning process and hypnosis. He postulated that during conditioning the one area of the brain most directly affected by the CS became the center of an inhibitory process which spread to other parts of the brain, so long as the CS was presented monotonously and without reinforcement. The final stage of this process of inhibition was

* Reprinted from the *Journal of Abnormal Psychology*, 1965, Vol. 70, No. 5, pages 378–381. Copyright 1965 by the American Psychological Association. Reprinted by permission.

sleep, and one of the stages prior to sleep was what Pavlov termed hypnosis. Pavlov's concepts such as "cortical inhibition," "cortical irradiation," and cortical localization with respect to specific stimuli have been utilized as the predominant interpretive framework employed by subsequent Russian investigators in the hypnosis field. The generalized conclusions of certain of the Russian studies on hypnosis may not bear a close relation to the empirical findings; on the other hand, they may be considered in their own right, without reference to the theoretical framework.

There has been considerable disagreement over the effects of hypnosis on CRs. Russian workers have long viewed hypnosis as a valid field for experimental investigation and have devoted considerable attention to the measurement of physiological responses. Most Russian investigators have reported that a CR established during the waking state shows a diminution during hypnosis (Korotkin and Suslova, 1951, 1959, 1960; Levin, 1959; Pen and Jigarov, 1959; Povorinsky, 1959; Povorinsky and Traugott, 1959). That the CR may be restored upon termination of hypnosis, has been reported by Korotkin and Suslova (1951). Among Russian investigators reporting no effect of hypnosis on CR extinction has been Livshits (1959). In general, the reports of Russian experimentation have been characterized by a lack of attention to control groups, use of a very small number of subjects, and a minimal use of statistics. Procedures, both conditioning and hypnotic, often appear poorly standardized and are rarely reported in the detail which would permit adequate replications.

Many of these criticisms of the Russian work can, unfortunately, be applied with equal relevance to American studies. In contrast to the general Soviet findings of inhibition of CR under hypnosis, Americans have more frequently reported no change in the CR (McCrainie and Crasilneck, 1955; Scott, 1930). Other American investigators, reporting that CR changes were due to age regression (Le Cron, 1956) or to such postulated effects as hypnotic blindness (Ludholm, 1928) or deafness (Erickson, 1944) have clearly assumed that hypnosis per se has no effect on the CR.

No clear-cut conclusion as to the fate of a previously established CR following the induction of hypnosis seems justified from the above studies. Contradictory findings could be explained largely in terms of different methodologies and the use of different CRs. There is some evidence (Livshits, 1959; McCrainie and Crasilneck, 1955) that hypnosis may have an inhibiting effect on previously acquired vocabulary (or motor) CRs but not on involuntary (or perhaps more accurately, physiological) CRs. Finally, there has been insufficient use of controls, so that effects reported as attributable to hypnosis could be accounted for in terms of an increased state of relaxation in subjects, without introducing the more complex concept of hypnosis as an explanatory term (Orne, 1959).

The present study was designed to investigate one aspect of the problem: the effect of hypnosis on the extinction of a previously established motor CR. A control group was employed in an attempt to discover whether any obtained change in the CR could be attributed to hypnosis or simply to an increased state of relaxation. The experimental hypothesis was that during extinction trials following the establishment of a conditioned finger retraction response, subjects who had been hypnotized immediately prior to the start of the extinction period would produce CRs of significantly lesser magnitude and significantly greater latency than control subjects, who went through similar procedures but were simply asked to relax. It was further predicted that experimental subjects, when awakened and given a second set of extinction trials, would give CRs which did not differ significantly from those produced by control subjects in a parallel second extinction period.

METHOD

Subjects

From approximately thirty Washington University and Medical School volunteer students, twelve subjects were chosen and equally divided into experimental (hypnosis) and control groups. Fourteen of the original thirty were excluded because they were unable to meet the conditioning criterion; the others failed to keep their appointments.

Assignment of each subject to an experimental or control group was made on a random basis. Each group contained four females and two males, and the two groups were equated with respect to mean age (19) and years of education (14).

Apparatus

The conditioning apparatus consisted of (*a*) an Eico Model 377 Audio Generator, adjusted to deliver the CS (a 2000 cycle per second, 80 decibel sine wave) to an amplifier which was placed approximately three feet behind the subject, (*b*) a Burdick muscle stimulator (Model MS-2) which delivered an UCS of up to 60 miliamperes. The UCS was delivered to the subject through two silver electrodes attached to the middle finger of the subject's right hand. Finger movements resulted in variations in the light reaching selenium cells, and activated one channel of an Offner polygraph, resulting in pen deflections which bore a linear correspondence to the finger movements. All fingers on the subject's right hand except for his middle finger were strapped down firmly and another strap was placed around the subject's forearm. Marker pens recorded onset, duration, and cessation of CS and UCS. The corresponding time periods, as well as the duration of the interval between CS and UCS, were controlled by automatic Hunter timers. The conditioning apparatus was operated from a one-way mirrored room next to the one in which the subject was seated. A red spot (0.5-inch diameter), placed on the wall in front of the subject's chair, approximately three feet above his eye level, served as the "target" in the hypnosis induction procedure.

Procedure

Both groups received identical conditioning procedures. After each subject was seated in a comfortable chair electrodes were attached, a large base electrode at the wrist, and the shock electrode on the middle finger of the right hand. The thread which led to the finger retraction recording apparatus was attached to the subject's middle finger.

Next, conditioning instructions, modeled after those of Lindley and Moyer (1961) were read. No subject responded with finger retraction to the initial presentations of tone. The shock was then adjusted to the strongest level of intensity the subject could tolerate. Learning trials were then presented, one in every block of five trials being a CS-alone presentation (test trial). The CS was presented for .5 second, followed by a .5-second interval, followed in turn by the UCS which lasted for .2 second. If it appeared that the subject was adapting to the shock level its intensity was increased. Intertrial intervals were randomly scheduled between twenty to forty seconds. A CR was defined as a pen deflection of no less than one millimeter from the baseline, occurring within one second after the onset of the CS. The criterion of conditioning was that the subject should give four conditioned responses in five consecutive test trials.

After conditioning, experimental subjects were given the following sections of the Stanford Hypnotic Susceptibility Scale (SHSS), Form A (Weitzenhoffer and Hilgard, 1959): (*a*) eye closure, (*b*) hand lowering (left hand), (*c*) arm rigidity (left), (*d*) eye catalepsy. The standard instructions were read to the subject in a quiet, rhythmic voice, the experimenter being seated behind and to the left of the subject, out of his line of vision. On each of the items *a* thru *d* the subject's performance was scored one or zero. If the subject obtained a total score of zero he was not considered hypnotized; any score from one to four was accepted as indicating hypnosis. No experimental subject obtained a total hypnotic susceptibility score of zero; one obtained a score of one; one, three; and the three remaining subjects, scores of four.

Following the above induction procedures, hypnosis group subjects were given the following instructions:

> Remain deeply relaxed and pay close attention to what I am going to tell you. In a moment I will be leaving the room for a while. All the time I am gone you will remain just as deeply relaxed as you are now. You will not wake up until I return and give you the instructions to awake. Remember, all the time I am gone you will continue to remain in a very deep state of relaxation. You will hear me leave, and you may hear me in the next room, but you will continue to feel deeply, comfortably relaxed, and you will not awake until I return and give you the instructions to awake. Now I am going to leave.

Twelve extinction trials were then administered to the hypnotized subject, an extinction trial being defined as the presentation of a CS without the UCS. Next, the arousal instructions from the SHSS were read. After the subject had been awakened another twelve extinction trials were administered.

Control and experimental groups received the same conditioning and extinction procedures, but instead of the hypnosis induction procedures ("eye closure" section of the SHSS), controls received the following instructions after conditioning:

> Now we come to the second part of the experiment. You are *not* going to be hypnotized in this experiment. Instead, I am simply going to ask you to relax, get as comfortable as you can, and go through certain simple procedures as I tell you to. I just want you to quite consciously follow the instructions I am going to give you.

Controls were instructed to make themselves comfortable and close their eyes. After a period of twenty minutes they were told to perform voluntarily the behaviors described above for hypnosis subjects (beginning with item *b* of the SHSS) and then the first twelve extinction trials were administered. Following this, control subjects were instructed to open their eyes and sit up again, and finally the second twelve extinction trials were presented.

RESULTS

In general, the records of control and experimental subjects demonstrated that subjects who had been hypnotized immediately prior to the start of extinction produced significantly fewer CRs during this period than control subjects, and that when hypnosis was terminated experimental and control subjects did not differ significantly (see Figure 5–1). To test for initial differences between the two groups in number of trials to criterion, a Mann-Whitney U test was applied. No significant difference was obtained (M of 38.8 and 36.0). The extinction records of each subject were scored independently by the two experimenters with a high degree of correspondence between their results (Pearson $r = .95$). Figure 5–1 presents the number of subjects giving CRs on each extinction trial (for the two extinction periods). The maximum number of CRs possible for either group on any trial was six, one for each subject. The difference between experi-

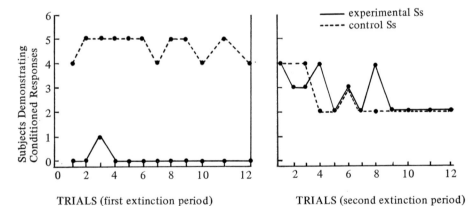

Figure 5–1. The number of subjects giving CRs on each extinction trial.

mental and control subjects during the first extinction period is clear. Only a single hypnosis subject responded at all to CS presentation during the first extinction period, while either four or five control subjects gave CRs on each trial. The sole hypnosis subject who responded was in fact that subject who obtained the lowest hypnotic susceptibility score, a score of one. During the second extinction period, after hypnosis subjects had been awakened, there was a reappearance of the CR for four experimental subjects on the initial trial and a subsequent gradual reduction in the number of CRs given. The groups were found not to differ significantly in number of CRs evoked during this second extinction period. A single experimental subject failed to respond during the second extinction period, and also one control subject failed to respond during either the first or second blocks of extinction trials. Since the CR was almost completely absent during the first extinction period for the experimental subjects, examination of the data in terms of CR amplitude and latency as had been originally proposed, was unnecessary.

DISCUSSION

If, as has been shown in this experiment, hypnosis does have an effect on the CR, it would seem that the type of response conditioned may be an important determinant of the effect obtained. The findings of a study by McCrainie and Crasilneck (1955) suggest such an inference. They found that all twelve subjects responded to the CS under hypnosis as they had in the normal state. Following age regression, the CR disappeared in the six subjects in whom a voluntary CR had been established, but failed to be influenced in the case of the six subjects in whom an involuntary response had been conditioned. Also relevant to the question of whether hypnosis has any effect on an established involuntary CR was the investigation by Livshits (1959), who conditioned differential vascular dilation and contraction responses to a buzzer and a bell before inducing hypnosis. Although he began with an impressive number of subjects (43), failures in conditioning and/or hypnosis reduced the N considerably (at least to 19), and the author presented his results mainly in intraindividual terms. Apparently there was much variation in the conditioning, and particularly in the hypnosis induction procedures used. Despite the general conclusion that "conditioned reflexes elaborated in the waking state were preserved in the state of hypnosis," clear evidence of this was presented only for a single subject.

Should a voluntary, but not an involuntary CR be inhibited during hypnosis, there is a strong possibility that this inhibition is part of an effect of hypnosis on the motor responsiveness of the subject, rather than being an interference with the ability to perceive the CS. And if, as seems to have been the case, most or all of the CRs which were reported to have disappeared or shown a reduction in amplitude under hypnosis were motor responses, it could be argued that the state of relaxation which accompanies hypnosis interferes with the generalized responsiveness of the subject. An adequate test of this possibility would necessitate the use of a control group who, though not hypnotized, were "relaxed" to the same extent as the hypnotized subjects. Investigation of the effects of employing such a control condition was one of the aims of the present study.

Since control subjects were presumably as relaxed as experimental subjects during first extinction period (they had sat with eyes closed for 20 minutes), the differences between the CRs produced by the two groups can be attributed to the specific hypnosis induction instructions received by the experimental group. Possibly, it was the repetitive, monotonous auditory stimulation from the experimenter which produced the differential effect on the CR, as would be suggested by the work of Dittborn and Kline (1958). Or it may have been the initial statement by the experimenter to experimental subjects that they were to be hypnotized and to control subjects that they were not to be, which led to the present results. The latter possibility would be consistent with the findings of Barber and Calverley (1964b) that subjects told they were in the hypnosis group were more responsive to suggestions than others told they were in the control group. Whether explanation of the present results is to be sought in terms of habituation resulting from repetitive stimulation or in the expectations of subjects, there is evidence here that the hypnotic state is not simply a point on a continuum from "alert wake-fulness" through "relaxation" to "sleep," as Pavlov and other Russian investigators have suggested. The present results also make necessary a reconsideration of certain conclusions regarding the effects of specific suggestions made to subjects during hyp-nosis. If hypnosis alone can result in the disappearance of a CR, this may help to explain some of the results of studies of "hyp-notic blindness," "hypnotic deafness," and "age regression" (Erickson, 1944; Le Cron, 1956; Lundholm, 1928). The need, in studying the effects of such hypnotic suggestions, for control groups of subjects who are simply hypnotized is thus underlined by the results of the present experiment.

Some questions may be raised about the adequacy of the pro-cedures used in the present investigation. The treatment of con-trol subjects during the interval which was intended to approxi-mate that of the hypnosis period for experimental subjects, may not have served its purpose adequately. Although it was at-tempted to match the two groups, control subjects differed in terms of receiving shorter, less repetitive introductory instruc-tions prior to performing the same behaviors as experimental subjects ("eye-closure" from the SHSS was omitted for controls). This fact makes it impossible to specify with complete assurance whether the behavior of experimental subjects during the first extinction period was due to "hypnosis" or simply to the longer and more detailed instructions they had received. In addition, the fact that the situation was defined to experimental (but not control) subjects as hypnosis, together with possible differential variations in experimenter's tone of voice, may have implied to experimental (but not to control) subjects that they were not expected to show the CR during the first extinction period. There is a need for further studies (e.g. Barber and Calverley, 1964a) which will vary systematically the instructions given to hypnosis and nonhypnosis groups, and also for investigations of the effects of hypnosis on voluntary as well as involuntary CRs. While cer-tain questions may be raised about the meaning of the present findings, there seems to be no doubt that extinction of a motor CR was clearly affected by hypnosis.

REFERENCES

Barber, T. X., and Calverley, D. S.: Effect of E's tone of voice on "hypnotic-like" suggestibility. *Psycho Rep, 15*:139–144, 1964a.

Barber, T. X., and Calverley, D. S.: Toward a theory of hypnotic behavior: Effects on suggestibility of defining the situation as hypnosis and defining response to suggestions as easy. *J Abnorm Soc Psychol, 68*:585–592, 1964b.

Dittborn, J. M., and Kline, M. V.: An instrument for the measurement of sleep induction. *J Psychol, 46*:277–278, 1958.

Erickson, M. H.: A study of clinical and experimental findings on hypnotic deafness. II Experimental findings with a conditioned response technique. *J Gen Psychol, 31*:191–212, 1944.

Korotkin, I. I., and Suslova, M. M.: *Zhurn Vyssh Nervn. Deyatel' Nosti,* Vol. I:(4), 1951.

Korotkin, I. I., and Suslova, M. M.: Changes in conditioned and unconditioned reflexes during suggestion states in hypnosis. In *The Central Nervous System and Human Behavior.* Princeton, N. J., Public Health Service, U. S. Department of Health, Education, and Welfare, 1959.

Korotkin, I. I., and Suslova, M. M.: Comparative effects of suggestion in the waking state and in hypnosis. *Pavlov Journal of Higher Nervous Activity, 10*:185–192, 1960.

Le Cron, L. M.: A study of age regression under hypnosis. In Le Cron, L. M. (Ed.): *Experimental hypnosis.* New York, Macmillan, 1956.

Levin, S.: In Platonov, K. (Ed.): *The Word as a Physiological and Therapeutic Factor.* Moscow, Foreign Languages Publishing House, 1959, p. 75.

Lindley, R. H., and Moyer, K. E.: Effects of instructions on the extinction of a conditioned finger-withdrawal response. *J Exp Psychol, 61*:82–88, 1961.

Livshits, L. S.: The investigation of the higher nervous activity of man in hypnosis in relation to chronic alcoholism. *Pavlov Journal of Higher Nervous Activity, 9*:745–753, 1959.

Lundholm, H.: An experimental study of functional anesthesias in hypnosis. *J Abnorm Soc Psychol, 23*:337–355, 1928.

McCrainie, E. J., and Crasilneck, H. B.: The conditioned reflex in hypnotic age regression. *J. Clin Psychol, 16*:120–123, 1955.

Orne, M. T.: The nature of hypnosis: Artifact and essence. *J Abnorm Soc Psychol, 58*:277–299, 1959.

Pavlov, I. P.: *Conditioned Reflexes.* London, Oxford Universities Press, 1927.

Pen, R., and Jigarov, M.: In Platonov, K. (Ed.): *The Word as a Physiological and Therapeutic Factor.* Moscow, Foreign Languages Publishing House, 1959, p. 75.

Povorinsky, Y.: (1937). In Platonov, K. (Ed.): *The Word as a Physiological and Therapeutic Factor.* Moscow, Foreign Languages Publishing House, 1959, p. 75.

Povorinsky, Y., and Traugott, N.: In Platonov, K. (Ed.): *The Word as a Physiological and Therapeutic Factor.* Moscow, Foreign Languages Publishing House, 1959, p. 75.

Scott, H. D.: Hypnosis and the conditioned reflex. *J Gen Psychol,* 4:113–129, 1930.

Weitzenhoffer, A. M., and Hilgard, E. R.: *Stanford Hypnotic Susceptibility Scale.* Palo Alto, Calif., Consulting Psychologists Press, 1959.

CHAPTER 6

POSTHYPNOTIC SUGGESTION AS HIGHER-ORDER CONDITIONING: A METHODOLOGICAL AND EXPERIMENTAL ANALYSIS*

ALFRED A. BARRIOS, PH.D.

Abstract: The hypothesis that hypnosis facilitates higher-order conditioning was tested. The results supported the three predictions made from the hypothesis: (a) The hypnosis group ($N = 43$) showed greater conditioning ($p < .01$) than the control group ($N = 42$); (b) the amount of conditioning for the hypnotic group was correlated with hypnotic depth ($p < .01$); and (c) this conditioned response, once formed, was a strong one, as evidenced by little extinction and the phenomenon of spontaneous recovery. The dependent variable, conditioned salivation, was measured by a unique procedure which allows large numbers of Ss to be measured simultaneously. The experimental design provided several innovative means for avoiding a number of shortcomings common to hypnosis experiments, including a most insidious one—the fact that most previous indicants of hypnosis have been misleading.

THEORY AND PURPOSE

THE PURPOSE of the present study is twofold: (a) to test the hypothesis that hypnosis facilitates higher-order conditioning; and (b) to suggest ways of overcoming some of the methodological shortcomings of previous hypnosis experiments.

In the theory of hypnosis proposed earlier by the present author (Barrios, 1969), changes produced by means of posthyp-

---

* This chapter is a shortened version of the original article, reprinted from the January 1973 *International Journal of Clinical and Experimental Hypnosis.* Copyrighted by The Society for Clinical and Experimental Hypnosis, January 1973.

notic suggestion (PHS) were explained as occurring through a process of higher-order conditioning (see also Barrios, 1970). As was pointed out by Pavlov (1927), words can act as conditioned stimuli and can thus be combined in sentences to produce higher-order conditioning (Mowrer, 1960). A posthypnotic suggestion sentence can then be considered a form of higher-order conditioning. Further, Barrios hypothesized that hypnosis facilitated such conditioning. Four sources of evidence supporting the latter hypothesis (referred to in the theory as hypothesis VII) were presented: (*a*) studies indicating that hypnosis facilitates first-order conditioning (Leuba, 1940; Scott, 1930); (*b*) successful use of PHS in medicine (Cangello, 1961; Crasilneck, Stirman, Wilson, McCranie, and Fogelman, 1955; Fogelman and Crasilneck, 1956; Kroger and DeLee, 1943; Marmer, 1956; Mason, 1955; Raginsky, 1951; Schneck, 1953); (*c*) successful use of PHS in psychotherapy (Abrams, 1963, 1964; Alexander, 1965; Biddle, 1967; Chong, 1964, 1966; Richardson, 1963; Stein, 1963); and (*d*) experimental studies on PHS (Edwards, 1963; Kellogg, 1929; Orne, 1963; Patten, 1930; Weitzenhoffer, 1950).

The main problem with the above studies, as well as with most hypnosis studies in general, is their methodological shortcomings. Several such shortcomings are reviewed below with reference to the way in which the present study attempts to eliminate them. (Shortcomings 1 to 4 will be familiar to most readers as those expounded upon recently by Barber [1969b] and Barber and Calverley [1966a].)

1. In many cases there was no comparison with a non-hypnotic control group. In such studies one could not be sure that presenting the suggestion without inducing hypnosis might not have achieved the same results. (This is especially true of the clinical studies.) In the present study not only was there a non-hypnosis group, but, in addition, each S acted as his own control.

2. When control Ss were used, the experimental Ss were usually pre-selected for their high hypnotic susceptibility, whereas controls were not, or, even worse, the controls were sometimes selected for their poor hypnotic susceptibility. In such cases one could not be sure that it was the actual hypnotic induction, and not the high initial level of suggestibility of the experimental Ss, that produced the difference in effect.

In the present study thare was *no* pre-selection of Ss for hypnotic susceptibility, directly or indirectly. The standard procedure for recruiting college Ss was followed, and Ss were randomly assigned to one of the two groups. It should be mentioned that still another often referred to shortcoming was eliminated by the design—there was no more time or special attention spent on the hypnotic Ss than on control Ss.

3. In experiments where hypnotic Ss have been used as their own controls it is usually obvious to these Ss which is the control state. As Barber (1962) points out, these Ss could ensure a worse performance in the control state, sensing that this is what *E* expects of them. This point was also brought out in the study by Scharf and Zamansky (1963). According to Orne (1959), the demand characteristics of an experiment may be particularly pronounced in hypnotic experiments because Ss recognize that they are expected to do better in hypnosis and, thus, we might also anticipate they are more likely to do poorer during the control phase (see also Barber, 1969b). In most hypnosis experiments this may very well be the case since the "own-control" session is run *after* the hypnosis session. In the current experiment the "own-control" session was run *first* for all Ss, and before they even knew hypnosis was to be involved.

4. In experiments where controls have been used, *E* has not usually controlled for difference in tone of voice or other subconscious differences in treatment of the groups, thus possibly biasing the results in favor of his hypothesis. That differences in tone of voice can have an effect was shown in a study by Barber and Calverley (1964). This shortcoming was taken care of in the current experiment by the extensive use of tapes.

5. Most of the responses used as the dependent variable in PHS experiments are highly subject to voluntary control. Such use of voluntary responses are more apt to lead to the criticism that S was faking—just performing the response to please the hypnotist. In the current experiment use was made of the salivary response, a response that is considerably less subject to voluntary control than most responses previously used in PHS experiments.

6. Controls have usually not been run for the effect of the hypnotic state, per se. Some might feel that the posthypnotic changes can be produced by just the state itself, rather than any

specific suggestion. This shortcoming was taken care of in the design by means of a neutral stimulus. If the salivary responses obtained were due solely to the effects of having been hypnotized, we should find no difference between the response to the conditioned stimulus and the response to the neutral stimulus. As can be seen by the results, this was not the case.

7. Perhaps the most prevalent, as well as the most insidious, of the shortcomings is that *the usual indicants of hypnosis are misleading.* This includes both (*a*) the *"antecedent"* type of indicant where *E* assumes that hypnosis has been induced because Ss have been put through a standard hypnotic induction, and (*b*) the *"consequent"* type of indicant where *E* concludes that hypnosis has been induced because of *S*'s responsiveness to a set of test suggestions given after *S* is hypnotized.

(*a*) The basic problem with the antecedent indicant is that it usually leads one to the incorrect conclusion that the results of the experiment hold for *hypnosis in general,* when actually they hold only for the *particular hypnotic induction* used. For example, many people seem to commit this error with regard to many of Barber's (1969b) experiments where he appears to operationally define hypnosis as a "standard 15-minute induction," and where he concludes that task motivating instructions (TMI) can produce hypnotic phenomena as effectively as a hypnotic induction. The use of such an antecedent indicant is quite acceptable as long as *E* makes it clear that any conclusions regarding hypnosis refer *only* to this narrow, operationally-defined band on the hypnosis continuum. Apparently this has not been done sufficiently, for many have mistakenly interpreted Barber as implying that *hypnosis* is not as effective as had previously been thought.*

Underlying such overgeneralizations are two basic assumptions, both subject to questioning. First, there is the assumption that hypnotic responsiveness is a fixed character-trait, heretofore ac-

---

* Actually, it seems that it is others more than Barber who tend to overgeneralize his findings. It would appear that what Barber is trying to point out is that it is the *standard hypnotic induction,* not *hypnosis in general* that is not uniquely effective. This is based on the observation that in recent studies (e.g. Barber, 1969a) he seems to be saying that hypnotic responsiveness could be increased if we first determine the variables playing the key roles in a hypnotic induction and then work on maximizing their effect.

cepted as fact. Recent studies (e.g. Barber, 1964) seem to indicate that such an assumption is not justified, and a considerable number of studies indicate that responsiveness can be increased with improved methods of hypnotic induction (Barber, 1969a; Baykushev, 1969; Dorcus, 1963; Klinger, 1968; Pascal and Salzberg, 1959; Sachs and Anderson, 1967; Wilson, 1967).

Thus, it is incumbent upon any *E* "testing the effectiveness of hypnosis" that he make it very clear that his experiment is merely testing the effectiveness of a *particular* hypnotic induction procedure and not hypnosis in general.

The second assumption open to questioning is that hypnotic induction primarily involves the giving of suggestions of relaxation, drowsiness, and sleep (after S has been properly motivated and a positive attitude and expectancy toward hypnosis established). According to the definition of hypnotic induction (discussed later in the paper) given in the theory proposed by the author (Barrios, 1969), this is just *one* form of hypnotic induction. *Barber's TMI followed by his test suggestions in ascending order of difficulty would also classify as a hypnotic induction.* Thus, when Barber states that his TMI are just as effective as hypnotic induction, one should realize that he is merely comparing the relative effectiveness of two forms of hypnotic induction.

Thus, it is also incumbent on *E* to let the reader know how he defines hypnosis and that results refer primarily to this definition and not "hypnosis in general."

(*b*) The trouble with the consequent type of indicant is that it is merely a measure of responsiveness, not *increase* in responsiveness. A truer indicant of how effective a hypnotic induction is (and the one used in the present study) would be the *difference* in response to test suggestions given both *after and before* S is hypnotized (T_2—T_1). Using T_2 alone as the indicant can be misleading in a number of ways. For example, a hypnotic induction could be ineffective and we could still get a high T_2 score if Ss were high responders to begin with. Conversely, a hypnotic induction could be effective but not show up as such if Ss were very low responders to begin with.[*]

---

[*] In cases where it would be difficult to give the pre-test suggestions, the next best thing is to have appropriate comparison control groups as described above.

OVERVIEW OF EXPERIMENT

The response to be conditioned was the salivary response produced by the suggestion of tasting a sour lemon. Two groups of Ss were compared. Prior to any hypnosis both groups were given the "posthypnotic suggestion" (hereafter referred to as the conditioning suggestion) that they would taste a sour lemon whenever they heard a particular symbol, and they were then tested for amount of conditioned salivation. Four days later the conditioning suggestion was repeated for both groups. However, prior to this repetition, the experimental group was hypnotized. In the case of the control group, the conditioning suggestion was repeated with no preceding hypnotic treatment. The change in amount of conditioning between the two sessions was compared for the two groups.

The experimental group was also put through an extinction series and a test for spontaneous recovery to see how the posthypnotic response holds up with continued presentation of the CS.

Both groups were given a set of five test suggestions in the first session. These same suggestions were repeated in the second session after hypnotic induction. (The control group was also hypnotized, but at the end of the second session.) The difference between the first and second session test suggestion scores (T_2—T_1) was used to determine S's hypnotic difference (HD); that is, the difference in responsiveness produced by the hypnotic induction.

Three predictions were made with regard to the hypothesis being tested (that hypnosis facilitates higher-order conditioning). First, it was predicted that the increase in conditioning of the experimental group would be statistically significantly greater than that of the control group; second, that the amount of increase for the experimental group would be positively correlated with the hypnotic difference (T_2—T_1); and third, that the CR for the hypnotic Ss would be a strong one, as indicated by little extinction and the phenomenon of spontaneous recovery.

HYPNOTIC INDUCTION (HI)

In the theory proposed by the present author (Barrios, 1969) *"Hypnotic induction is defined as . . . the giving of two or more suggestions in succession so that a positive response to one increases the probability of responding to the next one."* Also pointed out was the fact that hypnotic responsiveness is in addition affected by such factors as fears, attitudes, motivations, and expectations.

In the present study, then, there was first a pre-induction talk aimed at eliminating misconceptions, fears, and negative attitudes concerning hypnosis. The hypnotic induction itself consisted mainly of a series of suggestions starting with those felt to have a high probability of success. Three stages were used as opposed to one long series. This was done because it was felt that if S failed or did not do too well in the initial suggestions, he would be given a second and third chance to start over. In the pre-induction talk, failure was minimized. (See Barrios [1969], Appendix A, for the complete hypnotic induction.)

In designing the experiment no attempt was made to isolate the effect of the various factors involved in the HI. This we have left for future experiments.

RESULTS

Outcome of the Three Predictions

The mean increase in conditioning (CI) for the experimental group was 112.8 mg/min, and for the controls it was -35.8 mg/min ($F = 7.99$; df 1, 83, $p < .01$), thus confirming the prediction that the experimental group would show a greater increase in conditioning than the control.* (A complete compilation of data can be found in Barrios [1969], Appendix B.)

With regard to the second prediction made, there was a posi-

---

* The slight decrease (-35.8) for the control group is what Barber might have predicted for this group. In one of his studies (Barber and Calverley, 1966b), a straight repetition of the exact same set of suggestions over a series of sessions tended to produce boredom with consequent decrease in responsiveness *and* as early as the very first repeat session.

tive correlation (.38, $p < .01$) between the increase in conditioning (CI) and the hypnotic difference (HD) for the experimental
group. In other words, the greater the effect of the HI, the greater
the increase in conditioning, as predicted. *This means that as
methods of hypnotic induction are improved we should find even
greater differences between hypnotic and control groups.*

Now we come to the third prediction: CR would be strong
for the hypnotic Ss, as evidenced by the extinction and spontaneous recovery trials. With regard to extinction, we would expect
the strong CR, once formed, to maintain its level over a series of
extinction trials. In Figure 6–1 we see how the CI (directly pro-
portional to CR) remains fairly constant over seven non-rein-
forced trials for the experimental group (see also Barrios [1969],
Table C of Appendix B). An analysis of variance performed on

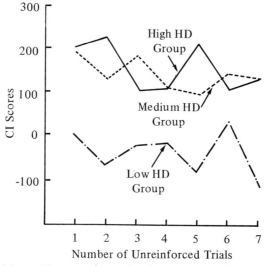

Figure 6.–1. Mean CI scores for each of seven unreinforced trials for the
group.*

* The responses of Trials 1 and 2 were those averaged to get mean CR
scores for second session. Trials 3 to 6 are the "extinction" trials. Trial 7
is the test for spontaneous recovery. These subgroups were formed by
simply dividing the experimental group on the basis of HD into the lower
third, middle third, and upper third.

the seven means showed that there were no significant differences among them ($F = 1.11$), thus supporting the prediction. A breakdown of this data into high, medium, and low HD groups indicates that each subgroup tended to maintain its own level.

An interesting and somewhat unexpected result shows up in Figure 6–1. We see that the medium group is almost at the same level as the high group. This would seem to imply that a medium level of hypnosis is sufficient to establish this particular conditioned response. However, it could be that under other circumstances greater differences might have shown up between the high and medium groups—a longer extinction series, perhaps.

It was expected that for the hypnotic Ss there would be evidence of spontaneous recovery from any initial extinction. Analysis of the data indicates this was true mainly for the high HD Ss. The opposite seemed to obtain for low HD Ss. A positive correlation of .37 ($p < .02$) was found between HD and amount of spontaneous recovery (CI_7—CI_6).

Discrimination

In addition to amplitude of response and resistance to extinction, there is yet another measure of conditioning one can look at in the current experiment—discrimination. It will be recalled that the measure of conditioning used here was not CR, but $\overline{CR\text{-}N}$ (salivation to conditioned stimulus minus salivation to neutral stimulus). Thus, it is conceivable that one might condition a strong CR and yet show no conditioning in this experiment. This would be the case if there was considerable generalization to the neutral stimulus. In order to lessen this possibility, part of the conditioning suggestion was aimed at decreasing generalization and increasing discrimination. That is, Ss were told not only that they would taste a sour lemon upon hearing their symbol, but also that this would happen *only* when they heard their symbol: "any other symbol would have no effect whatsoever."

In order to measure change in discrimination, the N scores before and after the hypnosis can be compared. We would expect to find a lower N score after hypnotic conditioning. Using N_1—N_2 as a measure of discrimination then, the mean N_1—N_2 score for the experimental group (485.2—414.4, or +70.8) is greater than the mean N_1—N_2 score for the control group (318.7—363.7, or —45.0); (.05 < p < .10). Also, the data revealed that discrimination for the experimental group was significantly correlated with HD ($r = .34$, $p < .02$).

An Additional Finding of Interest

Further analysis of the data discloses one additional finding of interest: hypothesis III of the author's theory (Barrios, 1969) contends that a positive response to a previous suggestion will increase, and a negative response will decrease, the probability of a positive response to a following suggestion. This contention is given some support by the data. The data most relevant here are the correlations between T_2 and D_2, the test suggestion scores and the indicant of conditioning, both from the second conditioning session. In the case of the experimental group we would predict a high correlation since the conditioning suggestion followed immediately after the test suggestions. For the control group we would predict a low correlation since the conditioning suggestion and the test suggestions were disconnected. It will be remembered that the controls were hypnotized considerably after the second conditioning suggestion; thus quite a bit of time passed between the conditioning suggestion and the test suggestions. Results show a correlation of .43 ($p < .01$) between T_2 and D_2 for the experimental group. For the control group we find no correlations ($r = —.06$).

In further support of hypothesis III is the low correlation between T_1 and D_1. It will be remembered that in the first session these two measures were disconnected for all Ss, in a manner similar to that used with the controls in the second session. Thus, we would also predict a low correlation here, and, in fact, this is what was obtained. (The correlations between T_1 and D_1 for both the experimental and the control groups were nonsignificant.)

Of course, since these are correlations, we would not be justified in making any definitive conclusions regarding causal effects of one variable on the other, although the positive correlations do lend some support to the hypothesis.

DISCUSSION

Implications of the Experimental Findings

The fact that the three predictions were upheld supports hypothesis VII of the present author's theory (Barrios, 1969)[*] that hypnosis facilitates higher-order conditioning. Now, what does this mean with regard to the theory?

One should first be aware that the present experiment was not run as a "critical test" of the theory. In science no one experiment can conclusively prove a hypothesis, let alone a theory. Nor, conversely, can we expect any one theory to uniquely account for the findings. Nothing is ever absolute in science. However, the results of the experiment *support* the theory. If, in time, a series of experiments are run testing various aspects of the theory and the preponderance of them support it, then the theory is a valid one. As for differentiating it from other theories, many theories can explain the same facts. What should be used to judge whether one theory is better than another are such criteria as the following: (a) which theory can explain or predict the most facts; (b) which theory is based on the least assumptions (law of parsimony) or can be broken down into the fewest postulates; and (c) which theory is most heuristic, stimulating the most worthwhile research. On the basis of such criteria, it is hoped that the present theory will prove to be a good one.

Regardless of whether the overall theory is or is not eventually "proven," it has at least stimulated the current study, leading to some rather interesting findings. The following are three of the more important implications supported by these findings:

1. Hypnotic behavior can be explained in terms of words acting as conditioned stimuli.
2. The changes produced by posthypnotic suggestion can be explained as occurring through a process of higher-order conditioning.
3. The greater the effectiveness of a hypnotic induction, the

---

[*] Copies of the theory can be had by writing the author. For the entire dissertation, including appendices and the complete hypnotic induction, see reference section.

more effective the conditioning produced by posthypnotic suggestion.

For those who might wonder what value there is in tying hypnosis in with conditioning, there seem to be at least three advantages: (*a*) tying hypnosis down to "known laws" takes away much of the usual mysticism associated with hypnosis (admittedly, theories of conditioning are not yet "laws," but they do seem somewhat closer than theories of hypnosis); (*b*) laws and facts relating to conditioning can be applied in developing new approaches in the investigation and understanding of hypnosis, as was done in the current study; and (*c*) laws and facts of hypnosis can be used to shed further light on the area of conditioning.

Methodological Implications

In addition to the above implications for a theory of hypnosis there are also certain important methodological implications of the study.

First of all, the experiment provides a simple format which can be used in other hypnosis experiments; one that will help avoid such methodological criticisms as those leveled by Barber.

Secondly, the experiment also provides a viable model for human conditioning studies. The current adaptation of Razran's (1935) technique has demonstrated that salivation appears to be a valid and highly reliable measure.* Further, with this adaptation there appears to be a distinct advantage over the current conditioning measures being used (e.g. GSR and eyeblink), in that with it Ss can more readily be run in large groups.

Finally, certain important flaws in the usual indicants of hyp-

---

* Judging from the outcome of the present experiment, one wonders why Razran's (1935) "cotton roll" technique has not been used more often in human conditioning experiments. Perhaps one reason for the hesitation has been that *E*s are somehow under the impression that salivation is not a reliable enough response when working with humans. Nothing could be further from the truth. In following the current adaptation of Razran's technique for use with large groups, we found the following correlations between first and second session salivation responses for each *S:* The correlation between N_1 and N_2 for the control group was .72, and for the experimental group was .55. The correlation between CR_1 and CR_2 for the control group was .87 and for the experimental group was .82. (All correlations, $p < .001$.)

nosis were pointed out, which it is hoped will help clear up such misconceptions as those that have arisen from much of Barber's (1969b) work. As has been pointed out, after reading many of Barber's studies one is liable to get the mistaken impression that *hypnosis* isn't as uniquely effective as many people seem to have thought. Students, experimenters, and clinicians relatively unfamiliar with hypnosis can be greatly influenced by such experiments and can easily conclude that since hypnosis has "been shown to be relatively ineffective" it is not worth investigating. This, it is felt, was definitely not Barber's intent. On the contrary, he has attempted to open up the field by trying to clear away the misconceptions associated with hypnosis and tie it down to known laws and facts. Unfortunately, it would appear that, for many, rather than explain hypnosis, he may have, instead, explained it away.

REFERENCES

Abrams, S.: Short-term hypnotherapy of a schizophrenic patient. *Am J Clin Hypn*, 5:237–247, 1963.

Abrams, S.: The use of hypnotic techniques with psychotics: A critical review. *Am J Psychother*, 18:79–94, 1964.

Alexander, L.: Clinical experiences with hypnosis in psychiatric therapy. *Am J Clin Hypn*, 7:190–206, 1965.

Barber, T. X.: Experimental controls and the phenomena of "hypnosis": A critique of hypnotic research methodology. *J Nerv Ment Dis, 134*:493–505, 1962.

Barber, T. X.: Hypnotizability, suggestibility, and personality: V. A critical review of research findings. *Psychol Rep, 14:*(Monograph Suppl. 3), 1964.

Barber, T. X.: An empirically-based formulation of hypnotism. *Am J Clin Hypn, 12*:100–130, 1969a.

Barber, T. X.: *Hypnosis: A Scientific Approach*. New York, Van Nostrand, 1969b.

Barber, T. X., and Calverley, D. S.: Effect of *E*'s tone of voice on "hypnotic-like" suggestibility. *Psychol Rep, 15*:139–144, 1964.

Barber, T. X., and Calverley, D. S.: Effects on recall of hypnotic induction, motivational suggestions, and suggested regression: A methodological and experimental analysis. *J Abnorm Psychol, 71*:169–180, 1966a.

Barber, T. X., and Calverley, D. S.: Toward a theory of hypnotic behavior: Experimental evaluation of Hull's postulate that hypnotic susceptibility is a habit phenomenon. *J Pers, 34*:416–433, 1966b.

Barrios, A. A.: *Toward Understanding the Effectiveness of Hypnotherapy:*

A Combined Clinical, Theoretical, and Experimental Approach. (Doctoral dissertation, University of California, Los Angeles) Ann Arbor, Michigan, University Microfilms, No. 69–14, 039, 1969.

Barrios, A. A.: Hypnotherapy: A reappraisal. *Psychother: Theor, Res Pract,* 7:2–7, 1970.

Baykushev, S. V.: Hyperventilation as an accelerated hypnotic induction technique. *Int J Clin Exp Hypn,* 17:20–24, 1969.

Biddle, W. E.: *Hypnosis in the Psychoses.* Springfield, Thomas, 1967.

Cangello, V. W.: The use of hypnotic suggestion for pain relief in malignant disease. *Int J Clin Exp Hypn,* 9:17–22, 1961.

Chong, T. M.: Hypnosis in general medical practice in Singapore. *Am J Clin Hypn,* 6:340–344, 1964.

Chong, T. M.: Psychosomatic medicine and hypnosis. *Am J Clin Hypn,* 8:173–177, 1966.

Crasilneck, H. B., Stirman, J. A., Wilson, B. J., McCranie, E. J., and Fogelman, M. J.: Use of hypnosis in the management of patients with burns. *JAMA,* 158:103–106, 1955.

Dorcus, R. M.: Fallacies in predictions of susceptibility to hypnosis based upon personality characteristics. *Am J Clin Hypn,* 5:163–170, 1963.

Edwards, G.: Duration of post-hypnotic effect. *Brit J Psychiat,* 109:259–266, 1963.

Fogelman, M. J., and Crasilneck, H. B.: Food intake and hypnosis. *J Am Diet Assoc,* 32:519–523, 1956.

Kellogg, E. R.: Duration of the effects of post-hypnotic suggestions. *J Exp Psychol,* 12:502–514, 1929.

Klinger, B. I.: The effects of peer model responsiveness and length of induction procedure on hypnotic responsiveness. Paper presented at the meeting of the East. Psychol. Assn., Washington, D. C., April, 1968.

Kroger, W. S., and DeLee, S. T.: The use of the hypnoidal state as an amnesic, analgesic and anesthetic agent in obstetrics. *Am J Obstet Gynec,* 46:655–661, 1943.

Leuba, C.: Images as conditioned sensations. *J Exp Psychol,* 26:345–351, 1940.

Marmer, M. J.: The role of hypnosis in anesthesiology. *JAMA,* 162:441–443, 1956.

Mason, A. A.: Surgery under hypnosis. *Anesthesia,* 10:295–302, 1955.

Mowrer, O. H.: *Learning Theory and the Symbolic Processes.* New York, Wiley, 1960.

Orne, M. T.: The nature of hypnosis: Artifact and essence. *J Abnorm Soc Psychol,* 58:277–299, 1959.

Orne, M. T.: The nature of the hypnotic phenomenon: Recent empirical studies. Paper presented at the meeting of the Amer. Psychol. Assn, Philadelphia, September, 1963.

Pascal, G. R., and Salzberg, H. C.: A systematic approach to inducing hypnotic behavior. *Int J Clin Exp Hypn,* 7:161–167, 1959.

Patten, E. F.: The duration of post-hypnotic suggestion. *J Abnorm Soc Psychol*, 25:319–334, 1930.

Pavlov, I. P.: *Conditioned Reflexes: An Investigation of the Psysiological Activity of the Cerebral Cortex.* (Re-issue of 1927 edition) New York, Dover, 1960.

Raginsky, B. B.: The use of hypnosis in anesthesiology. *J Pers.*, 1:340–348, 1951.

Razran, G. H. S.: Conditioned responses: An experimental study and a theoretical analysis. *Arch Psychol*, 28 (#191), 1935.

Richardson, T. A.: Hypnotherapy in frigidity. *Am J Clin Hypn*, 5:194–199, 1963.

Sachs, L. B., and Anderson, W. L.: Modification of hypnotic susceptibility. *Int J Clin Exp Hypn*, 15:172–180, 1967.

Scharf, B., and Zamansky, H. S.: Reduction of word-recognition threshold under hypnosis. *Percept Mot Skills*, 17:499–510, 1963.

Schneck, J. M.: *Hypnosis in Modern Medicine.* Springfield, Thomas, 1953.

Scott, H. D.: Hypnosis and the conditioned reflex. *J Gen Psychol*, 4:113–130, 1930.

Stein, C.: The clenched fist technique as a hypnotic procedure in clinical psychotherapy. *Am J Clin Hypn*, 6:113–119, 1963.

Weitzenhoffer, A. M.: A note on the persistence of hypnotic suggestion. *J Abnorm Soc Psychol*, 45:160–162, 1950.

Wilson, D. L.: The role of confirmation of expectancies in hypnotic induction. Unpublished doctoral dissertation, University of North Carolina, 1967.

CHAPTER 7

ACQUISITION OF VOLUNTARY CONTROL OVER AUTONOMIC NERVOUS FUNCTIONS BY CONDITIONING AND HYPNOSIS.

A. S. PATERSON, F. BRACCHI, D. PASSERINI, D. SPINELLI AND S. BLACK
From Psychiatric Laboratory West London Hospital (Charing Cross Group) London W6, England.

U P UNTIL THE PRESENT TIME, the study and treatment of the neuroses has been rather one-sided. The psychotherapist has been dependent for his knowledge of the nature of neurosis almost entirely on what the patient tells him, but it is obviously not satisfactory that our knowledge of an illness should be dependent merely on the description by the patient of his subjective symptoms. The present study represents an attempt to investigate neurotic symptoms chiefly from the objective standpoint. It is possible by a simple conditioning technique to produce a mild neurosis in a volunteer and to study the gradual appearance of a neurotic symptom as well as its disappearance under controlled conditions. (Alexander, 1958) In 1959 we constructed a five-channel polygraphic apparatus for recording the EEG (alpha rhythm), respiratory movements, heart rate (cardiotachymeter), galvanic skin reflex (GSR), and signals. The technique employed was for the human subject to be conditioned in such a way that

* Reprinted mostly from "Hypnosis and Psychosomatic Medicine," J. Lassner, (Ed.) Springer Verlag, Berlin, Heidelberg, New York, 1967. Proceedings of the International Congress for Hypnosis and Psychosomatic Medicine, Paris, 1965, pp. 236–241.

when a high tone (310 cycles) was presented to him for five seconds he received a painful shock to a finger on the fourth second. However when he heard a low tone (130 cycles) he never received a shock. After a week when he had five sessions, whenever he heard the high tone he showed a fear reaction, generally with acceleration of the heart, but when he heard the low tone he had a feeling of relaxation, often with slowing of the heart. (See Figures 7–1 a, b, c and d)

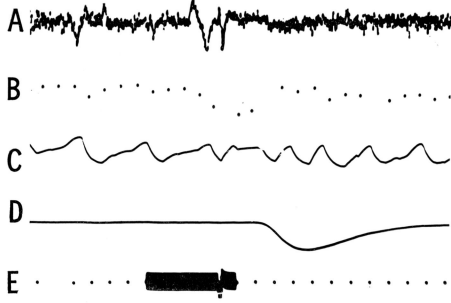

Figure 7–1a. *Reaction of unconditioned subject (S) to painful stimulus (unconditional stimulus, US)* Read from left to right.

A. EEG, fronto-occipital lead.

B. Cardiocyclometer, each dot represents the same point in the cardiac cycles. When the heart rate (HR) increases, the dots are closer together and the level of the line falls. The US causes an immediate acceleration and some missed beats (wide spaces between dots).

C. Respiration. Inspiration upwards. Note acceleration after US.

D. Galvanic Skin Reflex (GSR). Note reaction is marked and long lasting. A positive result is represented nearly always as a movement downwards, but may be upwards with this method. It is expressed in mV.

E. Time in seconds. The broad line represents the high tone (312 c.p.s.) lasting 6 seconds. The break in the line shows the US (Paterson et al., 1961).

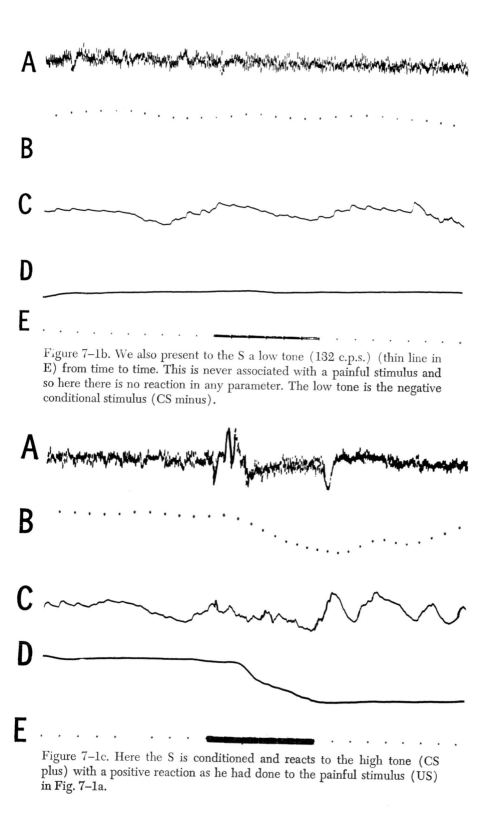

A

B

C

D

E

Figure 7–1b. We also present to the S a low tone (132 c.p.s.) (thin line in E) from time to time. This is never associated with a painful stimulus and so here there is no reaction in any parameter. The low tone is the negative conditional stimulus (CS minus).

A

B

C

D

E

Figure 7–1c. Here the S is conditioned and reacts to the high tone (CS plus) with a positive reaction as he had done to the painful stimulus (US) in Fig. 7–1a.

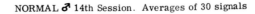

NORMAL ♂ 14th Session. Averages of 30 signals

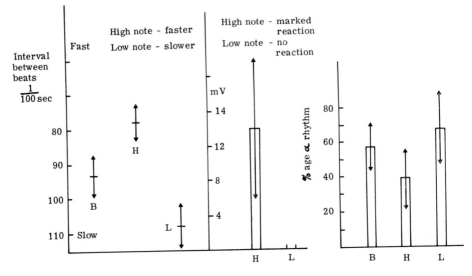

B - Before signals
H - High note un-reinforced. c.s.
L - Low note never reinforced.

H - alerting reaction
L - positive inhibition.

Figure 7–1d. The conditioning is recorded in another way. After 14 sessions, the S was tested on 30 occasions for heart rate, GSR and percentage of alpha rhythm in the EEG. The duration of the cardiac cycle diminishes greatly during the high tone (CS +) and lengthens during the low tone (CS −). Again the GSR shows a marked reaction to CS + and none to CS −.

The subject can now be said to have been given a mild experimental neurosis as he shows a fear reaction on hearing a specific tone for five seconds, even although it is not reinforced. (Of course, the subject is none the worse for this experience).

Extensive statistical studies were made on normal subjects regarding the extinction of the orienting reflex before conditioning began and of the number of subjects who could be conditioned in relation to the GSR and the heart rate. Eleven out of twelve were conditioned in the sphere of the GSR and five in the sphere of the heart rate (Passerini and Paterson, 1966).

It will be seen then that the experimenter has merely to sound a high tone even without presenting a painful stimulus and this will produce a fear reaction with acceleration of the heart rate, while the sounding of a low tone produces a feeling of relaxation in the patient, often with slowing of the pulse. It is possible to study how the reaction of fear in response to the high tone can be altered either by the action of drugs or by fresh conditioning or by the application of suggestion under hypnosis. We decided to use this technique to study the effects on autonomic functions such as the heart rate and GSR of suggestion under hypnosis. This was likely to have a significance for psychosomatic medicine. Many patients come to the doctor complaining that there is some malfunction of the autonomic nervous system such as that which occurs in migraine, enuresis or tachycardia, but the patient is unable to control this disturbed function by the exercise of the will (Black, 1969). However, by this technique we can measure exactly what effect suggestion under hypnosis is having on the heart rate and the skin resistance.

THE BLOCKING OF NEURAL TRANSMISSION BY SUGGESTION UNDER HYPNOSIS

The first experiment carried out was to anesthetise the subject's hand by hypnosis and then to attempt to condition him. If it were possible to condition the individual in spite of the anesthesia, one might suspect that the hypnotised subject is merely play-acting, but if no fear reaction develops then one might conclude that there is a definite block of the neural impulse at some point between the skin and the cerebral cortex. In fact, conditioning does not take place.

In a subject who has been conditioned and who has then been made deaf for CS + no fear reaction occurred in response to CS + (Black and Wigan, 1961).

From the clinical standpoint this sort of deafness is a fairly dramatic symptom. Although the individual is entirely deaf to the high tone, he can hear all other sounds quite clearly. In the audiogram, if he increases the amplitude of a number of tones beginning at the lower end of the scale and going up, he can hear most tones at a few decibels, but he becomes partially deaf for tones which are adjacent to the tone for which he has been made deaf, in this case 575 c.p.s. In order to try to hear the sound he increased the amplitude to sixty-seven decibels and was still un-

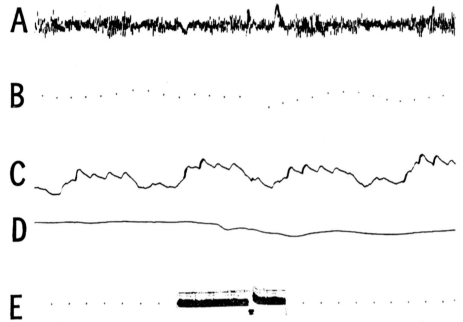

Figure 7–2. Here the S is hypnotised before a session and he is given the first of many posthypnotic suggestions that his left hand and forearm are insensitive to pain. This is demonstrated to him by administering the painful shock, which he does not feel. The fact that he does not become conditioned shows that hypnotic anaesthesia is "genuine." Compare with Fig. 7–1a. The only reaction here to the shock shown in E is a missed heart beat.

able to hear it. Two questions arise from this experiment: (Spinelli and Paterson, 1963)

    1. That from one point of view the subject could have "heard" the sound in fact although no sound has been perceived consciously. He must have "recognised" below the level of consciousness that the specific tone was the one to which he was deaf. How could this have happened?

    2. Where is the block located between the ear and the heart? Theoretically the site of the block could be situated on the afferent side, or in the cortex, or on the efferent side.

Our first experiment was devised to find out if the block was on the efferent side. Theoretically, suggestion under hypnosis could

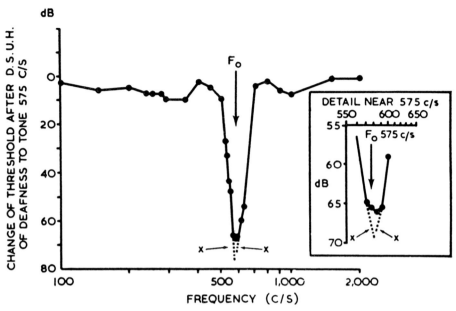

Figure 7–3a. After this S had been conditioned in the normal way, so that he reacted to the high tone (CS +) with acceleration of the heart, he was given a posthypnotic suggestion that he would be deaf to the high pitch but to no other pitch. This pitch was of 575 c.p.s. He found that he could hear pitches from 100 c.p.s. up to 550 c.p.s. at a few decibels, but he began to feel deaf about 500 c.p.s. while at 575 he was totally deaf, becoming normal again at about 580 c.p.s. (Black and Wigan, 1961)

cause an inhibition of the sympathetic system in such a way that no acceleration of the heart occurred.

It is, however, possible to devise an experiment in which deafness to a specific tone does not cause a slowing of the rhythm but an acceleration of the heart rate. For instance, we present to the patient a pattern of three specific tones lasting four seconds, followed by a second of silence followed in turn by the painful shock. This second of silence following the sequence of three notes was the conditional stimulus which indicated a painful shock. However, when the sequence of the same three tones was followed by a high pitch no shock ever occurred. The second of silence which indicated that a shock would occur was thus replaced by a high pitched sound which indicated that no shock

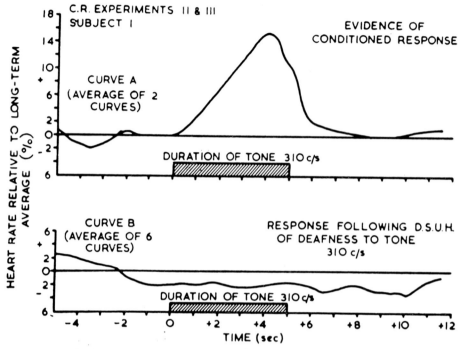

Figure 7–3b. S's reactions were then recorded when he was hypnotically deaf and we see that there is no cardiac response to the usual high tone (DSUH means direct suggestion under hypnosis). This demonstrates that the S was genuinely deaf. (Black and Wigan, 1961)

To recapitulate: it will be seen that in the above experiments the S, when in the normal state, showed acceleration of the heart in response to the conditional stimulus, which was a high tone. During the conditioning process this tone had lasted 6 seconds and on the 5th second a painful shock had been administered to the left index finger. However, when the S was made deaf under hypnosis he did not react to the high tone. This showed that there was a physiological block somewhere between the eardrum and the heart during hypnogenic deafness. Doctor D. Spinelli devised two experiments to find out whether the block was (1) between the ear and the cerebral cortex, or (2) in the cortex or (3) between the cortex and the heart.

In these experiments, with the present technique, hypnogenic deafness has caused inhibition of the heart, for when the S could hear, then the high tone caused acceleration, but when deaf there was no acceleration. Of the three possible sites mentioned above for the site of the block, one considered the third possibility first, that is, whether it was between the cortex and the heart. If, however, one could devise an experiment in which deafness would cause not an inhibition of the heart, that is to say, a sort of functional paralysis of the heart, but an acceleration, the block could not be in the efferent sympathetic supply of the heart.

would take place. When, therefore, the subject was made deaf by hypnosis to the high pitch, the negative conditional stimulus was replaced by a subjectively experienced moment of silence which indicated for the subject the positive conditional stimulus, and so there was an increase of heart rate. (Figs. 7–3 c, d and e)

In these circumstances then, there cannot be any inhibition or so to speak a functional paralysis of the sympathetic because the consequence of the suggested deafness is an acceleration of the heart and not a slowing.

Since it appears then that the inhibition is not on the efferent side, we sought further to establish whether the block was in the cortex itself or on the afferent side. For this purpose we used an apparatus which records what is known as "the averaged evoked response" to an auditory stimulus. The technique is described in

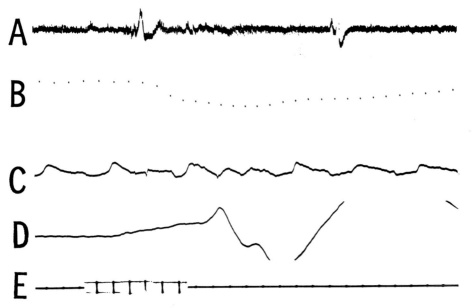

Figures 7–3c, d and e, show the technique whereby deafness caused not an inhibition but an acceleration. The technique is the same as before, except that CS + is no longer the high tone. It is shown in line E. It consists of a pattern of 3 tones in 4 seconds followed by a second of silence. This last silent 5th second is the essence of the signal which had regularly preceded the painful shock. Note the strong positive reaction in heart and GSR.

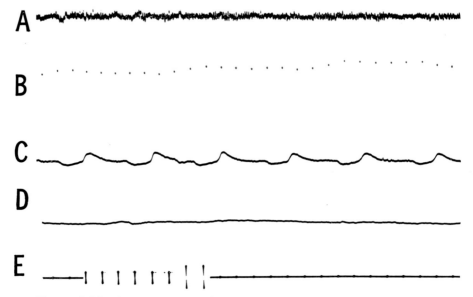

Figure 7–3d. The negative signal seen in line E consists of a pattern of 3 notes, but instead of the second of silence in the 5th second of the signal, there is a high pitched whistle. This is indicated by a widening of the line 2 seconds later. This constitutes the negative conditional stimulus and so there is no reaction.

the small print caption to Figure 7–3f on page 94. The conclusion is that the site of the block between eardrum and heart is not in the cortex, because the S was deaf to the high tone and so could not pay attention to the clicks. It is, therefore, in the afferent pathway, and other studies, e.g. Hernandez-Peón et al., 1956, suggest that the cochlear nucleus is the most likely site. Ref.: Hernandez-Peón, R., Sheher, H., and Jouvet, M. (1956) *Science, 123:*331.

This subcortical center then, which is probably situated in the cochlear nucleus, possesses a relative independence with regard to the cortex. This may be supposed to function as a sort of filter. A controlling center can cause a block at the level of the cochlear nucleus in such a way that the impulse caused by a specific tone cannot pass to the cortex even when impulses caused by other tones can do so. Many people have heard the story of the woman who during the war fell asleep in a shelter during a raid. Throughout the night she was able to sleep and did not hear any noise

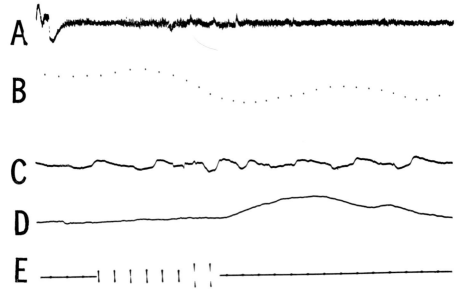

Figure 7–3e. Here the S is hypnotised and made deaf to the high pitched whistle, but to no other sound. He experiences instead a second of silence, which constitutes for him CS + and so there is a positive reaction especially in the heart rate and GSR. In the latter, with this technique, a movement up or down is positive (Spinelli and Paterson, 1963).

caused by the bombs dropping, but as soon as her baby began to cry she woke at once. One may suppose that a block has occurred on the afferent side and that the organ where the block occurs acts as a filter so that the impulse caused by the baby crying passes to the cortex while the impulses from all other sounds are blocked.

Similarly, we suppose that hypnosis has caused a block probably at the level of the cochlear nucleus which has prevented the impulse from the auditory signal from passing beyond the cochlear nucleus to the cortex.

The same mechanism explains how we can answer the first question. By means of the auditory mechanism situated peripherally to the cochlear nucleus, the individual has been able to "recognise" the specific tone and to react to it although the impulse did not reach the cortex. In this way he was unable to hear the sound consciously.

EVOKED POTENTIAL PHOTOGRAMS

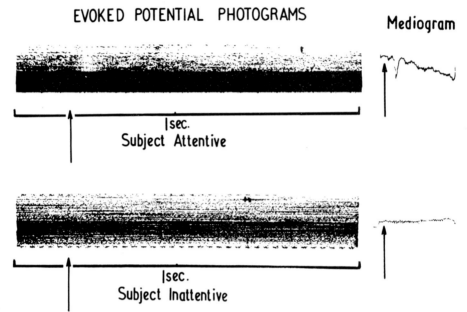

Figure 7–3f. This shows an apparatus, the purpose of which is to record impulses from an acoustic stimulus, such as a click, when they reach the auditory area in the cortex. In this experiment a click is sounded every two seconds and if the S persistently pays attention to it, the apparatus shows a change of potential in the cortex, but if his attention is directed elsewhere, no impulse is recorded. We see in the upper picture, the record of a S who is counting the clicks and so attending to them. A conventional EEG does not show a change of potential when a single click is sounded, because on each occasion other adventitious changes of potential obscure the record of the click. However, when 200 clicks are sounded the records of adventitious impulses cancel each other out and the averaged evoked potential shows up. In the two pictures there is a circular photographic band, which revolves once every 2 seconds and each click is sounded always at the same point (see arrow). The reaction to each click is recorded as an alteration of the brightness of the spot of light. This shot moves gradually upwards over half the width of the screen of the oscilloscope. The film shows 200 lines of this type of EEG. The impulses caused by clicks are recorded as a vertical line when the S is attentive (upper picture), but no impulses are recorded when he is inattentive (lower picture).

One also directs the rays of a lamp through the film so that they influence a photoelectric cell which transforms the variations of energy into a "mediogram." This records the average of the evoked potentials. The click is recorded as a downward spike in the upper picture, but in the lower there is no reaction.

RELATION OF CONDITIONING TO HYPNOSIS

In the above experiments hypnosis was used to inhibit conditioned responses, first the unconditioned response and secondly the conditioned response. However hypnosis could be used not only to inhibit but also to facilitate conditioned responses. If a subject failed to condition for any reason, for instance through having a high threshold to pain, it was found possible to condition the individual at one session through hypnosis. One suggested to the subject that when he heard the high tone he would feel very frightened but that when he heard the low tone he would have a pleasurable feeling of relaxation. The apparent conditioning which resulted from hypnosis did not appear to differ in character from ordinary conditioning. Conditioning produced in this way was still found to be present after a lapse of as long as three months (Paterson et al, 1965).

Our observations suggested a close relationship between the mechanism employed when autonomic responses were altered by suggestion under hypnosis and the mechanism by which new conditioned reflexes were formed. One could measure the relative strength of a newly formed conditioned reflex and the strength of a suggestion given under hypnosis. For instance, one could condition a subject, as we have seen, to increase the heart rate in response to a specific auditory signal but at the same time give a suggestion under hypnosis that the acceleration would not occur. In nearly every case the suggestion under hypnosis was stronger than the conditioned reflex.

VOLUNTARY CONTROL OVER AUTONOMIC NERVOUS FUNCTIONS

F. Bracchi made observations on some individuals who had been subjected both to conditioning and hypnosis over a period. One of these subjects formed the subject of a series of experiments carried out in our laboratory. This was a professional woman aged thirty-two. Although the normal rate of her heart was about sixty per minute, she could raise it to ninety or more within the space of three beats. The subject stated that her surprising sensation when she first voluntarily raised her heart rate

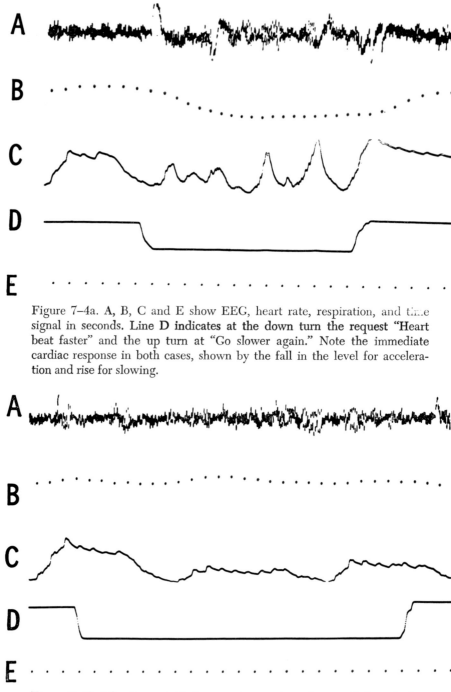

Figure 7–4a. A, B, C and E show EEG, heart rate, respiration, and time signal in seconds. Line **D** indicates at the down turn the request "Heart beat faster" and the up turn at "Go slower again." Note the immediate cardiac response in both cases, shown by the fall in the level for acceleration and rise for slowing.

Figure 7–4b. The S was told that on six occasions she would be asked to accelerate the heart voluntarily. She was asked to refuse to do so on one of the six occasions and this occasion was to be chosen by herself. The figure shows the refusal.

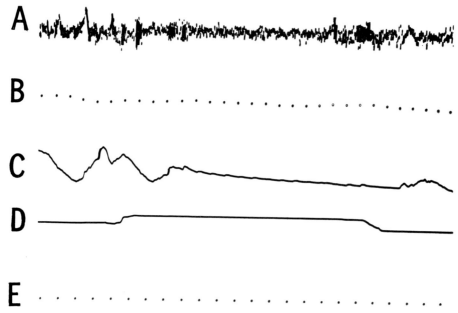

Figure 7–4c. The rise in the level of line D indicates the request "Make your heart go slow." Note there is no response. The S can make her heart go slow only to make it return to normal after it has been going fast.

might be described as one of "anguish." Nevertheless she did not imagine something terrifying in order to make her heart increase in rate. After a short time the increase of rate was achieved by a voluntary act like that of raising her hand. An experiment was carried out to see whether the increase of rate was merely a reflex response to the operator's voice. The subject was asked to increase her heart on five occasions but she was told beforehand that on one of these five occasions to be chosen by herself she was to refuse to increase it. She could do this easily. (Figures 7–4 a and b)

She could maintain the increased rate for several minutes but at any time during that period she could make the rate return to normal when she was given the appropriate command. She could not, however, make the heart go slower unless there had been a previous acceleration. (Fig. 7–4) It was noticed that when the

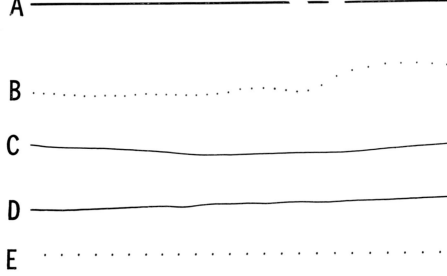

Figure 7–4d. To make sure that the cardiac acceleration was not due to increased rate of breathing, the S was asked to hold her breath throughout the experiment. The figure shows the end of the period of acceleration (shown in B) when the signal "return to normal" is shown in line A as a double break. Note breath-holding in C. D shows GSR.
Conclusion. The S who learned to control her heart rate did not do so by breathing faster. During these experiments the S could accelerate both heart and respiration at the beginning but later became more selective and could accelerate the heart only. (Paterson and Bracchi, 1962)

heart rate was increased there was a concomitant increase in the respiratory rate together with a diminution of amplitude. However, the voluntary control of respiration did not appear to be the mechanism by which the heart was voluntarily controlled because the increase occurred even when the subject was holding her breath. Furthermore, when the respiratory muscles were to some extent paralysed by curare this made no difference to the increase in heart rate.

It was therefore concluded that both the respiratory response and the cardiac response were controlled by the same mechanism, but the respiratory function could not be used voluntarily to control the heart rate. It is of interest that the subject was not able to make her heart go slower in response to a command by the operator except when terminating a suggested acceleration. This subject attained to a remarkable degree of voluntary control over her heart rate. The fluorescent screen of an oscilloscope was so prepared that she could observe on a scale the beat of her heart and when the operator pointed for instance to the figure ninety she could increase her heart from sixty to ninety and back to seventy, and so on.

DEGREES OF VOLUNTARY CONTROL OVER CONDITIONAL RESPONSES

D. Passerini investigated in our laboratory the ability of awake subjects to control autonomic nervous functions. In the first type of experiment he reversed the significance of the two auditory conditioned stimuli so that the subject was told that in future the high tone would never be associated with the shock but that the low tone might be. Of ten subjects examined, only four were able partially to reverse the pattern of their previous conditioning at will. In three out of the four only the GSR was reversed while the fourth case reversed the cardiac conditioning as well. Three more subjects, while not reversing the response, nevertheless showed a diminished response to the high tone. The remaining three subjects out of ten simply inhibited all the responses. Another individual was able to reverse the conditioning only when given suggestions under hypnosis that the high tone would be associated with security and tranquillity but that the low tone would signify danger. When these experiments are carried out on a larger scale it will be interesting to see with what personality traits the ability to reverse conditioning and the total inhibition of all responses correlate.

In another experiment the subjects instead of being presented with the usual high tone or low tone were asked to respond to the words high tone and low tone. In every case the subjects reacted in the sphere of GSR in the same way as to the real high tone

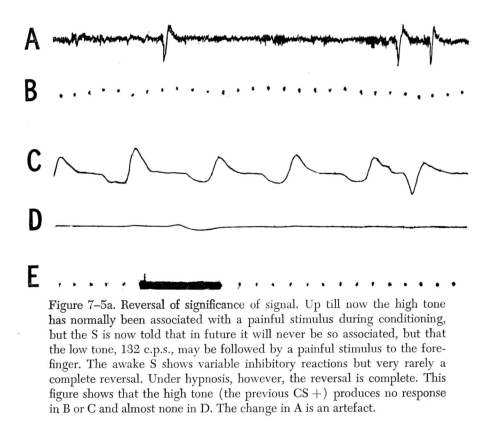

Figure 7–5a. Reversal of significance of signal. Up till now the high tone
has normally been associated with a painful stimulus during conditioning,
but the S is now told that in future it will never be so associated, but that
the low tone, 132 c.p.s., may be followed by a painful stimulus to the forefinger. The awake S shows variable inhibitory reactions but very rarely a
complete reversal. Under hypnosis, however, the reversal is complete. This
figure shows that the high tone (the previous CS +) produces no response
in B or C and almost none in D. The change in A is an artefact.

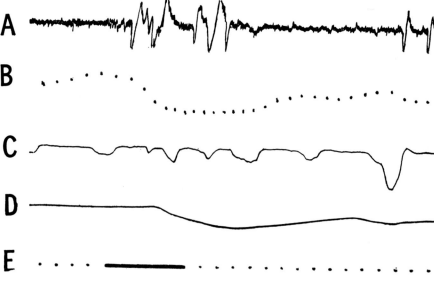

Figure 7–5b. Here the low tone (CS −) produces a reaction which hitherto
has been typical of the high tone (CS +). *Conclusion.* The hypnotised S
can control his ANS reactions in a way seldom possible in the waking state.

and the real low tone. However, the reactions were less marked, but the differentiation was more complete (Figures 7–5a and b).

Hypnosis and the Reticular Formation of the Midbrain

The spinal reflexes are the simplest in the central nervous system, yet most of these involve a concatenation of many neurones. There are, however, some spinal reflexes in which only two neurones are involved, the sensory and the motor neurone, with one synapse between, and so they are called monosynaptic reflexes. There is one condition at least in which such a reflex is totally inhibited and that is the so-called paradoxical or REM (rapid eye movement) sleep. We know further that it is the sensory part of the reflex arc which is inhibited, because the motor neurone can still be stimulated by way of the pyramidal tracts even when the inhibition is total.

The EEG in REM sleep shows "beta" waves which are of low voltage and relatively rapid. This is the deepest form of sleep and is generally associated with dreaming. A similar tracing is found in the individual who is awake and attending to a simple problem and would also, one might expect, occur in the individual under hypnosis, whose attention is also concentrated on a particular subject. Many of the phenomena in hypnosis are related to inhibition such as in pain, hearing and vision. It was therefore decided to investigate whether the monosynaptic spinal reflex was inhibited during hypnosis as occurs in REM sleep. The caption in Fig. 7–6a describes the first half of the experiment. (Bracchi and Paterson, 1965)

In order to study further the question of possible inhibition in this reflex, a comparison was made between the waking state and the hypnotic state by a method designed to test further the degree of inhibition affecting the monosynaptic reflex (Fig. 7–6b). Here the sciatic nerve is stimulated and the stimulation is repeated after an interval which varies from about 93 m secs. down to about 50 m secs. The amplitude of the response in the second reflex (b2) depends on the degree of spinal inhibition. Normally, the response in the second reflex is totally inhibited if the second stimulus occurs about 50 m secs. after the first, whereas the amplitude of the second response is 100 percent of

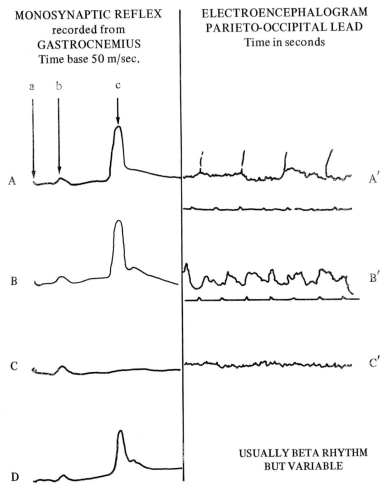

MONOSYNAPTIC REFLEX
recorded from
GASTROCNEMIUS
Time base 50 m/sec.

ELECTROENCEPHALOGRAM
PARIETO-OCCIPITAL LEAD
Time in seconds

a   b   c

A   A′

B   B′

C   C′

D

USUALLY BETA RHYTHM
BUT VARIABLE

Figure 7–6a. This shows the electromyographic (EMG) response, Ac, of the gastrocnemius muscle when the sciatic nerve is stimulated in the popliteal space from the skin surface. "a" shows the stimulus and b the response given by stimulation of *efferent* fibres (direct stimulation) and c shows the response of the monosynaptic reflex in which the same stimulus has also involved the *afferent* fibres, and so the impulse has passed to the muscle via a centre in the spinal cord. In A the reflex is present in the waking state. A′ shows beta rhythm. The four vertical strokes are artefacts. In B the reflex is present in delta sleep, the delta waves being shown in B′. (Time signal in seconds) In C note the absence of the reflex in REM (rapid eye movement) sleep where there is beta rhythm seen in C′. In D where the S is deeply hypnotised, the reflex is present. Compare with 7–6b and see comment in text. The EEG, not shown, can be variable, beta waves predominating.

TIME INTERVAL BETWEEN STIMULI in m/sec.

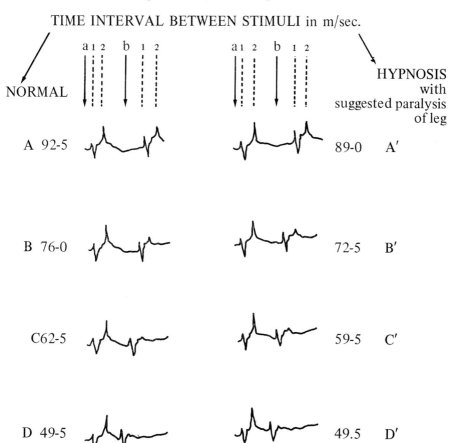

NORMAL

HYPNOSIS
with
suggested paralysis
of leg

A 92-5   89-0   A′

B 76-0   72-5   B′

C62-5   59-5   C′

D 49-5   49.5   D′

Fig. 7–6b. a, b stimuli – a1 direct response to the first stimulus, a2 first indirect response (first monosynaptic reflex). b1 direct response to the second stimulus. 62 indirect response (second monosynaptic reflex).
In the waking state (left hand half of diagram) the interval between the two stimuli in A, B, C and D diminishes from 92.5 m/secs. to 49.5 m/secs. Note that the amplitude of the reflex response b2 diminishes gradually and disappears in D. Note that in A′, B′, C′ and D′ Hypnosis the findings are same as in the waking state, A, B, C and D.

the first response if the second stimulus is about 100 m secs. after the first, i.e. after the refractory period. In the Fig. 7–6b, the spike marked b2 in the normal subject is seen to diminish progressively in the diagrams A, B and C and to disappear in D, showing the gradual disappearance of the reflex. Note that the spike b2 diminishes and disappears in almost exactly the same manner in the four diagrams showing the reactions of the hypnotised subject in the right hand column. (See A', B', C' and **D'**.

Conclusion: Figs. 7–6a and b illustrate experiments carried out by F. Bracchi in our laboratory. These have considerable importance for the relationship between hypnosis, REM sleep and delta sleep. James Braid was the first to use the word hypnosis. It meant literally "putting to sleep." With the development of EEG's many writers contrasted hypnosis with sleep, by which they meant delta sleep. However, when paradoxical or REM sleep was discovered, it was expected that hypnosis would be found physiologically to resemble REM sleep more than delta sleep. It is therefore surprising that hypnosis, which can enable an individual to inhibit for instance pain, or vision or hearing, is found unable to produce a state of generalised inhibition in the same manner as REM sleep does, even when the hypnosis is deep and when additional suggestions are given that the subject cannot move the lower limbs. Hypnosis in this case resembled delta sleep more than REM sleep. However, in scientific investigation, it often happens that an unexpected result in one experiment leads on to more extensive study and eventually to a better understanding of the problem. This may be what will happen as a result of this investigation.

CONCLUSION

1. This chapter gives a brief account of six years of experimental work on the relationship between conditioning and hypnosis. These are two methods which enable an individual to gain voluntary control over autonomic nervous functions. The two methods employ to a certain extent the same physiological mechanism. Hypnosis, however, is found to be more potent and more rapid in achieving results. The effects can be just as lasting.

2. Reference is made to a preliminary account of the technique of conditioning the human heart in respect of its frequency. This can be achieved in about 66 percent of cases. The galvanic skin reflex (GSR) can be conditioned in nearly 100 percent of cases.

3. The method was to link a high tone (310 cps) to a painful

stimulus applied to the index finger while a low tone (130 cps) was never associated with the painful shock. This was presented intermittently. It was therefore possible to cause a rapid heart rate by presenting a high tone and generally a slowing of the heart by presenting the low tone. Such conditioned subjects' cardiac reactions were then studied during various hypnotic procedures.

4. If a new volunteer were subjected to conditioning, but if on each occasion he were first hypnotized so that his hand was made anaesthetic by suggestion, then he did not become conditioned, thus showing that the anaesthesia was "genuine." Again, if a subject who was already conditioned was made hypnotically deaf to the high tone, then no conditioning occurred. This showed that the suggested deafness was also genuine. Thus, both the unconditional and the conditional stimulus could be abolished by hypnosis, and therefore the conditional reaction.

5. Hypnotic deafness posed several problems, the solution of which necessitated some sophisticated experiments. These threw light on various problems such as the difference between cortical and subcortical awareness, the site of the block of incoming auditory impulses during hypnotic deafness, and the concept of a subcortical center as a "filter of information."

6. As a test of the relative strength of cortical (voluntary) control and that of the conditioning process, ten subjects were told that the significance of the high tone and of the low tone would be reversed. The high tone would from now on never be associated with the painful stimulus but the low might be. Of ten subjects, only four were able partially to reverse the pattern of the previous conditioning at will. Three could reverse only the GSR, while the fourth reversed the cardiac conditioning by an act of will as well. Three more subjects, while not reversing their reactions, nevertheless showed a diminished response to the high tone. The three remaining subjects simply inhibited all responses. Complete reversal could be achieved under hypnosis.

7. Some volunteers who had been subjected to a course of conditioning and hypnosis could acquire a remarkable control over the heart rate and the GSR. The control of the heart rate was achieved not by increasing or decreasing the rate of respiration,

for the heart could be accelerated while the subject held his or her breath. The subject could not slow the heart rate except after a recent acceleration.

8. Instead of the operator presenting the high tone or the low tone to the subject he substituted the words "high tone" or "low tone," and the results were almost the same. This finding can act as a basis of discussion regarding the far reaching effects produced by the human voice and their relationship to conditioning.

9. An account is given of how an inhibitory state supposedly originating from the reticular formation of the midbrain could be measured, when it affects a monosynaptic spinal reflex during four different conditions, (1) the waking state, (2) delta sleep, (3) REM sleep, and (4) hypnosis. The inhibition of the reflex occurred only in REM sleep. However, further work in this important field is indicated.

REFERENCES

Alexander, L.: Apparatus and method for the study of conditional reflexes in man. *Arch Neur Psychiatry.* 80:629–649, 1958.

Black, S.: *Mind and Body.* London, Kimber, 1969.

Black, S., and Wigan, E. R.: An investigation of selective deafness produced by direct suggestion under hypnosis. *Brit Med J,* 2:736–741, 1961.

Bracchi, F., and Paterson, A. S.: Comparison of hypnosis with sleep in relation to reflex spinal activity in man (French). *C R Congr Psychiat Neur,* 62:519–523, 1965.

Passerini, D., and Paterson, A. S.: A study of cardiac conditioning in man. *Cond Reflex,* 1, 2:90–103, 1966.

Paterson, A. S., Bracchi, F., and Passerini, D.: A comparison of learning by conditioning and learning by suggestion under hypnosis (French). *C R Congr Psychiat Neur,* 63:490–497, 1965.

Paterson, A. S., and Bracchi, F.: Study of the voluntary control of the heart rate (French). *C R Congr Psychiat Neur,* 60:271–273, 1962.

Paterson, A. S., Passerini, D., Bracchi, F., and Black, S.: Study of Hypnosis by means of conditional reflexes in man (French). *C R Congr Psychiat Neur,* 69:336–345, 1961.

Spinelli, D., and Paterson, A. S.: Deafness caused by suggestion under hypnosis (French). *C R Congr Psychiat Neur,* 61:326–332, 1963.

CHAPTER **8**

OBJECTIVE ASSESSMENT OF HYPNOTICALLY INDUCED TIME DISTORTION*

PHILIP G. ZIMBARDO, PH.D.
GARY MARSHALL, M.A.
CHRISTINA MASLACH, PH.D.
GREG WHITE, M.A.

Abstract. The objective precision of operant conditioning methodology validates the power of hypnosis to induce alterations in time perception. Personal tempo was systematically modified by instructions to trained hypnotic subjects, with significant behavioral effects observed on a variety of response rate measures.

TIME PERCEPTION is one of the most important, although least studied, consequences of the socialization process. Infants and children, whose behavior is primarily under the control of biological and situational exigencies, must be taught to develop a temporal perspective in which the immediacy of the experienced reality of the present is constrained by the hypothetical constructs of past and future. Society thereby transforms idiosyncratic, impulsive, and potentially disruptive behavior into approved, predictable, controllable reactions through the time-bound mechanisms of responsibility, obligation, guilt, incentive, and delayed gratification (Mischel, 1966). The social acceptability of such reactions often depends on their rate of emission as much as upon other qualitative aspects. Thus, we develop, in addition to a sense of temporal perspective, a time sense of personal tempo,

* Reprinted from *Science*, 20 July 1973, Volume 181, pages 282–284. Copyright 1973 by the American Association for the Advancement of Science.

which involves both the estimation of the rate at which events are (or should be) occurring and affective reactions to different rates of stimulus input (Ornstein, 1966; Dürr, 1966).

The learned correspondence between our subjective time sense and objective clock time can be disrupted by the physiological and psychological changes that accompany some types of mental illness, emotional arousal, body temperature variations, and drug-induced reactions (Fischer, 1967; Cohen, 1967; Newell, 1971). However, it is possible to modify either temporal perspective or tempo within a controlled experimental paradigm by means of hypnosis. Our previous research demonstrates the marked changes in cognition, affect, and action that result when hypnotized subjects internalize the instruction to experience a sense of "expanded present" (Zimbardo et al, 1971). However, the data used to document such changes in this and related studies (Cooper and Erickson, 1950; Edmondston and Erbeck, 1967; Barber and Calverley, 1964) have been too subjective and gross. In the present study we attempted to alter personal tempo and measure the behavioral consequences with precise, objective techniques.

The experience of tempo was systematically varied (speeded up or slowed down) by time-distorting instructions administered to hypnotic subjects and controls. If effective, such a manipulation should generate asynchronicity between clock time and the subjective passage of time. This asynchronous responding was assessed by means of the objective precision of a specially designed operant conditioning and recording apparatus. As predicted, the operant behavior of these hypnotized subjects was significantly altered relative to their own normal baseline and also to that of subjects in two control conditions.

The volunteer subjects were thirty-six Stanford University undergraduates of both sexes, who were selected from among the high scorers on a modified version of the Harvard group scale of hypnotic susceptibility. (Shor and Orne, 1962) administered in their introductory psychology class. They were each randomly assigned to one of three treatments: hypnosis, hypnotic role-playing, and waking nonhypnotized controls. Before the experiment, the hypnosis group underwent a ten-hour training program designed to teach them to relax deeply; to concentrate; to ex-

perience distortions in perception, memory, and causal attribu-
tion; and to induce autohypnosis. The other subjects received no
prior training. During the experiment, the testing procedure was
identical for all subjects; an experimenter who was unaware of
the experimental treatment delivered the standardized instructions to the subject, who sat isolated in an acoustic chamber. A
second experimenter induced a state of hypnotic relaxation in
the hypnosis group and instructed the hypnotic role-playing subjects to try their best to simulate the reactions of hypnotic subjects, to behave as if they were really hypnotized throughout the
study. The waking controls were told only to relax for a period
of time equivalent to that given to subjects in the other two
treatments.

Subjects were taught to press a telegraph key at different rates
in order to illuminate various target lights in an array of ten
colored lights. In the first of five two-minute trials, a comfortable
operant rate of responding was established, and it became obvious to the subject that the sequential onset and offset of the
lights was controlled by response rate. The functional relationship
between response rate and change in the light stimulus was determined by relay circuits in the apparatus and can be characterized as a "conjugate" schedule of reinforcement (Lindsley, 1957;
Zimbardo et al, 1974). This schedule creates a dynamic interplay
between behavior and a selected environmental event—the
stimulus event changing continually as response rate varies.
Pressing the key at a faster or slower rate than that required to
illuminate the target stimulus light turned on one of the other
lights in the array. It was only by empirically determining the
rate appropriate to reach a particular target and then by maintaining that rate consistently that a subject could satisfy the task
demand, "to keep light X illuminated as long as possible."

Of the remaining four trials, the first and third were baseline
and the second and fourth were experimental. On one baseline
trial, each subject was instructed to keep the red light illuminated, which required three presses per second. On the other
baseline trial a faster rate of six responses per second was required to maintain the illumination of a blue light. Interspersed
between these baseline trials and the experimental trials were

the instructions to modify personal tempo. After being told about the differences between clock and subjective time, all subjects were instructed to alter their perception of tempo, by experiencing time as slowing down ("so that a second will seem like a minute, and a minute will seem like an hour"), and also by experiencing time as speeding up. Between these two tempo modification instructions, subjects were told to normalize their experience of time. The order in which these two tempo instructions (slower and faster) were given to each subject was counterbalanced across conditions (and did not have a significant effect upon the task behavior). A cumulative recorder provided an ongoing display of the subject's response rate and indicated whether responding was on- or off-target. In addition, an event recorder and electronic timers indicated to the experimenter the sequence and duration of the stimulus light levels being activated by variations in rate of responding.

The reinforcer for maintaining a particular target light level is probably the sense of competence a subject feels in being able to satisfy the experimenter's demand to do so. Knowledge of being off-target should serve as a negative reinforcer and guide efforts to modify responding to achieve the positive consequences of on-target performance. Such performance depends primarily upon two variables: a stable, veridical sense of personal tempo and the environmental feedback necessary for monitoring the effects of different response rates. Our tempo instructions, in conjunction with hypnosis, were designed to alter the first of these, and variation in feedback was introduced to alter the second. Within our repeated-measurements factorial design, the array of lights remained functional during the experimental periods for half the subjects (objective feedback), and they were extinguished during the experimental periods for the other subjects in each of the three conditions (no feedback). Those in the no feedback condition had to rely entirely on their memory of the previously appropriate baseline rates that they were asked to reproduce in the experimental periods, while objective feedback subjects had direct access to the external information provided by the illuminated array.

Since the electronic relay circuits in the apparatus function on fixed, real-time parameters, a subject operating on a subjective time dimension not in synchrony with clock time would have difficulty satisfying the task demand of achieving and maintaining a particular state of the apparatus. The absence of feedback frees task behavior from reality demands, thereby generating considerable asynchronous responding. But off-target responding can result from either intentionally altering response rate (without changing time sense) or altering personal tempo and thus indirectly affecting response rate. Feedback serves as a reality monitor to create a conflict only in subjects motivated to change their response rate voluntarily while also being motivated to maintain the target light level. For those who have internalized an altered sense of tempo, there is not a conflict between two competing motivations but rather an inability to successfully perform the task because of their altered cognitive state. They should continue to respond asynchronously even in the presence of feedback; the intentional responders should resolve their conflict in the direction of the most salient reinforcer—being on-target.

Only the hypnotic subjects were reliably able to translate the verbal suggestion of asynchronicity between clock time and personal time into behavioral "reality." This is shown in comparisons of mean rates of response, percentage of total time on- and off-target, mean deviation in individual response rates from baseline to experimental response levels, and in even the more subtle measures of variability—in displacement of the entire response distribution.

The sequence of responding for a typical hypnotic subject is shown in the cumulative response curves in Fig. 8–1. From an initially low operant level, the subject responds appropriately to the rate demands imposed by target levels three and six, being on target most of the time. Instructions to speed up time result in a steeper slope, while instructions to slow tempo lower the response rate. In this case, the slopes of the response curves for the two altered time periods almost converge. The substantial percentage of time the subject is responding at off-target rate levels reveals the extent of asynchronicity between his altered

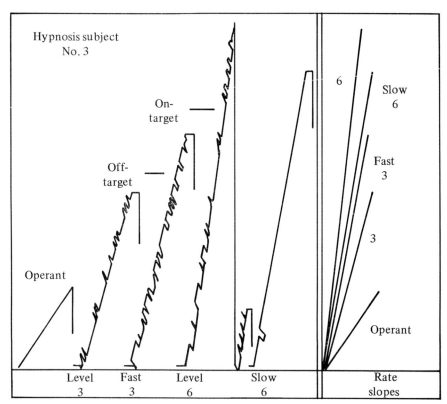

Figure 8–1. Cumulative records of representative hypnotized subject during each of five 2-minute test periods. The slope of the curve indicates rate of responding. Superimposed on this curve are upward and downward deflections; downward deflections signify when response rate is synchronized with target stimulus rate (*on-target* arrow), and upward deflections indicate asynchrony (*off-target* arrow).

experience of tempo and the constant rate requirements programmed into the apparatus.

Our research design permits both within- and between-subject comparisons. During baseline trials, there were no reliable differences on any measure between groups. An analysis of variance performed on the mean deviation in operant rate from baseline to experimental responding (Table 8–I) demonstrates a highly significant treatment effect ($P < .001$), and also a feedback ef-

TABLE 8–I

TEMPO MODIFICATION: DATA ARE MEAN DEVIATIONS IN
THE RATE FROM BASELINE PERFORMANCE

Treatment	N	No feedback	Objective feedback	Combined
Hypnotized	12	.534	.233	.38 *
Role players	12	.299	.004	.15 †
Waking controls	12	.023	.043	.03
		$P < .025$	$P < .005$	$P < .001$

* $P < .01$ for comparison with role players; $P < .001$ for comparison with
waking controls.   † Comparison with waking controls not significant.

fect ($P < .001$).* Deviation from target level (combined across
feedback conditions) significantly differentiated between the
hypnotized subjects and those in the other two conditions. The
marked deviations from target levels in the no feedback condition were attenuated by providing external feedback. However,
as predicted, this feedback served primarily to differentiate between the hypnotized and role-playing subjects. It totally eliminated the asynchrony in responding among the role-players,
but the reduced asynchrony of the hypnotized subjects was still
substantially different from the other two controls ($P < .005$).
Any volitional effect of responding to the tempo instructions as if
they were direct suggestions to vary response rate thus appears
limited to the no feedback condition. When confronted with information about the consequences of one's behavior, the controls
responded with appropriate synchrony, the hypnotized subjects
did not. Neither direction of tempo modification (slower or
faster) nor target light response level (low or high) was significant.

Perhaps the most convincing data of the extent to which hypnotic subjects altered their sense of personal tempo come from
analyses of the pattern of off-target response variability. This
measure of variability is the frequency of recorded shifts from
one stimulus level to another. The underlying variability in response rate could lead to shifts either around the target level

* Analysis of this data was performed by Perry Gluckman of the Center for
Advanced Study in the Behavioral Sciences (CASBS) by using Anovar BMDO
6V and 2V computer programs. The statistical advice of Lincoln Moses is also
gratefully acknowledged.

or to shifts around off-target levels. For example, if the target level were six, shifts to levels five or seven or from them back to six would represent around-target shifts. Off-target shifts would be between seven and higher levels (faster tempo) and between five and lower levels (slower tempo). There are no overall differences in total variation between treatments. However, there are significant differences between the hypnotized subjects and controls in the specific pattern of variability ($P < .001$, by Scheffé multiple t-test comparisons). The response distribution for the hypnotized subjects was displaced to off-target stimulus levels (in the experimentally appropriate direction), while that of the controls stabilized around the target levels. Thus, in the no feedback condition in which response variability was greatest, subtracting each subject's frequency of off-target shifts from baseline trials to experimental trials resulted in a group mean of $+31.0$ for the hypnosis condition, but only $+1.5$ for role-players and -5.0 for nonhypnotized waking controls.

To underscore the critical role of hypnosis in creating a cognitive state receptive to this time distortion manipulation, a subgroup of the role-playing subjects was subsequently given our program of hypnotic training and retested with the hypnotic induction. Four of the five subjects showed sizable changes in the suggested direction. While there were no differences in their standard baseline performance between earlier role-playing trials and these hypnosis trials, there were significant experimental trial differences due to the greater effectiveness of the time-distorting instructions when they were hypnotized (mean deviation in rate: $+.51$ for level 6, $P < .05$; and $+.38$ for level 3, $P < .10$).

Interviews and questionnaire responses of the hypnotic subjects indicated that they indeed tried to satisfy the experimenter's demand to keep the target light illuminated, but found they were unable to do so effectively. Their modified sense of personal tempo became a stable reference against which they judged environmental changes. As a result, they believed that the experimenters were covertly altering the apparatus to make their task more difficult (a situational error). By contrast, in an earlier study (Craik and Sarbin, 1963) in which clock time had been covertly altered by the researchers, subjects attributed discrepancies between clock and personal time to their own lack of ability in time estimation (a dispositional error).

We believe that a wide range of behaviors and physiological reactions which are under temporal control, such as drug addiction, depression, emotional arousal, and hypertension, may be modified by altering one's sense of personal tempo.

REFERENCES

Aaronson, B. S.: In Yaker, H., Osmond, H., and Cheek, F. (Eds.): *The Future of Time.* New York, Doubleday, 1971, pp. 405–436.

Barber, T. X. and Calverley, D. S.: *Arch Gen Psychiatry, 10:*209, 1964.

Cohen, J.: *Psychological Time in Health and Disease.* Springfield, Thomas, 1967.

Cooper, L. F., and Erickson, M. H.: *Bull Georgetown Med Cent, 4:*50, 1950.

Craik, K. H., and Sarbin, T. R.: *Percept Mot Skills, 16:*597, 1963.

Dürr, W.: In Fraser, J. T. (Ed.): *The Voices of Time.* New York, Braziller, 1966, pp. 180–200.

Edmonston, W. E., Jr.; and Erbeck, J. R.: *Am J Clin Hypn, 10:*79, 1967.

Fischer, R.: In Fisher, R. (Ed.): "Interdisciplinary perspectives of time," *Annual New York Academy of Science, 138:*440–488, 1967.

Lindsley, O. R.: *Science, 126:*1290, 1957.

Mischel, W.: *Prog Exp Pers Res, 3:*85, 1966.

Newell, S.: In Yaker, H., Osmond, H., and Cheek, F. (Eds.): *The Future of Time.* New York, Doubleday, 1971, pp. 351–388.

Ornstein, R. E.: *On the Experience of Time.* Baltimore, Penguin, 1970.

Shor, R. E., and Orne, E. C.: *The Harvard Group Scale of Hypnotic Susceptibility, Form A.* Palo Alto, California, Consulting Psychologists, 1962.

Zimbardo, P. G., Ebbesen, E. B., and Fraser, S. C.: Unpubl. M.S. Stanford University, 1974.

Zimbardo, P. G., Marshall, G., and Maslach, C.: *J Appl Soc Psychol, 1:*305, 1972.

CHAPTER *9*

STRATEGIES WITHIN HYPNOSIS FOR REDUCING PHOBIC BEHAVIOR*

SUZANNE L. HOROWITZ, PH.D.

INTRODUCTION

Three methods for reducing fear of snakes were compared using S's approach behavior and self-report anxiety measures. The methods, all involving hypnosis, were: (*a*) relaxation while recalling fearful snake-related events, (*b*) fear arousal during similar recall, and (*c*) posthypnotic suggestion about the disappearance of the snake phobia. All methods led to a significant decrease in fear as measured by overt behavior and self-report instruments, while no-treatment controls showed little change. Because fear arousal within treatment had no advantage over other methods, some doubt is cast on abreaction as essential to therapy of fears. Hypnotizability was positively related to degree of final approach behavior, and S's self-report of depth of hypnosis was positively related to degree of improvement. No S had ever experienced a harmful contact with snakes; the role of cognitive elaborations in the development of persistent fears was noted.

PROBLEMS in the theory and practice of psychotherapy have been of interest both to the academic world and to the general public for over seventy-five years. The present study is designed to investigate three contrasting therapeutic techniques for reducing phobic responses: relaxation, fear arousal, and suggestion.

Until recently, the major schools of psychotherapy were geared to the uncovering of mental processes hidden from the patient himself. These therapies have all emphasized emotional arousal

* Reprinted from J Abnorm Psychol, 1970, Volume 75, No. 1, 104–112. Copyright 1970 by the American Psychological Association. Reprinted by Permission.

as an important component. Freud (1955) stated that catharsis, or full reexperiencing of early affect, was a necessary but not sufficient event for obtaining good therapeutic results. Grinker and Spiegel (1945) treated large numbers of phobias in soldiers by means of an abreaction technique involving sodium pentothal. They claimed that treatment was successful only when a very high level of physiological and emotional arousal was reached. A recently developed therapy which makes extensive use of emotional arousal is Stampfl's "implosive therapy" (Stampfl, 1967).

Watson and Raynor (1920) and Guthrie both stated the notion that continued arousal of some response, such as fear, leads eventually to a state of exhaustion in the organism, at which time a new response to the fear producing cues may be learned. The Hullian concept of reactive inhibition is a related construct.

Such an "exhaustion" technique was applied directly in the therapy of a student with examination panic (Malleson, 1959) with good results. Using a fear hierarchy like Wolpe's, the student was instructed to go up gradually, and with each step to feel more and more afraid, until he was exhausted. Similar recent work using an anxiety "flooding" technique indicates that exposing phobic Ss to frightening stimuli can be effective in reducing fears (Hogan and Kirchner, 1967; Kirchner and Hogan, 1966; Strahley, 1966; Wolpin and Raines, 1966).

Within the past two decades, a different, behavior-oriented therapeutic approach has emerged, which derives from a Pavlovian stimulus (S)-response (R) position and draws on the work of Pavlov, Hull, Thorndike, Watson, Guthrie, and Skinner. Symptoms are regarded as conditioned responses which reflect nothing but maladaptive learning. Underlying psychic processes are considered irrelevant, if indeed their existence is admitted at all. Current examples of this viewpoint include Wolpe's (1958) reciprocal inhibition and systematic desensitization, Salter's (1949) conditioned reflex therapy, Krasner and Ullman's (1965) operant conditioning of verbal behavior, and others.

Behavior therapists view the phobia as a learned avoidance response vis-à-vis anxiety-arousing stimuli, where the stimuli have come to elicit anxiety through conditioning. Treatment, therefore, involves a counterconditioning procedure in which responses incompatible with anxiety, such as relaxation, are made to occur in the presence of anxiety-evoking cues (Bandura, 1961; Wolpe, 1958). The usual technique is to expose the patient to a graded series of cues, moving gradually from those which elicit little fear to those which are highly fear provoking.

Thus, relaxation seems to be implied by classical learning theory as the optimum strategy for reducing phobic behavior. This strategy contrasts with emotional arousal which is suggested by some of the same theorists (e.g. Guthrie). The present study was partly designed to compare these two strategies.

Both psychodynamic and behavior therapies involve an element of suggestion. It is well known that faith in the therapist and self-suggestion can sometimes be dramatically effective, as in the case of faith healing (Frank, 1961; Rosenthal and Frank, 1956). Therefore, therapeutic techniques need to be evaluated relative to the direct effects of suggestion; the third strategy employed in the present study, then, is posthypnotic suggestion regarding the disappearance of S's fear.

"Suggestion" therapy, especially in the form of hypnotherapy, antedates psychoanalysis as a therapeutic tool (Kaufman, 1961). Anecdotal accounts of hypnotherapy with phobias are scattered in the literature, and only one experimental study has been located (Clyde, 1947). Using a relaxation technique, Clyde had hypnotized, relaxed, phobic Ss recall the earliest traumatic experience related to their fear. All Ss showed a sharp decrease in anxiety immediately after treatment, with breathing rate used as the anxiety measure. Lang and others have used hypnosis as a technique adjunctive to relaxation in the treatment of snake phobics (Lang, Lazovik, and Reynolds, 1965). They found that success in desensitization was unrelated to S's hypnotizability. However, in Schubot's (1967) study of desensitization with snake phobics, hypnotic susceptibility was positively related to degree of improvement, among highly anxious Ss. Information regarding the role of hypnosis in therapies of this kind awaits further experimental test.

In view of the contrasting techniques offered by psychodynamic, behavior, and suggestion therapies, further studies on the sub-processes involved in psychotherapy are needed. In the present investigation, hypnosis was used as a vehicle of treatment in the study of the therapeutic effects of relaxation and arousal and the effects of direct suggestions of symptom disappearance.

METHOD

Subjects

The Ss were thirty-six adult female snake phobics recruited from a predominantly middle-class community through newspaper advertisements. They ranged in age from late teens to late sixties. At the pretest assessment of approach behavior, no S was able to touch a live, harmless snake. Each S served individually. There was no payment for participation.

Design

On Day One, each S was pretested to measure the strength of the phobia. First, self-ratings of anxiety were obtained through the Manifest Anxiety Scale (MAS) and a fear checklist (FCL), where S rated herself on the intensity of thirty-eight common fears. Then, the degree of phobic anxiety was directly assessed by asking S to approach as closely as possible to a harmless, live snake in a glass cage with a sliding screen top. Finally, a brief interview followed where S was asked to relate her encounters with snakes, both early and recent, and to discuss the extent to which the snake phobia interfered with her life.

On Day Two, Form A of the Stanford Hypnotic Susceptibility Scale (SHSS; Weitzenhoffer and Hilgard, 1959) was administered to each S to measure her hypnotizability.

The S was assigned to one of four conditions: Group R (relaxation), Group A (fear arousal), Group PH (posthypnotic suggestion), or a control group. For each condition, $n = 9$. The first twenty-seven Ss were randomly assigned to groups. To equate groups for initial snake-approach behavior, the last nine Ss recruited were assigned so as to equalize the means on the snake-approach measure (approach scale).

Each S in the three experimental groups was hypnotized and given the assigned therapy for nine successive sessions (Days Three to Eleven). Then, on Day Eleven, after completing the hypnosis series, S took part in a posttest procedure. Finally, after a no-treatment interval of nine to thirty-four days, a follow-up posttest was administered (Day Twelve).

Control Ss were seen only on Days One, Two, Eleven, and Twelve, with no treatment following the pretest. The interval between Day Two and Day Eleven lasted two to three weeks, comparable in length to the treatment period of the experimental groups. On Day Eleven, control Ss were posttested, and a follow-up testing (Day Twelve) was administered nine to twenty-five days after that. All testings for all groups were identical and occurred at comparable intervals. Experimental Ss were seen twelve times; control Ss were seen four times.

Procedure

Testing procedures: Day One. All Ss first filled out two self-report anxiety measures: (*a*) the FCL, composed of thirty-eight common fears on which S rated the intensity of her fear on a seven-point scale (S's score was the sum of the ratings for each item); and (*b*) a modified form of the MAS (McCreary and Bendig, 1954). Next, S's overt approach behavior toward the feared object was measured on a twenty-seven-point approach scale, derived from behaviors actually observed. A score of zero meant that S refused to go to the experimental room where the snake was kept and look through the doorway. A score of ten meant that S advanced a distance of eight to nine feet into the room and remained there for ten seconds. The highest score possible was twenty-six, achieved when S picked up the snake and held it clear of the cage floor for more than six seconds. During this test, E served as a model for fearless behavior, carrying out only the behavior that was next in S's approach hierarchy. The snake employed for testing was a California Rosy Boa, twenty-four in. long, selected for its harmlessness and extreme docility. Finally, S was interviewed about her phobia (prethet only). Any events during which S had been frightened by snakes were recorded.

Day Two. Susceptibility to hypnosis was measured by testing all Ss on Form A of the SHSS.

Days Three to Eleven. Treatment procedures for the experimental groups were carried out under hypnosis. Control Ss were not seen during this period.

Day Eleven. All four groups were post-tested with a procedure identical to the pretest, including self-report anxiety measures and the direct test of approach behavior of Day One.

Day Twelve. The follow-up posttest, which was administered to all Ss nine to thirty-four days after the posttest, was identical to that of Days One and Eleven.

Group R. The S was hypnotized and asked to imagine a pleasant scene for thirty seconds, in order to facilitate recall of other events under hypnosis. Then S was instructed to recall a specific snake-related event that she had reported during the pretest interview and to remain entirely calm and relaxed during recall. Over treatment sessions, six scenes in all were reinstated under relaxation, two events per session. The events were not arranged in a hierarchy, but were presented in reverse chronological order. On Days Three and Four, the two most recent events were recalled. On Days Five, Six, and Seven, two earlier events were used, and on Days Eight, Nine, Ten, and Eleven, the two earliest events were recalled. The S was allowed to recall each scene for thirty seconds and was then asked to describe the experience. The trance was then terminated with the suggestion that S would remember everything that had occurred during the session.

Group A. The procedure was exactly parallel to the relaxation condition except for the hypnotically requested emotion. Arousal Ss were instructed to recall and to reexperience their early fear as fully as possible.

Group PH. The S was hypnotized and asked to perform various (irrelevant) hypnotic tasks for about fifteen minutes in order to become involved in hypnotic behavior. Tasks of various difficulty levels were selected so that all Ss should have experienced the hypnotic effect at least some of the time. Following the trance-deepening tasks, a posthypnotic suggestion was administered to the effect that S would no longer be frightened by harmless snakes; Ss were also told they would remember everything that had occurred while hypnotized.

All experimental Ss were trained to report the depth of their hypnotic state on an eleven-point scale. They were asked for a "state report" twice during each hypnosis session—after induction and before trance termination.

All Ss were given a rationale for the particular treatment method employed and informed that this method would be helpful to them in overcoming their fear of snakes. Control Ss were told that repeated exposure to snakes in a controlled setting was effective in reducing snake phobias.

RESULTS

Instrument Characteristics

Table 9–I presents the intercorrelations among anxiety and approach measures. The upper entry in each pair relates the pre-test scores, the lower entry the follow-up posttest scores. Both sets of r's are similar.

All correlations between approach measures and anxiety measures were negative and small, in the expected direction, while a

TABLE 9–I

PRE- AND FOLLOW-UP POSTTEST CORRELATIONS FOR
APPROACH AND ANXIETY MEASURES

Measure	Approach scale	Fear check list	Manifest anxiety scale
Fear checklist			
Pretest	−.04		
Follow-up	−.03		
Snake item, fear checklist			
Pretest	−.39 *	.32 *	.40 **
Follow-up	−.29 *	.49 **	.53 **
Manifest Anxiety Scale			
Pretest	−.13	.57 **	
Follow-up	−.07	.45 **	

Note.—$N = 36$.
* $p < .05$, minimum $r = ±.28$.
** $p < .01$, minimum $r = ±.39$.

positive relationship existed between the two anxiety measures. Since intercorrelations between the two kinds of measures (approach and anxiety) tended to be low, but were high within the two sets, it appears that two different dimensions of avoidance behavior were being tapped. Hence, information about avoidance behavior is increased by using both direct measures of S's approach and by indirect, self-report anxiety measures.

Treatment Effects

Since groups were matched on the basis of pretest approach scale scores, an analysis of variance was used to establish their comparability on the other measures. One-way analyses of variance revealed no significant differences between groups on any of the other pretest scores, all $Fs \leq 1.56$, $p > .10 < .25$.

Self-report Anxiety Measures

An analysis of variance was performed on each measure to test the effect of different experimental conditions, the effect of the three trials (pre-, post-, and follow-up testing), and their interaction. This analysis showed a powerful trials effect for all self-report measures except the MAS (Fs are shown in Table 9–II). Irrespective of experimental condition, S's behavior showed decreasing anxiety with succeeding trials. The MAS is a more gen-

TABLE 9–II

ANALYSIS OF VARIANCE ON PRE-, POST-, AND
FOLLOW-UP TESTINGS

		Measures					
		Fear checklist (38 items)		Fear checklist (snake item only)		Manifest anxiety scale	
Source	df	MS	F	MS	F	MS	F
Between Ss	35						
Conditions (A)	3	1511.0	1.17	10.91	4.72 **	100.70	0.59
Error	32	1292.0		2.31		170.40	
Within Ss	72						
Trials (B)	2	1064.0	26.05 ***	22.69	34.46 ***	5.08	0.65
(3 testings)							
A × B	6	42.0	1.03	2.26	3.41 *	8.85	1.13
Error	64	40.85		0.66		7.86	

    * $p < .05$.
    ** $p < .01$.
    *** $p < .001$.

eralized anxiety measure than the others and may reflect an
enduring predisposition to anxiety rather than anxiety specific to
the experimental situation.

The only measure sensitive to the experimental condition was
the FCL snake item. The differences were strong enough to yield
a significant main effect and, since groups did not differ on pretest, the interaction with trials was also significant.

Approach Scale

Approach scale measures showed a significant interaction between trials and conditions, $F = 2.86$, $df = 6/64$, $p < .05$. Figure 9–1 depicts the interaction in graphic form for approach
scale scores. Because the groups were deliberately matched on
the basis of pretest approach scale scores, an analysis of variance,
strictly speaking, should not use the raw scores of Trial 1 to yield
estimates of error variance. Therefore, simple analyses of covariance were performed for post- and follow-up tests (Trials 2 and
3) on the approach scale, partialing out the initial level of performance. The error terms thus obtained were used to compute t
tests comparing groups on approach scores. For corrected Trial 2
means, a t test of the difference between the lowest experimental
group mean (arousal) and the control was significant at $p < .05$

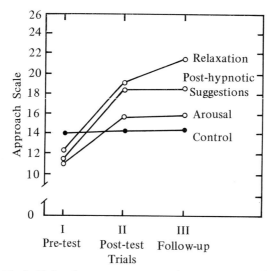

Figure 9–1. Trials X Conditions interactions for approach scale scores.

(one-tailed test), while there were no differences among experimental group means. For corrected Trial 3 means, the difference between Group A and the control dropped below significance. However, both Groups R and PH means remained significantly higher than the control mean, $p < .025$ for the smallest difference (one-tailed test). Again, experimental group means did not differ from each other.

The analysis of covariance (basic data are in Table 9–III) on Trial 2 approach scores showed $F = 4.25$, $p < .025$; for follow-up scores $F = 3.01$, $p < .05$. These results are identical to those obtained for change scores (Trial 2–1 and Trial 3–1). Both sets of change scores showed a significant treatment effect: the former $F = 4.68$, $df = 3/32$, $p < .01$, and the latter $F = 3.15$, $df = 3/32$, $p < .05$. The two posttests themselves, though, did not differ significantly, $F = .63$, $df = 3/32$.

At follow-up testing, the arousal group's change score (Trial 3–1) fell to the level of the control group's. This is due to a "relapse" effect found for three arousal Ss, who together totalled twenty units of increased avoidance from Trial 2 to 3. Other arousal Ss did not show this effect, however, so that overall,

TABLE 9-III
MEANS AND STANDARD DEVIATIONS ON PRE-, POST-, AND FOLLOW-UP MEASURES FOR EACH GROUP

Group	Measure									
	Approach scale		Fear checklist		Fear checklist snake item		MAS		SHSS Form A	
	M	SD	M	SD	M	SD	M	SD	M	SD
Relaxation										
Pretest	12.11	6.55	44.19	28.37	5.81	0.35	19.33	11.21	5.78	2.25
Posttest	18.89	4.06	32.06	22.48	4.50	1.24	18.11	7.09		
Follow-up	21.56	4.61	29.14	23.35	3.92	0.83	17.89	8.75		
Arousal										
Pretest	11.11	6.49	41.36	27.24	5.89	0.33	19.56	6.77	6.33	2.91
Posttest	15.78	6.83	39.04	22.82	5.17	0.94	19.89	7.94		
Follow-up	15.89	10.36	33.08	24.25	4.69	1.77	21.44	7.67		
Posthypnotic Suggestion										
Pretest	11.67	7.25	28.53	11.53	5.50	0.56	17.00	8.43	6.22	3.26
Posttest	18.44	6.00	22.28	16.45	3.50	1.35	15.89	6.98		
Follow-up	19.44	6.58	17.97	18.09	2.92	1.56	14.89	9.27		
Control										
Pretest	14.00	5.77	44.11	15.50	5.56	0.53	17.11	6.11	6.44	3.56
Posttest	14.11	6.30	39.44	18.81	5.61	0.66	17.44	5.19		
Follow-up	14.22	6.76	34.72	15.78	4.94	1.47	15.78	5.54		

Note.—MAS = Manifest Anxiety Scale; SHSS = Stanford Hypnotic Susceptibility Scale; n = 9 in each group.

Group A showed one unit of increased approach behavior from Trial 2 to 3. No relaxation S showed negative change, while Group PH and controls showed five and two units of relapse, respectively; these changes were smaller than overall group gains on the approach scale.

Comparisons within Therapeutic Treatments

Because of the theoretical importance of abreaction in the therapy of fears, it was of particular interest to compare improvement using the fear arousal strategy with that in the other groups using different techniques. In each experimental group, the four anxiety measures were inspected for change over trials in the direction of reduced fear. There were sixteen possible comparisons (four measures, two posttreatment trials, relaxation versus fear arousal, and posthypnotic suggestions versus fear arousal); in fourteen out of the sixteen comparisons, the posthypnotic suggestion and relaxation groups showed greater positive change than the arousal group, $p < .01$, using the binomial test.

Subject Characteristics

Hypnotizability and Anxiety

Hypnotizability as measured by the SHSS was not significantly related to initial approach scores $(r = .11)$; however, there was a significant negative relationship $(r = -.30)$ between hypnotizability and initial scores on the self-report anxiety measures. The subjective feeling of depth of hypnosis as reported by S (mean "state" score) was not related to any initial anxiety measures (largest $r = .12$).

Hypnotizability and Improvement

Hypnotizability appears to be related to reduction of phobic behavior when hypnosis is used as the vehicle of treatment. For experimental Ss $(n = 27)$, there was a significant positive relationship $(r = .39)$ between hypnotizability and posttreatment approach scores. The relationship was slightly stronger between these approach scores and S's state report $(r = .46)$. A significant positive relationship also occurred between state report and change scores both immediately after treatment and at follow-up (r's $= .31$ and $.33$, respectively). SHSS performance did show significant correlations with change scores, but they were all positive. There was a significant negative association between hypnotizability and all post-test self-report anxiety measures.

Interestingly, for the posthypnotic suggestion group ($n = 9$) in which improvement might be based on the effects of hypnosis only there was no relationship between hypnosis measures and any approach measures, suggesting that something was operating here besides the sheer effects of hypnotic suggestion.

Nonquantitative Findings

The degree to which the fear of snakes affected Ss' everyday living varied from a disinclination to hike or garden to a total avoidance of rural areas or outdoor family activities. All Ss reported physical symptoms associated with high anxiety on seeing a snake including accelerated pulse and respiration, dizziness, nausea, perspiring, trembling, and the impulse to flee. The great majority of snake-related experiences for these Ss were imaginal. No S reported ever having had a realistically dangerous experience with a snake, nor having been bitten by one. Apparently, for humans a long-lasting fear and stereotyped avoidance behavior can arise without the presence of physical pain.

DISCUSSION

Self-Report Measures of Anxiety

All pencil-and-paper anxiety measures showed a decrease in anxiety over trials. The greatest change was in Ss' self-rating of fear of snakes which showed a significant effect across trials, treatments, and their interaction. This result parallels findings by Paul (1965), Lang, Lazovik, and Reynolds (1965) and others that self-rated anxiety tends to decrease after treatment for a specific fear and that changes in self-rating behavior are related to more general behavior change.

Cognition and Phobias

Since no S reported any real, harmful experience with snakes, it appears that cognitive factors, in contrast with classical conditioning or instrumental learning, played a major part in the development of the fear. Although no experimental work has been published on the interrelationship of cognitions and the development of phobias, there have been a number of studies on verbal mediation and conditioned autonomic fear responses. Two early studies showed that S's expectations were more powerful than his experiences in establishing a conditioned galvanic skin response (GSR; Cook and Harris, 1937; Mowrer, 1938). The Ss showed GSRs when a light was presented if they expected the light to be followed by shock, although no Ss were shocked at any time; further, the GSRs were very resistant to extinction.

For a GSR conditioned to a word stimulus, autonomic response generalization can occur along dimensions of pleasantness (Baxter, 1962), hostility and similarity in meaning (Lang, Geer, and Hnatiow, 1963), and "rurality" (Lacey, Smith, and Green, 1955). The human ability to generalize along such abstract dimensions might augment the growth of conditioned phobic responses by providing more stimulus occasions to which the fear response may occur.

Another source of avoidance behavior in phobias is the fear of being afraid. Several Ss reported that they avoided contacts with snakes lest panic, which they found intensely unpleasant, overwhelm them.

Possibly a major component of successful fear therapies is the "self-dosage" of anxiety by S. Desensitization takes advantage of this, but even during "flooding" techniques, some Ss appear to maintain a tolerable anxiety level by "tuning out" incoming stimuli as needed.

Anxiety, Hypnotizability, and Conditioning

Conditioning is one component in the development of a phobia; most people are exposed to fear-producing stimuli but do not develop phobias, so that these phobic Ss may have been especially conditionable in some sense. A positive relationship between anxiety as measured by the MAS and the conditionability has been demonstrated (Spence and Spence, 1964; Taylor, 1953). In the present study, phobic Ss had higher MAS scores than an unselected group of normals, and these scores remained high across trials despite several anxiety-reducing influences.

A negative association was obtained between hypnotizability and anxiety as measured by initial self-report measures. A similar result was obtained by Lang et al. (1965), where hypnotizability was negatively related to anxiety as measured by both overt behavior and one self-rated fear measure. This finding seems plausible in light of the fact that the usual hypnotic induction calls for sleepiness, some abdication of control, and a relaxed state.

In contrast to earlier findings (Clyde, 1947; Lang et al., 1965), a positive relationship was found between improvement for experimental Ss and S's state report. Those Ss who felt more hypnotized benefited more from hypnotic treatment than Ss who did not experience the hypnotic effect as strongly. Similarly, Schubot (1967) found that hypnotic susceptibility and vividness of hypnotic imagery were positively related to reduction of fear in highly anxious Ss.

Treatment Outcomes

Immediately following treatment, all experimental groups improved significantly in approach behavior over the control group, while the experimental groups did not differ significantly among themselves. At follow-up, Ss in the experimental groups showed significantly more cases of improvement than those in the control group $(x^2 = 8.17, p < .01)$ The percentage of experimental group Ss improved was 81 percent, comparable with the usual findings in the behavior therapy literature. However, an overall analysis of variance of follow-up approach scores fell short of significance even though the change scores differed significantly, as did an analysis of covariance which partialed out initial approach scores.

Relaxation, fear arousal, and suggestion were all effective in increasing approach behavior, without personality exploration or attempts at gaining insight. The control group remained very stable across trials.

One explanation for the differences between experimental Ss and controls is that all experimental Ss had twelve treatment sessions, and their expectations for change may, therefore, have been high; controls were seen only four times, and so may have had correspondingly lower expectations for improvement, even though the number of actual exposures to the snake was the same for all Ss. It is also possible that the stability of controls was due to subtle cues communicated to these Ss by the *E,* who was not blind as to group assignments. The investigator was aware of this possibility, however, and made every effort to remain neutral with all Ss. The question of *E* bias can only be resolved by further research.

In addition to Ss' expectations, the efficacy of the relaxation procedure may lie in the substitution of relaxation responses to imaginal cues formerly evoking fear. Although systematic desensitization was not used, all Ss treated with the relaxation and recall technique improved.

Improvement in the posthypnotic suggestion group (seven out of nine Ss) was unrelated to any hypnotizability measures. One could conclude that even the very lightest stages of hypnosis are sufficient to promote the effectiveness of therapeutic suggestions (Gill and Brenman, 1959; Platonov, 1959). An alternative possibility is that during the nine hypnosis sessions, Ss were desensitizing themselves by thinking about the snake which they knew to be present in the building, while in a state of relaxation (Cautela, 1966).

Six fear arousal Ss showed increased approach scale scores. Explanations for their improvement must be speculative, as the present study was not designed to discriminate among the alternative possibilities. Catharsis of fear, desensitization during the reexperiencing of fear in a controlled setting, and learning to discriminate early experience from the present situation are all possible explanations that await further experimental test.

In other studies where arousal techniques were used (e.g. implosive therapy, Hogan and Kirchner, 1967) with subsequent improvement, the reduction in fear may have been due to a kind of exhaustion phenomenon. As Staub (1968) pointed out, sufficiently high arousal levels activate inhibitory mechanisms which ultimately repress anxiety, after which a kind of counterconditioning can rapidly occur. To achieve these high arousal levels, though, long exposure times to fearful stimuli are needed (ten minutes or more). In cases where arousal techniques have failed (e.g. Rachman, 1966), the exposure times were probably too short (Staub, 1968). The thirty-second exposure time used in the present study was less than that employed by Rachman and may have aroused insufficient anxiety for some Ss, so that exhaustion and relearning did not occur. This may explain why fear arousal was less effective than the other therapeutic strategies in reducing phobic behavior. Further, the relapse effect noted for some fear arousal Ss may be due to the repeated hypnotic instruction to reexperience their fear; Ss may have interpreted this as a suggestion that snakes were, in fact, harmful.

The small degree of behavior change found in the control group (two Ss improved) is consistent with the slight, nonsignificant improvement of control Ss found in other studies (Lang and Lazovik, 1963; Paul, 1965). The influence of being contacted to participate in a study, attention received during testing, and repeated exposure to the phobic object in a permissive context with a fearless model were not sufficient to produce substantial reductions in phobic behavior.

REFERENCES

Bandura, A.: Psychotherapy as a learning process. *Psychol Bull,* 68:143–159, 1961.

Baxter, J. C.: Mediated generalization as a function of semantic differential performance. *Am J Psychol,* 75:66–76, 1962.

Cautela, J.: Hypnosis and behavior therapy. *Behav Res Ther,* 4:219–224, 1966.

Clyde, D. J.: Hypnotherapy and phobias. Unpublished master's thesis, Pennsylvania State College, 1947.

Cofer, C. N., and Foley, J. P.: Mediated generalization and the interpretation of verbal behavior: I. Prolegomena. *Psychol Rev,* 49:513–540, 1942.

Cook, S. W., and Harris, R. E.: The verbal conditioning of the galvanic skin reflex. *J Exp Psychol,* 21:202–210, 1937.

Frank, J. D.: *Persuasion and Healing.* Baltimore, Maryland, Johns Hopkins Press, 1961.

Freud, S.: *The Standard Edition of the Complete Psychological Works of Sigmund Freud.* (Originally published 1895). London, Hogarth Press, 1955, vol. 2.

Gill, M. M., and Brenman, M.: *Hypnosis and Related States: Psychological Studies in Regression.* New York, International Universities Press, 1959.

Grinker, R., and Spiegel, J.: *Men Under Stress.* Philadelphia, Blakiston, 1945.

Hogan, R. A., and Kirchner, J. H.: Preliminary report of the extinction of learned fears via short-term implosive therapy. *J Abnorm Psychol*, 72:106–109, 1967.

Kaufman, M. R.: Hypnosis in psychotherapy today. *Arch Gen Psychiatry*, 4:30–39, 1961.

Kirchner, J. H., and Hogan, R. A.: therapist variable in the implosion of phobias. *Psychotherapy: Theory, Research and Practice*, 3:102–104, 1966.

Krasner, L., and Ullman, L. P., (Eds.): *Research In Behavior Modification*. New York, Holt, Rinehart and Winston, 1965.

Lacey, J., Smith, R., and Green, A.: Use of conditioned autonomic responses in the study of anxiety. *Psychosom Med*, 17:208–214, 1955.

Lang, P. J., Geer, J., and Hnatiow, M.: Semantic generalization of conditioned autonomic responses. *J Exp Psychol*, 69:552–558, 1963.

Lang, P. J., and Lazovik, A. D.: Experimental desensitization of a phobia. *J Abnorm Soc Psychol*, 66:519–525, 1963.

Lang, P. J., Lazovik, A. D., and Reynolds, D. J.: Desensitization, suggestibility, and pseudotherapy. *J Abnorm Psychol*, 70:395–402, 1965.

Malleson, N.: Panic and phobia: A possible method of treatment. *Lancet*, 1:225–227, 1959.

McCreary, J. B., and Bendig, A. W.: Comparison of two forms of the Manifest Anxiety Scale. *J Consult Psychol*, 18:206, 1954.

Mowrer, O. H.: Preparatory set (expectancy)—a determinant in motivation and learning. *Psychol Rev*, 45:62–91, 1938.

Paul, G. L.: *Insight Versus Desensitization in Psychotherapy: An Experiment in Anxiety Reduction*. Stanford, California, Stanford University Press, 1965.

Platonov, K. I.: *The Word As a Physiological and Therapeutic Factor*. Moscow: Foreign Languages Publication House, 1959.

Rachman, S.: Studies in desensitization: II. Flooding. *Behav Res Ther*, 4:1–6, 1966.

Rosenthal, D., and Frank J. D.: Psychotherapy and the placebo effect. *Psychol Bull*, 53:294–302, 1956.

Salter, A.: *Conditioned Reflex Therapy*. New York, Creative Age Press, 1949.

Schubot, E. D.: The influence of hypnotic and muscular relaxation in systematic desensitization of phobias. *Dissertation Abstracts*, 27:3681–3682, 1967.

Spence, K. W., and Spence, J. T.: Relation of eyelid conditioning to manifest anxiety, extraversion, and rigidity. *J Abnorm Soc Psychol*, 68:144–149, 1964.

Stampfl, T. G., and Levis, D. J.: A learning-theory-based psychodynamic behavioral therapy. *J Abnorm Psychol*, 72:496–502, 1967.

Staub, E.: Duration of stimulus exposure as determinant of the efficacy of flooding procedures in the elimination of fear. *Behav Res Ther*, 6:131–132, 1968.

Strahley, D. F.: Systematic desensitization and counterphobic treatment of an irrational fear of snakes. *Dissertation Abstracts, 27*:973, 1966.

Taylor, J. A.: A personality scale of manifest anxiety. *J Abnorm Soc Psychol, 48*:285–290, 1953.

Watson, J. B., and Raynor, R.: Continued emotional reactions. *J Exp Psychol, 3*:1–14, 1920.

Weitzenhoffer, A. M., and Hilgard, E. R.: *Stanford Hypnotic Susceptibility Scale, Forms A and B.* Palo Alto, California, Consulting Psychologists Press, 1959.

Wolpe, J.: *Psychotherapy by Reciprocal Inhibition.* Stanford, California, Stanford University Press, 1958.

Wolpin, M., and Raines, J.: Visual imagery, expected roles and extinction as possible factors in reducing fear and avoidance behavior. *Behav Res Ther, 4*:25–37, 1966.

CHAPTER 10

THE EFFECT OF HYPNOSIS ON CONDITIONABILITY*

Milton V. Kline, Ed. D.

IN THE MAIN, contemporary hypnosis emphasizes the emerging distinction between the hypnotic state and the hypnotic relationship. This permits a clarified awareness of the process of hypnotic response and the alterations in behavior organizing mechanisms which may accompany this response formation. Hypnosis is not so much a unitary phenomenon as a process of adaptation within which there are varied and selective shifts in receptor and effector mechanisms (Kline, 1961, 1963, 1965, 1967).

One concept which emerges in present-day thinking about hypnosis is that the multiphasic aspects of the hypnotic process and of hypnotic behavior which result from a fundamentally central process take on the form of the behavioral structure within which the experience of hypnosis is organized. There can be as sharp a differential in response formation within the hypnotic process as outside, thus obviating the recognition of the nature of hypnosis via the expression of simplistic or one dimensional responses. The nature of hypnosis is inherently bound up with the meaning or function of the experience. Experiential involvement in the hypnotic process must be studied from both the intra-psychic and inter-personal levels of involvement. It is not unlikely that, at the present time, different theories of hypnosis represent operational examples of different mechanisms of function within the hypnotic process.

Ultimately, all who use hypnosis must face a basic problem: the relationship of hypnosis to other facets of behavior. For example, what is the relationship of hypnosis to conditioning? Clini-

* Original manuscript.

cal observations suggest that, when one deals with human conditioning and examines the effects of human conditioning, it is not infrequent that one may be observing the results of a hypnotic experience and of a hypnotic process underlying this aspect of behavior. The basic process of conditioning and of the induction of a conditioned response is by its repetitiousness and reinforcement similar to and suggestive of hypnotic procedure. On the other hand, the conditioned response which is acquired in a laboratory situation may show sharply different characteristics.

A conditioned response of a nonhypnotic type shows a pattern of extinction, tends to go into somewhat more rapid extinction, whereas the "conditioned" response which appears to be the result of hypnosis frequently displays much greater strength and tenacity.

In an earlier study of the reactions of amputees to prosthetic adjustment, the writer (Kline, 1959) became concerned with the problem of conditioning and found that it was difficult to produce relatively simple conditioned responses in human subjects, but when the same approach was utilized within a hypnotic situation, conditioning appeared to have been achieved rapidly, and, in a number of instances, could not be extinguished quickly even though this was the experimental objective (Kline, 1952). There has not been a great deal of systematic work dealing with the effect of hypnosis upon conditionability either in experimental settings or in relation to therapeutic applications. Drawing upon Pavlovian theory, Russian investigators have extended concepts of conditioning and conditionability in relation to hypnotherapy in a wide range of applications. Unfortunately, due to differences in definition of terms and interpretation of theoretical constructs, the data are not readily applicable to the manner in which hypnosis may be viewed and utilized in behavioral science studies in countries outside the Soviet sphere (Kline, 1959).

Edmonston (1972) has presented the most distinct and comprehensive data on the effects of neutral hypnosis on conditioned responses which bear some relation to the main issues under discussion here. In reviewing his data, Edmonston essentially presents an experimental analysis of Pavlov's cortical inhibition theory of hypnosis. This points out that, as hypnosis deepens, there is interference with the voluntary but not with the involuntary components of conditioned responses, due to a progressive spread of cortical inhibition. Edmonston clearly points out that earlier experimental work on this prediction has been sparse and inconclusive. On his own part, in a series of carefully and methodically converging studies, he analyzes and interprets the complexities, the experimental flaws and the inaccurate interpretations inherent in research that has centered on the Pavlovian position.

In the main, his conclusion is that hypnotic studies have been concerned primarily with the effects of complex hypnotic phenomena such as amnesia and age regression on conditioned responses or the effects of hypnotic induction on complex motor and verbal learning. Conditioned responses and their relation to hypnosis have been of primary concern to the Russian investigators. In his early work, Pavlov (1927) concluded that hypnosis brought about a prolonged, monotonous and environmental stimulation, and created in the cells of the cortex a state of radiated inhibition. In this respect, he was quite clear that the portion of the central nervous system involved in hypnosis, the cortex, was such that he said, "We are dealing with a complete inhibition confined exclusively to the cortex, without a concurrent dissent of the inhibition that centers regularly in the equilibrium and maintenance of posture." He further added, "Thus in the form of sleep (hypnosis) the plane of demarcation between inhibited regions of the brain and the regions which are free from inhibitions seem to pass just beneath the cerebral cortex." Edmonston's conclusion from his survey of the scanty experimental data is that there is "no clear cut conclusion as to the fate of previously established conditioned responses following the induction of hypnosis." (Plapp and Edmonston, 1965)

Based on his own work, Edmonston (1972) further concluded that, just as Pavlov indicated they would be, voluntary motor functions are inhibited by hypnotic induction and nonvoluntary functions appear not to be. Clinical experience utilizing a variety of sensory-motor techniques in hypnotherapy (Kline, 1971) have indicated that a wide range of symptomatic responses which are on an involuntary level and function in many respects like conditioned responses can be readily altered, modified and removed without alteration in the homeostatic equilibrium of the patient. Likewise, it has been observed in a number of situations that hypnotically induced responses and modifications or alterations in behavior can be induced directly. Through self hypnotic reinforcement they can be maintained over long periods of time and thus they assume many of the characteristics of an acquired conditioned response.

Thus, to all intents and purposes, without going into some of the involved and overly determined methodological issues relative to conditioning and its roles in both neurotic behavior and psychotherapy, there is strong evidence that the process of conditionability is one which can be influenced by hypnosis and one to which hypnosis has an inherent relationship. As such, it can readily be incorporated into the therapeutic process. Thus, the entire sphere of communication theory within psychotherapy must be considered as an aspect of the conditionability process.

While the Soviet work, were it to be reviewed and analyzed in detail, would constitute a study of its own, it is nevertheless interesting to make references to various aspects of what they refer to as cortical dynamics, particularly the co-activity and interactivity of the first and second signaling systems during hypnosis. R. M. Pen and M. P. Dzhagarov (1936) researched the formation of conditioned responses during hypnosis and concluded that the establishment of a new conditioned response was not readily obtained in deep hypnotic states but was very possible during light hypnotic states although characterized by some difficulties. The conditioned response which was established was, in their observations, characterized by a certain amount of frailty. At the same time, these investigators succeeded in observing a state of hypnosis within which a disappearance of conditioned reactions to verbal stimuli occurred while the direct stimuli were maintained. The details of the hypnotic procedures and aspects of the hypnotic relationship are either lacking or obscured by semantics and different therapeutic orientations. Nevertheless they seem to be consistent with our clinical observations. Symptom formation which becomes autonomous, like a conditioned response, can be altered relatively permanently by hypnotic procedures, and newly acquired conditioned responses involving involuntary behavior can be brought about more readily, when at all possible, in lighter hypnotic states rather than in deeper ones. This is of considerable interest and warrants further investigation in relation to therapeutic application.

In connection with the differences noted between the levels of hypnosis and conditionability, Soviet investigators (1955) reported that the latent period of the conditioned motor reactions during light stages of hypnosis varied within normal limits or else somewhat exceeded them, and amounted to 0.8 to 1.8 seconds. In the deeper stages of hypnosis, it fluctuated from four to ten seconds. This differential is of considerable significance and, should it be confirmed by more detailed studies and observations, has clear implications for therapeutic technique as well as theory. The writers also reported that, in the hypnotic condition, they were able, with the aid of verbal reinforcement, to form conditioned reactions in the form of one autonomic reaction or another, such that even a complex autonomic reaction as the act of vomiting could be elucidated. Thus, with hypnosis, they had the feeling that they could create new conditioned responses with various stimuli and autonomic reaction; their observation being that it was necessary for the patient in hypnosis to know the verbal designation of this autonomic reaction. This is consistent with our own experience in which, in eliminating symptoms of pain, organ system dysfunction, and the creation or maintenance of states of well being, it is very important for the patient in hypnotherapy to have a clearly defined designation of what the organ system response is expected to be like and to be able to conceive of it. In instances of treating patients with functional bladder disturbances and in a number of cases of functional disorders of the uterus and urethral tract, rapid and permanent relief could be afforded when the patient was able to visualize the designated organs and the response that was being suggested during the hypnotic session. The Soviet authors (1955) concluded in their observations that autonomic conditioned reactions, when formed and consolidated upon verbal reinforcement during hypnosis, were found to be maintained from one and a half to four years.

More in relation to technique, although obviously related to an interacting process, these investigators found that the manner in which verbal suggestions were given, particularly the loudness of the voice of the therapist, played a significant role in the effectiveness of establishing conditioned responses. On the basis of their investigations with a large number of patients it was felt that it was essential to revise what they considered to be obsolescent conceptions existing in the field of hypnotherapy and that it was necessary to adopt a more viable method of conducting verbal suggestions, almost always in a low voice. Based on extensive studies, they concluded that the elaborations and consolidation during hypnosis of new conditioned responses can be carried out in light stages of hypnosis. They also observed that these conditioned responses are preserved in the waking state. The latent period of conditioned responses considerably increased during hypnosis in the majority of subjects. They felt that in hypnosis the formation and consolidation of autonomic conditioned reactions was very effective and relatively easily produced when the subject knew the verbal designation of the reactions. In effect, he was able to form new conditioned responses between any given stimulus and autonomic reaction with the sole aid of verbal reinforcement.

In considering the importance of hypnosis on conditionability, we are obviously dealing with one of the important variables in the modification of behavior disorders. In keeping with Wolpe's (1971) consideration of the use of hypnosis and behavior therapy, wherein he considers behavior therapy to be clearly defined as the application of experimentally established principles of learning to the purpose of changing unadaptive habits, it is clear that the ability to influence conditionability is a prime element in developing a viable system of behavior therapy. In Wolpe's own words: "Where neurotic responses are conditioned to situations involving direct interpersonal relations, the essence of reciprocal inhibition therapy has been to inhibit anxiety by the instigation of patterns of behavior that express other feelings that are relevant." While the concept of conditionability and the conditioning process have to be redefined and expanded somewhat within the framework of human neurosis and the behavioral modification of such neurosis, it is clear that the ability to alter involuntary mechanisms as well as to bring about new responses which have the strength of a conditioned response is an integral part of the therapeutic procedure. In this respect, and under circumstances which now remain to be delineated as well as defined, hypnosis appears to be a potent and readily available condition for submitting to therapy.

In attempting to synthesize the available data on the effects of hypnosis on conditioning, as well as the limited work that has been done on hypnosis and conditionability, it would appear that the degree to which hypnosis can be utilized in relation to the conditioning process must be based on the nature of the hypnotic or the hypnotherapeutic experience, the means for achieving this, and from both dynamic and theoretical points of view, the function which hypnosis assumes in this connection. Insufficient attention has been paid in contemporary work with hypnosis to the function of hypnosis. It has been noted from clinical experience that the function of hypnosis varies according to the role involvement (Kline, 1953), or, as Orne (1969) has so clearly stated, the "demand characteristics of the hypnotic situation." In being able to bring about functional alterations in the role that hypnosis plays for the individual, different therapeutic potentialities and outcomes become possible. Without sufficient recognition and structuring of this functional role of hypnosis, such therapeutic outcomes may not be at all possible.

In a report describing primate-like behavior in a hypnotic subject (Kline, 1952), it was noted that apparent "unlearned" responses could be elucidated in such a state. In later publications (Kline, 1960; 1963), this led to the theoretical position that studies of the learning and adaptive mechanisms in subjects in deeply regressed hypnotic states reflect a shift in response formation from chronological levels to levels composed of elements of ontogenic regression (Kline, 1960).

For example, in a deeply regressed state in many subjects the presentation of a dental click will produce erotic arousal which may result in frenzy and spontaneous orgasm or it may lead to involuntary sexual acting out. This is a reaction which has been observed in infraprimates as well.

Hypnotic alterations of consciousness may be considered to

fall into two major categories: (1) that which is produced by the particular level of hypnosis achieved by the subject and, (2) that which is produced by the hypnotic instrumentation being employed, and this relates to the function of the hypnosis and particularly to the function of the hypnotic relationship. Hypnosis is clearly neither a simple nor singular reaction, but rather a compactly agglutinated state within which stimulus function may become radically altered and reality mechanisms become more flexible and capable of multifunctional transformation. Perceptual constancy may be replaced by a multiplicity of perceptual organizing devices. For this reason, present day findings and observation with hypnosis may contain seemingly paradoxical and conflicting results.

The often expressed idea that everything observed or produced on a hypnotic level can be observed or produced on a nonhypnotic level is both true and meaningless at the same time, unless one can establish definitive criteria for what constitutes hypnotic and nonhypnotic. We can differentiate between the deliberate induction of the hypnotic state and the state in which no deliberate induction has been made. But this does not rule out the presence of a hypnotic process, either spontaneously or indirectly.

The acceptance of hypnotically induced behavior would appear dynamically to be consistent with the implication that hypnosis involves a degree of self-exclusion and the capacity to accept subjective responses without the necessity for critical evaluation by the self. This may permit the structuring of hypnotic perception and behavior on a pre-logical level which would be consistent with greater interaction with the process of conditionability.

In considering the total dynamics that may be involved in creating the hypnotic basis for altering both the existence of certain involuntary or conditioned responses and allowing for accessibility to newly acquired conditioned responses, it is essential to consider the fact that the form or level of hypnotic interaction that is created in the treatment situation follows the function that has been designated in the interpersonal relationship. Thus, form follows function but that function must be one of the most clearly designated goals in the process of therapeutic communication.

Without this basis, the form of hypnosis which evolves can vary from one which permits only relatively simplistic enhancement of suggestibility to one that provides less accessibility than may be present in the waking state.

From the point of view of psychological activity, the basis for the appearance of a functional level of hypnosis that permits accessibility to the conditioning process may be considered as the construction of invariance or the concepts of the self through conservation * (Piaget, 1954).

Conservation may be equated on a behavioral level with the activating element behind reality appraisal, structuring body image and awareness of self in relation to externalized symbols. In this respect, conservation is the process of logical organization even though it may deal with illogical components. It may well be that much of what happens within the reconstruction-conservation process in hypnosis is very similar to what goes on in the condensation-reconstruction process in dreaming. The process of conservation might therefore be considered as the result of operational reversability. Operational reversability is based upon Piaget's (1957) genetic model of the development of logical structures in the mental development of children, and relates to the capacity to manipulate observations through the logical associations of externalized connections as compared with the capacity to deal with observations linked to internalized associations. Response mechanisms relate to modality functions of tension, awareness and the gradations of consciousness as they may be viewed in terms of criticalness and vigilance. Operational reversability, in this sense, is a structural process within which cognitive and perceptual mechanisms develop and emerge.

Based upon these underlying observations, concepts and implications, the writer has, during the past number of years, utilized hypnosis in relation to symptom modification approaches in psychotherapy in which the goal has been the direct alteration of focal symptoms in brief hypnotherapeutic contacts, reinforced through the use of self hypnosis and the utilization of audio tape recordings (Kline, 1970, 1972).

* Conservation as a cognitive perceptual process is here used in the way Piaget utilized it in his concept of the development of logical structures.

For the greater part, patients who have been seen in such treatment sessions are seen only two or three times, with the average length of the treatment session being two hours. The emphasis has been upon the utilization of dissociative and conditioning techniques along with specific training in the utilization of self hypnosis, which—as taught—incorporates vivid recall and revivification of the hypnotherapy experience through the use of audio tape recordings. In each instance, specific tape recordings are made for each patient, and are made during the sessions. They are designed to reinforce therapeutic goals and, at the same time, to facilitate the use of self hypnosis spontaneously at designated times without having to rely on self-induction or formalized induction at all.

A variety of therapeutic techniques have been employed which, for the greater part, are based on the use of some degree of dissociation, time distortion and the development of imagery which becomes linked with the therapeutic goal. Each tape recording has been specifically prepared in keeping with the individual needs of the patient and the circumstances surrounding the history and difficulties presented for treatment.

In some instances, a series of tapes are prepared and the proper sequence of utilization is outlined and discussed with the patient. In a number of instances, patients have been seen on only one occasion, but usually three sessions are more typical. Case illustrations have included problems of insomnia, smoking habituation, a broad range of psychosomatic and psychophysiological disorders, frigidity, impotence, pain and anxiety problems relating to forthcoming surgery, and special adaptation requirements in relation to specific organic disorders. Particularly responsive have been problems of obesity and drug dependence.

Brief Clinical Illustrations

A number of patients presenting long histories of psoriasis have been significantly helped and, in a number of instances, the psoriasis completely eliminated by inducing, under hypnosis, various sensations in each and every area of the body where the lesions of psoriasis have been present (Kline, 1954). The more intense the experience, the more likely the therapeutic outcome.

In several instances, following two or three sessions, and with daily use of audio tape recording, patients have reported that, for the next six to eight months, sensations of warmth have appeared spontaneously ten to fifteen times a day in each affected area of the body. Frequently, rapid improvement is noted and is continuous and progressive.

In cases of migraine, patients have been taught, by touching the painful area of the head, to experience a sense of ease and a feeling of lightness and, at times, a sensation designated and created by the patient's own description of what to them is the "most normal, comfortable feeling about the head." Frequently, this is tied in with the ability to visualize the self, pain free, and again reinforced through visual imagery and audio tape recordings.

A number of patients with functional disorders of the urethra which had required continuous dilation with minimal therapeutic results were helped within two or three hypnotherapy sessions, by being able to experience the feeling or sensation of dilation which they then could bring about merely by thinking about it in the waking state. Symptomatic improvement occurred within three or four days and in ten such cases that have been followed for a year, there has been no return of the symptom. The sensations of dilation continue to occur spontaneously so long as the patient uses the self-hypnosis via audio tape as a reinforcement at least once a day for an average period of four to five minutes.

The function of hypnosis and the incorporation of sensory motor and imagery activity appears to assume the characteristic of "new learning" which effects the conditionability of the acquired symptomatic behavior and leads to rapid and effective improvement through a process which may be linked to or connected with conditioning. The dynamics and mechanisms of this type of hypnotherapeutic procedure and its relationship to conditioning theory demands a great deal more experimental research for a fuller understanding of its substance. On the clinical level, it is quite clear that a viable and rapid means of dealing with a broad range of functional disorders within a brief period of treatment is both possible and, in terms of the durability of the results, justified.

REFERENCES

Edmonston, W. E., Jr.: The effects of neutral hypnosis on conditioned responses in hypnosis. In Fromm, E. and Shor, R. (Eds.): *Responses in Hypnosis: Research Developments and Perspectives.* New York/Chicago, Aldine-Atherton, 1972.

Kline, M. V.: A note on primate-like behavior induced through hypnosis: a case report. *J Gen Psychol, 81*:125, 1952.

Kline, M. V.: Hypnotic retrogression: a neuropsychological theory of age regression and progression. *J Clin Exp Hypn, 1*:21, 1953.

Kline, M. V.: Psoriasis and hypnotherapy: a case report. *J Clin Exp Hypn, 2*:318, 1954.

Kline, M. V.: Soviet and western trends in hypnosis research. *Int J Parapsychol, 1*:89, 1959.

Kline, M. V.: Hypnotic age regression and psychotherapy: clinical and theoretical observations. *Int J Clin Exp Hypn, 8*:17, 1960.

Kline, M. V. (Ed.): *The Nature of Hypnosis: Contemporary Theoretical Approaches.* New York, The Institute for Research in Hypnosis and the Postgraduate Center for Psychotherapy, 1961.

Kline, M. V. (Ed.): *Clinical Correlations of Experimental Hypnosis.* Springfield, Thomas, 1963.

Kline, M. V.: Hypnotherapy. In Wolman, B. (Ed.): *The Handbook of Clinical Psychology.* New York, McGraw-Hill, 1965.

Kline, M. V. (Ed.): *Psychodynamics and Hypnosis: New Contributions to the Practice and Theory of Hypnotherapy.* Springfield, Thomas, 1967.

Kline, M. V.: The use of extended group hypnotherapy sessions in controlling cigarette habituation. *Int J Clin Exp Hypn, 18*:270, 1970.

Kline, M. V.: Research in hypnotherapy: studies in behavior organization. In Bilz, R., and Petrilowitsch, N. (Eds.): *Akt Fragen Psychiat Neurol.,* Basel, Karger, Vol. 11, 1971.

Kline, M. V.: Hypnosis and therapeutic education in the treatment of obesity: the control of visceral responses through cognitive motivation and operant conditioning. In Langen, Z. (Ed.): *Hypnose und Psychosomatische Medizin.* Stuttgart, Hippokrates Verlag, 1972.

Orne, M. T.: Demand characteristics and the concept of quasi-controls. In Rosenthal, R., and Rosnow, R. L. (Eds.): *Artifact in Behavioral Research.* New York, Academic Press, 1969.

Pavlov, I. P.: *Conditioned Reflexes.* London, Oxford University Press, 1927.

Pen, R. M., and Dzhagarov, M. P.: The formation of conditioned connections during hypnotic sleep. *Arkh Biol Nauk, 9*:1, 1936.

Piaget, J.: *The Construction of Reality in the Child.* New York, Basic Books, 1954.

Piaget, J.: *Logic and Psychology.* New York, Basic Books, 1957.

Plapp, J. M., and Edmonston, W. E., Jr.: Extinction of a conditioned motor response following hypnosis. *J Abnorm Soc Psychol, 70*:378, 1965.

Smolenskii-Ivanov, A. G.: *Works of the Institute of Higher Nervous Activity.* Pathophysiological series, Vol. 1. Moscow, The Academy of Sciences of the U.S.S.R., 1955.

Wolpe, J.: The use of hypnosis in behavior therapy. Paper presented at the 1971 meeting of the American Psychological Association, Washington, D. C.

USES OF HYPNOSIS IN BEHAVIOR THERAPY

IN ANY THERAPEUTIC SITUATION, there are important nonspecific variables which help to mediate behavioral change. In this section, Spanos, De Moor and Barber describe the nonspecific variables employed in and common to both hypnosis and behavior therapy, and Lazarus investigates the importance of expectancy as a nonspecific variable in the use of hypnosis with behavior therapy. Originally one of the more prolific behavioral writers on the use of hypnotic techniques (Lazarus, 1958, 1960, 1963, 1971), over the years Lazarus has enlarged his therapeutic sphere, to develop first his notion of broad-spectrum behavior therapy and then his multimodal format (see Chapter 1).

The use of hypnosis with specific behavioral techniques is limited only by the ingenuity of the therapist. Cautela's covert conditioning procedures have been used by hypnotherapists from time immemorial, but he organizes them into a more efficient framework, into which methodological rigor may be introduced. Interestingly, other authors (Foreyt and Hagen, 1973) state that the results obtained by covert sensitization may just as easily be interpreted in terms of suggestion and attention conditioning per se. Glick illustrates the clinical usefulness of hypnosis to enhance aversive imagery in a covert sensitization situation.

Using the principle of reciprocal inhibition, Rubin delineates

145

the manner in which hypnosis facilitates behavioral change by directly suggesting alternative adaptive responses to the client while hypnotized. Todd and Kelley further illustrate the utility of hypnosis in facilitating the substitution of relaxation for tension responses. They also emphasize the manner in which hypnosis can enhance imagery, facilitate conditioning and help maintain new response patterns through posthypnotic suggestion. Scott describes the use of desensitization under hypnosis for the treatment of bird phobia, together with his use of hypnosis for behavioral diagnosis and assertive training.

Krippner uses posthypnotic suggestion to facilitate adaptive behavioral changes in education, in the improvement of study habits, the reformation of test-taking behavior, and the strengthening of academic motivation. Other authors (e.g. Jampolsky, 1972) have used similar techniques for educational purposes, such as helping children with reading problems.

Rothman, Carroll, and Rothman discuss the use of a combined program of behavioral homework and self-hypnosis to reinforce newly acquired behavior.

Both Bell and Fromm illustrate the ingenuity of the hypnotherapist who introduces creative, novel ways of changing behavior; ways that the behavior therapist would do well to mimic when treating patients. Bell discusses the uses of behavioral techniques in hypnotherapy within the framework of a humanistic and existential approach. Fromm combines desensization, assertive and role playing techniques from a psychoanalytic perspective.

REFERENCES

Foreyt, J. P., and Hagen, R. L.: Covert sensitization: conditioning or suggestion? *J Abnorm Psychol,* 82:17, 1973.

Jampolsky, G. D.: A special suggestive and auto-suggestive technique in helping children with reading problems. Presented at the VIth International Congress of Hypnosis, Uppsala, Sweden, July 1 to 4, 1973.

Lazarus, A. A.: Some clinical applications of autohypnosis. *Med Proc,* 4:848, 1958.

Lazarus, A. A.: New methods in psychotherapy: a case study. In Eysenck, H. J. (Ed.): *Behavior Therapy and the Neuroses.* New York, Pergamon, 1960.

Lazarus, A. A.: Sensory deprivation under hypnosis in the treatment of pervasive ("free-floating") anxiety: a preliminary impression, S *Afr Med J*, 37:136, 1963.

Lazarus, A. A.: *Behavior Therapy and Beyond.* New York, McGraw-Hill, 1971.

CHAPTER 11

HYPNOSIS AND BEHAVIOR THERAPY: COMMON DENOMINATORS*

Nicholas P. Spanos, Ph.D.
Wilfried Demoor, Ph.D.
Theodore X. Barber, Ph.D.

INTRODUCTION

In this paper, the relationships between hypnosis and behavior therapy are examined on two levels. First, the authors consider the contention that a "hypnotic state" mediates some of the therapeutic changes that are seen in behavior therapy. Logical and empirical problems pertaining to the hypothetical construct "hypnotic state" or "trance" are specified and it is concluded that the construct is not useful in explaining the changes in behavior observed in either hypnotic situations or in behavior therapy situations. Secondly, the authors focus on parallels between hypnotic situations and those behavior therapy situations that make subjects' imaginings the pivot of therapeutic change. Four sets of variables are delineated that appear to play a role in mediating the changes in behavior seen in both hypnotic and behavior therapy situations: (a) motivational variables, (b) attitudinal and expectancy variables, (c) the specific wording of the suggestions or instructions, and (d) circumscribed cognitive processes (e.g. goal-directed imagining) occurring in response to the suggestions or instructions.

B EHAVIOR THERAPISTS have at times used hypnotic induction procedures to produce relaxation and to facilitate imagery (Lang, Lazovik and Reynolds, 1965; Larsen, 1966; Lazarus, 1971;

* Originally published in *The American Journal of Clinical Hypnosis*, Volume 16, Number 1, July 1973, pages 45–64. Copyright 1973 by the American Society of Clinical Hypnosis.

Wolpe, 1958; Wolpe and Lazarus, 1966). Consequently, writers such as Litvak (1970) and Murray (1963) have tried to explain some of the successful results of systematic desensitization and other behavior therapy procedures in terms of hypnosis and suggestions. In fact, Litvak (1970) has suggested that a hypnotic state may be an important factor in mediating therapeutic change during systematic desensitization even when a formal hypnotic induction procedure is not used. According to Litvak, subjects undergoing desensitization may, unbeknown to the therapist, enter a hypnotic state which mediates therapeutic gain.

Other writers seem to believe that "hypnosis" is helpful, but not necessary, during systematic desensitization. For instance, Wolpe and Lazarus (1966) used hypnotic induction procedures in about one-third of their desensitization sessions and they stated that the hypnotic trance state may "enable certain patients to achieve more vivid and realistic images, and/or deeper and more satisfactory levels of relaxation [p. 135]." Wolpe (1958) had also written previously that "Those who cannot or will not be hypnotized but who can relax will make progress, although apparently more slowly when hypnosis is used [p. 141].*

In this paper, we shall take issue with the notion that the construct "hypnotic state" or "trance" is useful for explaining the results of any behavior therapy. In fact, we shall argue that the hypothetical construct "hypnotic state" or "trance" has little scientific utility in explaining even hypnotic phenomena, let alone the changes in behavior achieved by behavior therapists. However, we shall also argue that the hypnotic *situation* (as opposed to the hypothetical "hypnotic state") shares several variables in common with many behavior therapy *situations*, and that these common variables are important in producing behavior change in both types of situations.

While there are a wide range of procedures included under the term *behavior therapy*, we shall consider parallels between hypnosis and only those behavioral techniques that employ the subjects' imaginings as part of the therapeutic procedure. Spe-

---

* However, during recent years, Wolpe has apparently become more and more disenchanted with the use of hypnosis and has limited its use to about 10 percent of his current patients (Wolpe, 1969).

cifically, we shall deal with similarities between hypnosis and systematic desensitization (Wolpe, 1958), implosion therapy (Stampfl and Levis, 1967, 1968), and Cautela's (1967, 1969, 1970, 1971) covert techniques which include covert sensitization, covert reinforcement, and covert extinction. Because systematic desensitization has been more extensively investigated than the other behavior therapies, much of our discussion will focus on this procedure. We shall not be concerned with behavior therapies that do not ask the subject to imagine (e.g. electrical or chemical aversion therapy or operant conditioning). We shall turn first to a logical and empirical analysis of the "hypnotic state" construct, and then to an analysis of the commonalities in hypnotic and behavior therapy situations.

THE "HYPNOTIC STATE" CONSTRUCT: LOGICAL AND EMPIRICAL CONSIDERATIONS

The hypothetical construct *hypnotic state* or *trance* has served as an explanation of hypnotic phenomena for well over a century. According to the traditional formulation, susceptible subjects enter an altered state of consciousness ("hypnotic state") when they are exposed to procedures labeled as *hypnotic inductions* (Evans, 1968; Hilgard, 1965; Orne, 1966, 1969, 1970, 1971). These procedures, although varying widely in content, usually include interrelated suggestions that the subject will become increasingly relaxed, will enter an unusual or special state ("hypnotic state" or "trance"), and will be able to respond well to further suggestions. The "altered state" that is said to be produced by hypnotic induction procedures is thought to possess certain special properties that lead to "hypnotic behaviors." Historically, "hypnotic behaviors" have included the following: (a) heightened responsiveness to suggestions for limb or body rigidity, analgesia, age regression, hallucination, amnesia, and the like (Hilgard, 1965; Hilgard and Tart, 1966), (b) "hypnotic appearance" (e.g. relaxation, lethargy or passivity, and fixity of gaze), (c) reports of unusual experiences (e.g. illogical thinking, distortions of perception) (Orne, 1959, 1966), and (d) reports of having been hypnotized (Hilgard and Tart, 1966). Despite the longevity and wide acceptance of the "hypnotic state" notion in recent years the scientific utility of this construct has become increasingly suspect on both logical and empirical grounds.

Logical Considerations

One major difficulty with the "hypnotic state" construct is that it is often denoted by the very behaviors it purports to explain (Barber, 1964, 1969; Chaves, 1968; McPeake, 1968; Spanos, 1970; Spanos and Chaves, 1970, 1971). For example, the "hypnotic trance state" is said to be present when subjects respond to suggestions for limb rigidity, analgesia, or amnesia, and, turning around circularly, these responses to suggestions are "explained" by positing a "hypnotic trance state." Of course, this kind of circularity explains nothing and retards theory development in science.

In recent years, advocates of the "hypnotic state" notion have, themselves, become aware of the constructs' circularity and have tried to circumvent the difficulty by using multiple indices to converge on the "trance state" (Hilgard, 1965, 1969). The two indices most commonly used are heightened response to suggestions and reports of having been hypnotized. However, the use of these two indices quickly leads to difficulties for advocates of the "hypnotic state"; namely, subjects' response to suggestions and their reports of having been hypnotized can vary independently of one another. In other words, subjects can respond well to suggestions while stating that they were not hypnotized and, conversely, they may state that they were hypnotized but fail to respond to suggestions (Barber, 1969, 1970a; Conn and Conn, 1967). Furthermore, subjects' reports that they were or were not hypnotized can be easily manipulated by varying the wording of the questions used to elicit their reports (Barber, Dalal, and Calverley, 1968).

Other common indices of "hypnotic trance," such as "hypnotic appearance," have also been shown to vary independently of response to suggestions. Subjects who appear to be hypnotized— e.g. who appear lethargic, move slowly, and stare fixedly—may respond poorly to suggestions for limb rigidity, analgesia, amnesia, and the like. Conversely, subjects who appear wide awake may respond well to suggestions (Barber, 1969). Attempts have also been made to find neurophysiological indices of the "hypnotic trance state." A critical analysis of the available data, however, shows that such physiological indices are not available (Barber, 1970a, pp. 184–187). In short, the various indices of "hypnotic trance" fail to converge satisfactorily and thus fail to provide a parsimonious account of hypnotic phenomena (Spanos and Chaves, 1969).

A related criticism of the "hypnotic state" notion has been proposed by Sarbin and Coe (1972). They have pointed out that hypothetical constructs such as "hypnotic state," "trance," or "hypnotic trance state" function primarily as reified pseudo-explanations to fill gaps in empirical knowledge. Such constructs develop when complex behavior cannot be readily explained in terms of proximal and easily observable antecedent variables. As empirical information about the phenomena in question becomes available, such constructs usually drop out of scientific discourse. Unfortunately, while they persist, explanations in terms of reified unobservables such as "trance" can produce detrimental effects by lulling investigators into a false sense of believing that they have explained what they, in fact, do not understand. Even Hilgard (1971), who has been a major advocate of the "hypnotic state" notion during the past decade, has recently declared that the term "hypnotic state" or "trance state" is merely a convenient label for denoting an interrelated set of empirical phenomena, and should not be used as an explanation of the phenomena.

Empirical Considerations

Traditionally, the notion that a special state—"hypnotic trance"—can explain hypnotic behavior has been fostered by the beliefs that (a) hypnotic subjects exhibit markedly higher levels of suggestibility than control subjects and (b) hypnotic induction procedures lead to unique and unusual experiences. However, research carried out during the last decade calls both of these propositions into serious question.

An extensive series of studies carried out primarily by Barber and his associates (Barber, 1969, 1970a, 1970b) has clearly indicated that increments in suggestibility achieved by administering a hypnotic induction procedure can be matched by giving control

subjects short instructions designed to motivate their performance ("task motivational instructions"). For example, in one extensive study (Barber, 1965), the eight standardized test suggestions of the Barber Suggestibility Scale (BSS) were administered
to subjects who had been exposed to a hypnotic induction procedure and also to subjects who had received brief task motivational instructions. The BSS assesses subjects' objective performance on test suggestions for arm levitation, inability to unclasp
hands, body immobility, post-experimental response, amnesia,
and the like. This scale also provides for the quantification of
subjective responses to the test suggestions; that is, the extent to
which subjects report experiencing the suggested effects. The
results of the study indicated that hypnotic and task motivated
subjects did not differ in either their objective or subjective responses to the BSS. Similar results have also been obtained when
hypnotic and task motivated subjects have been tested on suggestions not included in the BSS. For instance, Barber and Hahn
(1962) found that suggestions given to hypnotic and task motivated subjects gave rise to equivalent reductions in physiological
and verbal report measures of pain produced by immersion of a
hand in ice water. Similarly, Spanos, Barber, and Lang (1969)
found that suggestions of anesthesia were equally effective in reducing pain in hypnotic subjects and task motivated controls.
Further, when given suggestions for auditory and visual hallucinations or suggestions for amnesia, hypnotic and task motivated subjects have shown equally high levels of responsiveness
(Barber and Calverley, 1964a, 1966a; Spanos and Barber, 1968;
Spanos, Ham, and Barber, 1973). In short, the data indicate that
brief task motivational instructions are generally as effective as
hypnotic induction procedures in producing a high level of responsiveness to suggestions of the type that have been traditionally thought to be associated with "hypnotic trance" (Barber,
1969; Barber and Calverley, 1968; Spanos, 1970).

Writers on hypnosis have commonly stated that hypnotic induction procedures give rise to unique and unusual experiences.
Contemporary proponents of this view hold that the "hypnotic
trance state" produces distortions of perception and memory and
also gives rise to an illogical pattern of thinking labeled as "trance

logic" (Evans, 1968, Hilgard, 1965; Orne, 1959, 1966). However, the evidence in favor of this view is largely anecdotal. Recent studies employing appropriate control groups (Blum and Graef, 1971; Johnson, Maher, and Barber, 1972; Spanos and Ham, 1972; Spanos, Ham, and Barber, 1973) indicate that the subjective reports of hypnotic subjects and of task motivated control subjects concerning the experiences of perceptual and memory distortions are highly similar. These studies also indicate that reports of "trance logic" occur as frequently among control subjects as they do among hypnotic subjects.

An example of the similarities in the subjective reports of hypnotic and task motivated subjects is provided by Spanos, Ham, and Barber (1973). These investigators gave subjects a visual hallucination suggestion and later questioned them in depth concerning the nature of their experiences. Information was gathered on the vividness and reality of the suggested hallucination and on the following dimensions of the subjects' visual imagery: subjective location (whether subjects experienced the suggested hallucination as being "out there" or inside of their heads); vividness; transparency, and differential clarity (whether or not the suggested hallucination or image was uniformly clear and detailed). Hypnotic and task motivated subjects did not differ in the reported vividness or reality of their hallucination experience. Also, the two groups of subjects did not differ on any of the dimensions of visual imagery that were assessed. In a related study, Spanos and Ham (1972) questioned hypnotic and task motivated subjects in depth concerning what they experienced when they were given a suggestion for selective amnesia. The two groups of subjects could not be distinguished from one another either in terms of their subjective reports or their overt behavior.

Taken together, logical and empirical considerations indicate that the construct "hypnotic state" or "trance" is an inadequate conceptual tool for organizing the available data in the area of hypnotic research. Consequently, an *ad hoc* extension of this construct to "explain" data accrued by behavior therapists would appear to be unparsimonious at best.

The above considerations should not be taken to mean that hypnotic induction procedures fail to produce changes in behavior such as increments in reported hallucinations and amnesia. Instead, these considerations indicate that the behavioral changes that are observed are not a unique function of hypnotic induction procedures and are not readily explicable by postulating a "hypnotic state" or "trance" as a causal variable. Hypnotic induction procedures give rise to changes in subjects' private experiences and overt behaviors because they include specific antecedent variables that tend to enhance the subjects' attitudes, motivations, and expectancies toward the situation and that tend to produce a willingness to think and imagine with those things that are suggested (Barber, 1970b; Barber, Spanos, and Chaves, 1974).* Below, we shall contend that the occurrence of hypnotic behaviors is explicable in terms of cognitive variables—thinking and imagining with those things that are suggested—that are engendered by specific suggestions and instructions and that are fostered by subjects' motivations, attitudes, and expectancies toward the tasks they are asked to perform. We shall also suggest that these factors are important in achieving positive behavior change with those behavior therapy techniques that utilize subjects' imaginings as an integral part of the therapeutic procedure.

A COMPARISON OF HYPNOTIC AND BEHAVIOR THERAPY SITUATIONS

A comparison of the typical hypnotic situation and many behavior therapy situations indicates a number of interesting parallels. Specification of these parallels may help to elucidate the processes responsible for behavior change in both types of situations. In this section, we shall suggest that the behavior changes occurring in a hypnotic situation and in those behavior therapy situations that utilize the subjects' imaginings are in part, a function of the following variables: (a) subjects' motivations toward

---

* These antecedent variables which are commonly found in hypnotic induction procedures include the following: defining the situation as unusual (as "hypnosis") and as one in which high response to suggestions is desired and expected; securing cooperation; maximizing the wording and the vocal characteristics of suggestions; coupling suggestions with naturally-occurring events; stimulating goal-directed imagining; and preventing or reinterpreting the failure of suggestions (Barber and DeMoor, 1972).

both the general situation and the specific suggestions to which they are exposed, (b) subjects' attitudes and expectancies with regard to the suggestions they receive, (c) the wording of the specific suggestions that are administered, and (d) subjects' involvement in circumscribed patterns of imagining that are congruent with the specific suggestions or instructions that are received.*

It is important to point out that we are *not* suggesting that these are the only variables important in producing therapeutic change. Each of the behavior therapy techniques is comprised of a highly complex composite of interacting variables. The effects of these variables are only beginning to be delineated and, as yet, cannot be specified with any certainty. Some of the variables important in producing therapeutic benefits may turn out to have little relationship to the variables found in hypnotic situations. We are simply calling attention to the fact that there are common factors in hypnotic situations and in some behavior therapy situations and that these common factors may be important in understanding at least some of the behavioral changes that occur in each situation.

Before we specify the overlapping variables that are found in both hypnosis and in behavior therapy that are responsible for behavior change, it is necessary to discuss an overlapping variable —suggestions or instructions for relaxation—that does *not* seem to be a critical variable in producing the changes in behavior.

Effects of Relaxation Instructions in Hypnosis and Behavior Therapy

The tendency to suggest relationships between hypnosis and behavior therapy seems to be related to the fact that both hypnosis and systematic desensitization usually include relaxation instructions. Therefore, it is important to point out that response to hypnotic suggestions is not seriously affected when relaxation

---

* Some of the major *differences* between hypnosis and behavior therapy have been specified in an earlier paper by Cautela (1966b). In a second paper, Cautela (1966a) presented a series of arguments which suggest that the therapeutic benefits that occur in the hypnotic treatment of phobias are due not to a presumed "trance state" but, instead, to the use of *un*-systematic desensitization.

instructions are deleted from hypnotic induction procedures (Barber, 1969). Also, an impressive number of reports indicate that successful desensitization can be accomplished without first relaxing the subjects (Agras, Leitenberg, Barlow, Curtis, Edwards, and Wright, 1971; Lazarus, 1971; LoPiccolo, 1971; McGlynn and Davis, 1971; Myerhoff, 1967; Rachman, 1968; Sue, 1972; Vodde and Gilner, 1971; Wilkins, 1971; Wolpin, 1966; Wolpin and Raines, 1966). Although relaxation is not *necessary* for successful desensitization, it may play a role in some cases in reducing subjects' fears (Brown, 1970; Davison, 1968; Howlett and Nawas, 1971; Lomont and Edwards, 1967; Rachman, 1966). Although there are many complex issues here (Agras et al., 1971; Budzynski and Stoyva, in press; Farmer and Wright, 1971; Land, 1969; Persely and Leventhal, 1972; Schubot, 1966), the available data suggest that relaxation may not be crucial in eliciting the behavior change seen in either hypnotic or desensitization situations. We shall now consider some of the variables common to hypnosis and to behavior therapy that appear to be more closely related to behavior change.

Motivational Factors in Hypnosis and Behavior Therapy

Subjects' motivation appears to be one important factor determining response to suggestions and instructions in both hypnotic and behavior therapy situations. An extensive series of studies, reviewed elsewhere (Barber, 1969; Spanos and Chaves, 1970, 1971), indicates that response to suggestions is enhanced when subjects are first exposed to instructions that aim to motivate their performance. As pointed out earlier, brief task motivational instructions given to control subjects are generally as effective as a lengthy hypnotic induction procedure in heightening response to suggestions.

The task motivational instructions used in the experiments mentioned above typically consisted of statements such as the following: ". . . try to imagine and to visualize the things I will ask you to imagine . . . What I ask is your cooperation . . . try to imagine vividly what I describe to you . . . [Barber, 1969, p. 46]." Behavior therapists often use very similar instructions to motivate subjects to become involved in their imaginings. For example, rather than simply asking subjects to passively imagine a particular situation during covert sensitization or covert reinforcement, Cautela (1970, 1971) exhorts subjects to perform maximally with statements such as the following: "try to imagine everything as vividly as possible, as if you were really there [Cautela, 1970]," and "try to imagine the scene I am going to describe. Try to imagine that you are really there. Try not to imagine that you are simply seeing what I describe; try to use your other senses as well . . . the main point is you are actually there experiencing everything [Cautela, 1971, p. 192]." Subjects undergoing desensitization (Wolpe, 1958) and implosion therapy (DeMoor, 1969) are often exposed to similar exhortations. The use of motivational instructions in both hypnotic situations and various types of behavior therapy situations suggests that (a) subjects' motivations may be important in determining response to the procedures administered and (b) subjects' motivations may be effectively manipulated to enhance their performance.

Additional data also suggest the importance of subjects' motivations in behavior therapy. Clinical reports indicate that subjects who are not motivated to change their maladaptive behavior often do not improve when exposed to procedures such as desensitization (Davison, 1969; Lazarus, 1971). For example, Lazarus (1971) noted that desensitization is effective only with subjects "who do not derive too many primary or secondary gains from their avoidance behavior" and "who are not strongly averse to the method [p. 95]." However, motivation is not the only variable mediating change in hypnotic and behavior therapy situations. Attitudes and expectations may also play an important role. We will examine these variables next.

Attitudes and Expectancies in Hypnosis and Behavior Therapy

Evidence converging from several sources indicates that certain kinds of attitudes and expectancies may also be important factors in mediating response to suggestions and instructions in both hypnotic situations and behavior therapy situations. The effect of subjects' attitudes and expectancies on their hypnotic performance has been determined in two ways. First, subjects' attitudes and expectancies have been assessed with various scales and subsequently correlated with their hypnotic suggestibility. Second, subjects' attitudes and expectancies have been experimentally manipulated and then related to their hypnotic performance. We shall briefly discuss each of these kinds of studies in turn.

Studies correlating subjects' attitudes toward hypnosis with their hypnotic performance indicate that subjects holding positive attitudes toward hypnosis achieve higher scores on suggestibility tests than subjects holding negative attitudes (Barber & Calverley, 1966b; London, Cooper, and Johnson, 1962; Melei and Hilgard, 1964; Shor, Orne, and O'Connell, 1966). Similar results have also been obtained with regard to subjects' expectations of their hypnotic performance and their actual hypnotic performance. Subjects expecting that they would respond well to hypnosis were more responsive than those expecting that they would not respond well (Barber and Calverley, 1969; Melei and Hilgard, 1964; Shor, 1971).

Several experiments have demonstrated that hypnotic performance can be influenced by manipulating subjects' attitudes and expectancies toward hypnosis. For example, in a recent experiment (Cronin, Spanos, and Barber, 1971), one group of randomly selected subjects was given information that aimed to correct misconceptions and to produce positive attitudes and expectancies toward hypnosis and a second randomized group was not given such information. Subjects given positive information manifested greater hypnotic suggestibility than the no information group. Diamond (1971) obtained the same pattern of results in a comparable experiment.

In two related experiments, Barber and Calverley (1964b, 1964c) found that subjects' response to suggestions can be markedly reduced if subjects are led to develop negative attitudes toward the experimental situation. In one of these experiments (Barber and Calverley, 1964c), for example, a group of randomly selected subjects was informed that they were to be given a test of *gullibility*. A second group of randomized subjects was told that they were to be tested for ability to imagine. Both groups were then tested for response to the same standardized suggestions. As expected, the group told that they were being tested for gullibility responded much more poorly than did the group told that they were being tested for ability to imagine. These studies, together with other studies reviewed in detail elsewhere (Barber, 1970b), indicate that subjects' attitudes and expectancies toward the test situation affect their response to suggesions. Let us turn to an examination of attitudes and expectancies in behavior therapy.

Although the study of subjects' attitudes and expectancies in conventional psychotherapy is a well established area of inquiry, relatively few studies have examined the role of these factors in behavior therapy. However, the importance of these factors has been implicitly recognized and taken into account in the clinical work of many behavior therapists. For example, Wolpe (1958) makes a special point of explaining the procedures he will use to each subject in great detail. While explaining the procedures, Wolpe (1969) (a) takes pains to correct any misconceptions that might give rise to negative attitudes toward the therapeutic techniques, (b) attempts to build positive attitudes and expectancies by presenting the subject with a learning theory rationale for the procedure he will undergo, and (c) points out the effectiveness of behavior therapy as compared to psychoanalytically oriented therapeutic techniques.

Observers of behavior therapy (Brown, 1967; Klein, Dittman, Parloff, and Gill, 1969) have also noted that behavior therapists typically manipulate their subjects' attitudes and expectancies. For example, Klein, et al. (1969), after observing Wolpe and his associates treat subjects, made the following observations:

> Perhaps the most striking impression we came away with was of how much use behavior therapists make of suggestion and of how much the patient's expectations and attitudes are manipulated . . . the therapist tells the patient at length about the power of the treatment method, pointing out that it has been successful with comparable patients and all but promising similar results for him too . . . treatment plans and goals were laid out in such a detail that the patient was taught precisely how things would proceed and what responses and changes were expected of him all along the way [Klein, et al., 1969, p. 262].

The importance of subjects' attitudes and expectancies in determining the success of behavior therapy procedures is also indicated by reports that subjects possessing negative attitudes and expectancies toward behavior therapy do not fare well from such treatment. For example, Lazarus (1971) has cited several instances in which subjects' negative attitudes and expectancies toward behavior therapy techniques interfered with the success of procedures such as desensitization.

The hypothesis that attitudes and expectancies play a role in determining the effects of behavior therapy has been tested in recent experiments. In one set of experiments (Leitenberg, Agras, Barlow, and Oliveau, 1969; Oliveau, Agras, Leitenberg, Moore, and Wright, 1969) subjects were exposed to a systematic desensitization procedure under two different sets of expectations. To one group of subjects desensitization was defined as therapy, and to another group it was defined as a technique for studying imagination. Thus, the former group was led to expect that desensitization would reduce their fears, whereas the latter group did not expect that it would do so. The results indicated that desensitization leads to fear reduction only when subjects expect that it will reduce fear. The subjects who underwent desensitization defined as an experiment in imagination did not manifest a reduction in their phobias.

Three other recent studies (Borkovec, 1972; Miller, 1972; Persely and Leventhal, 1972) also found that animal phobics exposed to desensitization defined as therapy tended to exhibit greater fear reduction on a behavioral approach task than phobics exposed to desensitization defined as a nontherapeutic procedure. The Borkovec study also compared phobics exposed to implosion defined as therapy with phobics who received implosion defined as an imagination experiment. Only subjects receiving implosion defined as therapy exhibited significant fear reduction on a behavioral approach task.

Jaffe (1968) carried out a similar experiment in which two groups of subjects received implosion therapy. Subjects in one of these groups were told that the procedure was an effective therapy for phobias, whereas subjects in the other group were told that they were receiving a control ("dummy") treatment. Although both groups received the same treatment, the group told that it was receiving therapy showed significantly greater reduction in both subjective and objective indices of fear than the group told that it was receiving the control treatment. With regard to those subjects receiving implosion defined as therapy, Jaffe (1968) found that subjects' pre-treatment expectations of therapeutic success were highly correlated ($r = .70$) with post-treatment approach to the feared object. Interestingly enough, he also found that pre-treatment expectations of success were highly correlated with fear reduction in a group of subjects exposed to a "pseudo-therapy" treatment; that is, a treatment in which subjects were deceived into believing that they were undergoing a counter-conditioning therapy.

Apparently contradicting the studies summarized above, recent studies by McGlynn (1971) and McGlynn, Reynolds, and Linder (1971a) found that desensitization defined to the subjects as therapy failed to produce greater fear reduction than desensitization defined as an experiment in imagination. However, in both of these experiments, the two desensitization treatments also failed to produce greater fear reduction than a pseudo therapy condition in which the subjects were instructed to imagine neutral scenes. These results do not disconfirm the conclusion of Leitenberg, et al. (1969), Oliveau, et al. (1969), Jaffe (1968) or Borkovec (1972) that subjects' expectations play an important role in mediating the effects of behavior therapy. On the contrary, the finding of McGlynn and his associates, that a pseudo therapy condition produced as much therapeutic gain as each of the desensitization conditions, suggests a hypothesis that should be tested in further experiments; namely, subjects' expectations may play an important role in mediating the fear reduction produced under each of these experimental conditions. The reasons for the failure of desensitization to produce greater fear reduction than pseudo therapy in these experiments is not clear. It may be that the phobic response chosen for study (fear of mice) is easily neutralized by a wide variety of procedures.[*]

[*] In the studies summarized above, a comparison was made between a group undergoing a behavior therapy procedure defined as *therapy* and a group undergoing the same procedure defined as something other than therapy (e.g. an experiment in imagination or a control procedure). A separate series of studies (Cataldo, 1970; Howlett and Nawas, 1971; Lomont and Brock, 1971; McGlynn,

The results of clinical studies with implosion therapy are also consistent with the notion that expectancies play a role in determining the effects of behavior therapy. For example, Rachman (1966) found that spider phobics showed no improvement after exposure to implosion, while Wolpin and Raines (1966) found that implosion was effective in reducing snake phobias. The discrepancy between these results may be due to differences in expectancies produced by preliminary instructions. Wolpin and Raines (1966) instructed their subjects to consider implosion as training for overcoming their fear and informed their subjects about the rationale of the method. None of Rachman's (1966) subjects received such information. They were, as Wilson (1967) put it, merely imagining frightening situations and rehearsing fear responses.

Of course, the results of behavior therapy cannot be attributed simply to subjects' attitudes and expectations. Although some investigators (Agras, et al., 1971; Marcia, Rubin, and Efran, 1969) have suggested that the effects of desensitization and other behavior therapies can be accounted for almost entirely in terms of subjects' expectations, other studies (Davison, 1968; Jaffe, 1968; Lang, Lazovic, and Reynolds, 1965; Paul, 1966) have shown that

---

1972; McGlynn & Mapp, 1970; McGlynn, Mealiea, and Nawas, 1969; McGlynn, Reynolds, and Linder, 1971b; McGlynn & Williams, 1970; Woy and Efran, 1972) has examined the effects of subjects' expectations in a different way. In these studies desensitization was *always* defined to the subjects as a therapy. However, instructions were administered to inculcate different groups with varying expectations concerning either (a) the effectiveness of the therapy (e.g., this treatment has been shown to be highly effective versus I do not think this treatment is going to work) or (b) subjects progress in therapy (e.g., your GSR indicates that you are improving versus your GSR indicates you are not improving). The results of these studies have been mixed. Some have found that expectation instructions have no effect, others indicate that such instructions have an effect, and in three studies (Cataldo, 1970; Howlett and Nawas, 1971; Lomont and Brock, 1971) the results appear to be equivocal.

The majority of these studies failed to assess the success of their attitude change manipulations in actually changing subjects' attitudes about the therapy they were to undergo. This is an important methodological deficiency because several reports (Cataldo, 1970; Marcia, Rubin, and Efran, 1969) indicated that subjects often forget or "cognitively neutralize" negative information about behavior therapy. Thus, the contradictions in the above studies may be due to an unequal effectiveness of the various attitude change manipulations in changing subjects' attitudes.

subjects given positive expectations and exposed to "pseudo therapy placebo conditions" do not usually improve to the same extent as subjects exposed to desensitization or implosion. However, the data reviewed above support the notion that subjects' attitudes and expectations play an important role in fostering at least some of the therapeutic gains seen in behavior therapy situations.

The Wording of Hypnotic and Behavior Therapy Suggestions

Subjects' general motivation, attitudes, and expectancies appear to be important in determining their responsiveness to suggestions. However, it is the wording of the suggestions themselves that provide specific information concerning the cognitive activity and overt behavior expected in both hypnotic and behavior therapy situations.

Typically, hypnotic suggestions and the suggestions or instructions used by behavior therapists do *not* directly tell subjects to engage in overt behavior. Instead, the suggestions usually provide subjects with a cognitive strategy that asks them to imagine a set of hypothetical events and implies that these imaginings will produce changes in behavior.

The following arm heaviness suggestion, from the Stanford Hypnotic Susceptibility Scale, is typical of those used in hypnotic situations:

> Imagine you are holding something heavy in your hand . . . Now the hand and arm feel heavy as if the [imagined] weight were pressing down . . . as it feels heavier and heavier and heavier the imagined weight begins to move down . . . [Weitzenhoffer and Hilgard, 1962, p. 17].

The wording of this suggestion clearly indicates that (a) arm lowering is expected as an overt response and (b) the arm lowering is expected to be experienced as an involuntary and unguided movement rather than as a self-guided volitional act. The wording of the suggestion also provides a cognitive strategy for meeting these expectations. It asks subjects to become involved in imagining a situation; that is, imagining a heavy weight pressing on the arm, which, if it were real rather than imaginary, would be expected to produce an involuntary arm lowering.

The instructions used by behavior therapists are often similar to hypnotic suggestions in the following ways. First, they clearly specify the overt behavioral change that is expected. Second, they ask subjects to imagine events which, if they actually existed, would give rise to the behavioral change. For instance, when carrying out covert sensitization with alcoholic patients, Cautela (1967, 1969) typically defines avoidance of alcohol as the specific behavioral change that is expected and he asks subjects to imagine themselves involved in a series of behavioral sequences culminating in the involutary avoidance of drinking (e.g., vomiting while lifting a glass of liquor to the lips). Other behavior therapy techniques, such as desensitization and covert reinforcement, also ask subjects to imagine structured sequences aimed at mediating specific overt behaviors. In short, behavior therapy suggestions, in the same way as hypnotic suggestions, provide a cognitive strategy for mediating overt behavior.

There are, of course, differences as well as similarities in the suggestions administered to hypnotic and behavior therapy subjects. In most hypnosis research, for example, subjects are seen in only a single session and, during that time, are exposed to suggestions asking them to imagine a series of relatively unrelated situations (e.g., imagine your arm is as heavy as lead, imagine your throat is in a vise so that you can't say your name, or imagine you are in a desert without water). In behavior therapy situations, subjects are typically seen over several sessions and they are usually asked to imagine a series of events relating to a single situational theme (e.g., imagining progressive approach responses to a phobic object). While differences such as these are obviously important in mediating the different types of behavior seen in hypnotic and behavior therapy situations, they should not obscure the fact of a basic similarity: in both types of situations suggestions are worded in a manner that instructs subjects to employ specific patterns of imagining for the purpose of achieving specific behavioral changes.

The suggestions used in hypnosis and in behavior therapy also possess other similarities. In both situations, for example, the suggestions often vary in how concretely they specify the situations the subjects are asked to imagine. Some hypnotic suggestions specify concrete situations in detail (e.g., asking subjects to imagine a cast on their arm that keeps their elbow from bending). Other suggestions specify only the behavior and experiences expected while leaving the details of the imaginings up to the subject (e.g., asking the subject to imagine a force moving his hands apart but failing to specify the nature of the force). Similarly, behavior therapy suggestions also vary along an abstract-concrete dimension. For example, desensitization hierarchies are sometimes highly individualized, asking subjects to imagine well-defined, specific situations. Oftentimes, however, standardized hierarchies are employed. In these cases subjects must tailor the relatively abstract instructions, in imagination, to suit their own specific circumstances.

The wording of hypnotic and behavior therapy suggestions provides subjects with more or less detailed strategies for using imaginary situations to mediate overt behavior. However, subjects in both situations differ widely in their responses to suggestions. Next, we shall examine how cognitive processes are related to responsiveness to suggestions.

Thinking and Imagining in Hypnosis and Behavior Therapy

Before examining the data relating to thinking and imagining in hypnosis and behavior therapy, it is important to look closely at the concept of imagining. Some behavior therapists treat subjects' imaginings as *stimuli* eliciting responses such as relaxation and anxiety. Our work in hypnosis has led us to adopt a somewhat different perspective. We believe it is more profitable to focus on the response aspects rather than the stimulus aspects of subjects' imaginings. More specifically, suggested imaginings often involve active, albeit covert, constructions of the hypothetical events referred to or implied by the suggestions. Imagining includes not only sensory imagery but also a more general change in cognitive focus. The subject who is imagining is employing his images and his self-indications (what he is thinking or saying to himself) to covertly construct hypothetical situations. The more a subject is involved in imagining, the more he fails to indicate to himself that his imaginings are not actual, external occurrences (Spanos, 1971; Spanos and Barber, 1972; Spanos, Ham, and

Barber, 1973). In these respects, involved imagining is more closely related to active role-rehearsal or involved play acting than to the passive reception of external events traditionally connoted by the term stimulus (Horowitz, 1970; Klinger, 1971; Pavio, 1971; Ryle, 1949; Sarbin, 1970; Skinner, 1953).

It will be recalled that the suggestions used in both hypnosis and behavior therapy often ask the subject to carry out *goal-directed imagining* or *goal-directed fantasy*. That is, subjects are asked to imagine a situation which, if it actually occurred, would give rise to the desired behavior. In both areas of investigation, evidence is accumulating that subjects tend to show the desired behavior when they carry out the goal-directed imagining which is implied or specifically stated in the suggestion. In one study, for example, hypnotic subjects who passed a suggestion that their arm was to become stiff, rigid, and unable to bend tended to imagine situations which, if they actually occurred, would lead to the desired arm rigidity. For example, they imagined that their arm was either in a cast, or between two boards, or held in place by a metal rod (Spanos, 1971). Other recent studies in hypnosis (Spanos and Barber, 1972; Spanos and Ham, 1972; Spanos, Ham, and Barber, 1973) also indicate that goal-directed imagining is commonly present when subjects are responsive to suggestions.

Hypnotic subjects who fail suggestions usually do not report goal-directed imagining. Instead, these subjects typically report that they were not motivated to pass the suggestions or they did not believe that they could pass. Some of these subjects, for example, report that they simply did not want to respond or that they thought the suggestions were silly. Others state that the suggestions were impossible to perform (Spanos, 1971). A few subjects who fail suggestions seem to continuously contradict the reality of their imaginings; that is, they repeatedly think or say to themselves that their imaginings are not actual occurrences.

A second line of evidence indicating the importance of subjects' thinking and imagining in hypnotic performance comes from studies that attempted to increase suggestibility in unresponsive subjects. A number of these reports (Sachs, 1969, 1971; Sachs and Anderson, 1967) indicate that suggestibility can be heightened substantially by training the subjects to engage in cognitive activity relevant to responding to suggestions. These training procedures consist of (a) teaching subjects to focus their attention on specific suggestion-related imaginings and to exclude competing thoughts and competing sensory input and (b) teaching them, through the use of direct instructions and of modeling procedures, to carry out the cognitive strategies called for by the suggestions and to have the subjective experiences implied by the suggestions. Taken together, the available data indicate that responsiveness to suggestions is closely related to a specific type of cognitive activity: subjects who respond to suggestions tend to think and imagine with the themes that are suggested, whereas those who are unresponsive fail to engage in suggestion-related thinking and imagining.

The role of subjects' thoughts and imaginings in mediating the behavior change seen in behavior therapy has only recently begun to receive research attention (D'Zurilla and Goldfried, 1971; Goldfried, 1971; Jacobs and Wolpin, 1971; Locke, 1971; Valins and Ray, 1967; Wilkins, 1971). However, the importance of these factors is hinted at by the insistence of behavior therapists that vivid and realistic imagery is a prerequisite to success in treatments such as desensitization (Cautela, 1971; Nawas, Meliea, and Fishman, 1971; Wolpe, 1958, 1969). Behavior therapists often employ the term *imagery* to refer to the broader concept of *involved imagining*. For example, implosion therapists (Stampfl and Levis, 1967, 1968) not only ask the subject to imagine a particular scene, they also ask him to play-act and to "live" the scene with genuine emotion. After repetition of a particular scene in imagination, the subject is given the opportunity to act out the scene and is encouraged to verbalize his own role-playing behavior. In addition, sound effects are at times used to make the subjects' imaginary experiences as realistic as possible (Kirchner and Hogan, 1966).

McLemore (1972) has presented data indicating that *imagery per se* is not as important in behavior therapy as is sometimes indicated. Along these lines, we suggest that it is the ability to engage in suggestion-related or instruction-related *involved imagining* that mediates behavior change in such situations. From our perspective, subjects who report imagery, but who are not involved in their imaginings, will tend to show little behavior change in treatments such as desensitization. Danaher and Thoresen (1972) have reached a similar conclusion: "Simply visualizing an imaginal scene is not sufficient in most therapeutic regimens; rather, actual involvement in the scene itself with patient-as-actor is more often required [p. 137]." Recent data provided by Janda and Rimm (1972) also suggest the importance of "involvement in the imagined scene" in behavior therapy. These investigators found a positive relationship ($r = .53$) between the extent that subjects undergoing covert sensitization rated feeling discomfort when they were imagining noxious scenes and the extent to which they showed improvement on the criterion measure (weight reduction).

It is important to note that both hypnotic subjects and behavior therapy subjects sometimes respond successfully to suggestions when they imagine situations which are quite different from those suggested. For example, hypnotic subjects who were given the suggestion that a helium filled balloon was tied to their wrist and was raising their arm tended to show arm levitation when they imagined one of the following situations: a gust of wind pushing the hand in the air; air being pumped into the hollowed-out arm; a rope tied to the wrist and to a pulley that is raising the arm; or a magnet attached to the arm which is attracted by a second magnet suspended above (Spanos, 1971). Although all of these imaginary situations differ from one another and from the situation described in the suggestion, they all fulfill the criteria for *goal-directed imagining* because they all involve imaginary situations which, if they existed in reality, would give rise to an involuntary raising of the arm.

In brief, the data available indicate that subjects tend to pass hypnotic suggestions when they engage in goal-directed imagining, regardless of whether or not their imaginings correspond closely to the specific imaginary situations described in the suggestion (Spanos, 1971; Spanos and Barber, 1972; Spanos and Ham, 1972). This is not to say that imaginings of any kind lead subjects to pass hypnotic suggestions. On the contrary, subjects whose imaginings are not related to the goals of the suggestions tend to fail. For example, subjects who were asked to imagine a balloon raising their arm, but who instead imagined situations unrelated to arm raising (e.g., imagining themselves standing quietly next to a tree) usually did not pass the suggestion (Spanos and Barber, 1972).

In the same way as with hypnotic subjects, the imaginings of subjects in behavior therapy can mediate change even when they differ considerably from the specific imaginary situations described by the suggestions or instructions. For example, in a study by Weitzman (1967), six patients who were undergoing systematic desensitization were interviewed about their imaginings. Weitzman reported that: "Without exception, when closely questioned, patients reported a flow of visual imagery. The initiating scene, once visualized, shifted and changed its form. Moreover, these transformations took place continuously and, when the imagining was terminated by the therapist, had produced images which were quite removed in their content from the intended stimulus [p. 305]". Similar findings have also been reported by Weinberg and Zaslove (1963), Brown (1967), and Barrett (1969). Spanos, Kosloff, and Chaves (1971) also found that subjects sometimes report experiences markedly different from what is suggested. For example, one of their desensitization subjects, simply asked to visualize herself approaching a snake at the end of a long corridor, instead imagined the following situation: "When you asked me to imagine the snake, I started thinking about millions of these little snakes coming up through the sand. When I thought about the millions of snakes, I was scared to death. I started to imagine the snake, but I was still on the beach and they all started crawling. Oh, it was terrible. It was crawling all over me." Data such as these indicate that behavior therapy subjects, in the same way as hypnotic subjects, at times imagine situations that differ markedly from those that are suggested.

Systematically gathered data are not available concerning the range of content in subjects' imaginings which is congruent with therapeutic change. It is interesting to note, however, that some behavior therapists (Wolpe, 1969) regularly question subjects about the content of their imaginings in order to insure that they have not strayed too far from the intention of the therapeutic suggestion. Coupled with the evidence available from hypnosis research, this indicates that imaginings may fail to produce therapeutic benefits when their contents are unrelated to or inconsistent with the intention of the suggestions.

Specific relationships between the wording of suggestions, the contents of subjects' imaginings, and overt behavioral change, are only beginning to be empirically delineated in either hypnotic or behavior therapy research. In our estimation, however, more precise delineation of such relationships constitute exciting problems for future research in both hypnosis and behavior therapy.

SUMMARY

This paper takes issue with the contention, proffered by a series of investigators, that a "hypnotic state" plays a role in mediating the behavioral changes associated with those behavior therapy procedures that ask the subject to imagine, e.g., systematic desensitization, implosion, covert sensitization, covert reinforcement and covert extinction. The hypothetical construct "hypnotic state" or "trance" involves a number of empirical and logical limitations that negate its utility for explaining even hypnotic phenomena, let alone the phenomena of behavior therapy. The empirical limitations of the construct are indicated by a series of recent studies which found that motivated control subjects are generally as responsive to suggestions as subjects who have been exposed to a hypnotic induction procedure and who are said to be in a "hypnotic state". The logical difficulties with the "hypnotic state" construct include the following: (a) The construct is often used circularly. (b) When multiple indices are used to denote the construct, they can be shown to vary independently of each other and, consequently, they fail to "converge" on the construct. (c). The construct represents a reified pseudo-explanation to "fill in" gaps in empirical knowledge.

Although it is not useful to posit a "hypnotic state" to explain the results obtained in either hypnotic situations or in behavior therapy situations, a review of research data indicates that the following four variables, found in both situations, play a role in mediating the changes in behavior:

1. *Motivational variables.* In both hypnotic situations and behavior therapy situations, (a) subjects are usually provided with motivational instructions asking them to **try** to imagine the events

that are described and (b) research data indicates that response to the suggestions or instructions is heightened by such motivational instructions.

2. *Attitudinal and expectancy variables.* Experimental studies in hypnosis and in behavior therapy indicate that subjects' responsiveness to the suggestions or instructions is related, in part, to their attitudes and expectancies toward the situation and toward the tasks they are asked to perform.

3. *Wording of suggestions or instructions.* The suggestions or instructions used in hypnotic and behavior therapy situations are often worded in similar ways. In both situations the suggestions (a) specify the specific overt and covert behaviors the subjects are expected to perform and (b) ask the subjects to engage in circumscribed patterns of imagining that are congruent with the intent of the suggestions.

4. *Circumscribed cognitive processes occurring in response to the suggestions or instructions.* Subjects in both hypnotic and behavior therapy situations tend to carry out the overt behaviors called for by the suggestions or instructions when they think and imagine with the themes described in the suggestions or become "involved" in imagining situations that are congruent with the intent of the suggestion (goal-directed imagining).

Of course, other variables, that do not overlap hypnotic and behavior therapy situations, are also important in determining the behavior change that occurs in these situations. However, the parallels that exist in hypnotic and behavior therapy situations suggest that a free flow of information between these two areas, unencumbered by the unnecessary notion of "hypnotic state" or "trance", can lead to a mutual theoretical enhancement.

REFERENCES

Agras, W. S., Leitenberg, H., Barlow, D. H., Curtis, N. A., Edwards, J., and Wright, D.: Relaxation in systematic desensitization. *Arch Gen Psychiatry, 25*:511–514, 1971.

Barber, T. X.: "Hypnosis" as a causal variable in present-day psychology: A critical analysis. *Psychol Rep, 14*:839–842, 1964.

Barber, T. X.: Measuring "hypnotic-like" suggestibility with and without "hypnotic induction"; psychometric properties, norms, and variables influencing response to the Barber Suggestibility Scale (BSS). *Psychol Rep, 16:*809–844, 1965.

Barber, T. X.: *Hypnosis: A Scientific Approach.* New York, Van Nostrand Reinhold, 1969.

Barber, T. X.: *LSD, Marihuana, Yoga, and Hypnosis.* Chicago, Aldine, 1970a.

Barber, T. X.: *Suggested ("hypnotic") Behavior: The Trance Paradigm Versus An Alternative Paradigm.* Harding, Massachusetts, Medfield Foundation, 1970b.

Barber, T. X., and Calverley, D. S.: An experimental study of "hypnotic" (auditory and visual) hallucinations. *J Abnorm Soc Psychol, 63:*13–20, 1964.

Barber, T. X., and Calverley, D. S.: Empirical evidence for a theory of "hypnotic" behavior: effects of pretest instructions on response to primary suggestions. *Psychol Rec, 14:*457–467, 1964b.

Barber, T. X., and Calverley, D. S.: The definition of the situation as a variable affecting "hypnoticlike" suggestibility. *J Clin Psychol, 20:*438–440, 1964c.

Barber, T. X., and Calverley, D. S.: Toward a theory of "hypnotic" behavior: Experimental analysis of suggested amnesia. *J Abnorm Psychol, 71:*95–107, 1966a.

Barber, T. X., and Calverley, D. S.: Toward a theory of "hypnotic" behavior: Experimental evaluation of Hull's postulate that hypnotic susceptibility is a habit phenomenon. *J Pers, 34:*416–433, 1966b.

Barber, T. X., and Calverley, D. S.: Toward a theory of "hypnotic" behavior: Replication and extension of experiments by Barber and co-workers (1962–65) and Hilgard and Tart (1966). *Int J Clin Exp Hypn, 16:*179–195, 1968.

Barber, T. X., and Calverley, D. S.: Multidimensional analysis of "hypnotic" behavior. *J Abnorm Psychol, 74:*209–220, 1969.

Barber, T. X., Dalal, A. S., and Calverley, D. S.: The subjective reports of hypnotic subjects. *Am J Clin Hypn, 11:*74–88, 1968.

Barber, T. X., and DeMoor, W.: A theory of hypnotic induction procedures. *Am J Clin Hypn, 15:*112–135, 1972.

Barber, T. X., and Hahn, K. W., Jr.: Physiological and subjective responses to pain-producing stimulation under hypnotically suggested and waking-imagined "analgesia." *J Abnorm Soc Psychol, 65:*411–418, 1962.

Barber, T. X., and Spanos, N. P., and Chaves, J. F.: *Hypnotism, Imagination, and Human Potentialities.* New York Pergamon, 1974.

Barrett, C. L.: Systematic desensitization versus implosive therapy. *J Abnorm Psychol, 74:*587–592, 1969.

Blum, G. S., and Graef, J. R.: The detection over time of subjects simulating hypnosis. *Int J Clin Exp Hypn, 14:*211–224, 1971.

Borkovec, T. D.: Effects of expectancy on the outcome of systematic desensitization and implosive treatments for analogue anxiety. *Behav Ther, 3:*29–40, 1972.

Brown, B. M.: Cognitive aspects of Wolpe's Behavior Therapy. *Am J Psychiatry, 124:*854–859, 1967.

Brown, H. A.: *Systematic desensitization: Counter-conditioning or expectancy manipulation?* Unpublished doctoral dissertation, State University of New York at Stony Brook, 1970.

Budzynski, T. H., and Stoyva, J. M.: *Biofeedback Techniques in Behavior Therapy.* In Birbaumer, N. (Ed.): Die Bewaltigung von Angst. Beitrage der Neuropsychologie zur Angstforschung. Reihe Fortschritte der Klinischen Psychologie, Bd. 4. Munchen, Wien, Verlag Urban and Schwarenberg, in press.

Cataldo, J. F.: *Systematic Desensitization: A Cognitive-Expectancy Approach.* Unpublished doctoral dissertation, State University of New York, at Buffalo, 1970.

Cautela, J. R.: Desensitization factors in the hypnotic treatment of phobias. *J Psychol, 64:*277–288, 1966.

Cautela, J. R.: Hypnosis and behavior therapy. *Behav Res Ther, 4:*219–224, 1966b.

Cautela, J. R.: Covert sensitization. *Psychol Rec, 20:*459–468, 1967.

Cautela, J. R.: Behavior Therapy and Self-control: Techniques and Implications. In Franks, C. (Ed.): *Behavior Therapy: Appraisal and Status.* New York, McGraw-Hill, pp. 323–340, 1969.

Cautela, J. R.: Covert reinforcement. *Behav Ther, 1:*33–50, 1970.

Cautela, J. R.: Covert extinction. *Behav Ther, 2:*192–200, 1971.

Chaves, J. F.: Hypnosis reconceptualized: An overview of Barber's theoretical and empirical work. *Psychol Rep, 22:*587–608, 1968.

Conn, J. H., and Conn, R. N.: Discussion of T. X. Barber's "Hypnosis as a causal variable in present-day psychology: A critical analysis." *Int J Clin Exp Hypn, 15:*106–110, 1967.

Cronin, D. M., Spanos, N. P., and Barber, T. X.: Augmenting hypnotic suggestibility by providing favorable information about hypnosis. *Am J Clin Hypn, 13:*259–264, 1971.

Danaher, B. G., and Thoresen, C. E.: Imagery assessment by self-report and behavioral measures. *Behav Res Ther, 10:*131–138, 1972.

Davison, G. C.: Systematic desensitization as a counterconditioning process. *J Abnorm Psychol, 73:*91–99, 1968.

Davison, G. C.: Appraisal of behavior modification techniques with adults in institutional settings. In Franks, C. (Ed.): *Behavior Therapy: Appraisal and Status.* New York, McGraw-Hill, pp. 220–278, 1968.

DeMoor, W.: *Reciprocal Inhibition Versus Unreinforced Response Evocation in Behavior Therapy.* Unpublished Ph.D. dissertation, Katholieke Universiteit te Leuven, 1969.

Diamond, M. J.: *The Use of Observationally-presented information to Modify Hypnotic Susceptibility.* Paper presented at Eastern Psychological Association, New York, April, 1971.

D'Zurilla, T. J., and Goldfried, M. R.: Problem solving and behavior modification. *J Abnorm Psychol*, 78:107–126, 1971.

Evans, F. J.: Recent trends in experimental hypnosis. *Behav Sci*, 13:477–487, 1968.

Farmer, R. G., and Wright, J. M. C.: Muscular reactivity and systematic desensitization. *Behav Ther*, 2:1–10, 1971.

Goldfried, M. R.: Systematic desensitization as training in self-control. *J Consult Clin Psychol*, 37:228–234, 1971.

Hilgard, E. R.: *Hypnotic Susceptibility*. New York, Harcourt, Brace and World, 1965.

Hilgard, E. R.: Altered states of awareness. *J Nerv Ment Dis*, 149:68–79, 1969.

Hilgard, E. R.: Hypnotic phenomena: The struggle for scientific acceptance. *Am Sci*, 59:567–577, 1971.

Hilgard, E. R., and Tart, C. T.: Responsiveness to suggestions following waking and imagination instructions and following induction of hypnosis. *J Abnorm Psychol*, 71:196–208, 1966.

Horowitz, M. J.: *Image Formation and Cognition*. New York, Appleton-Century-Crofts, 1970.

Howlett, S. C., and Nawas, M. M.: Exposure to aversive imagery and suggestion in systematic desensitization. In Rubin, R. D., Fensterheim, H., Lazarus, A. A., and Franks, C., (Eds.): *Advances in Behavior Therapy*. New York, Academic Press, 1971, pp. 123–135.

Jacobs, A., and Wolpin, M.: A second look at systematic desensitization. In Jacobs, A., Sachs, L. B. (Eds.): *The Psychology of Private Events*. New York, Academic Press, 1971, pp. 78–108.

Jaffe, L. W.: *Non-specific Treatment Factors and Deconditioning in Fear Reduction*. Unpublished doctoral dissertation, University of Southern California, 1968.

Janda, L. H., and Rimm, D. C.: Covert sensitization in the treatment of obesity. *J Abnorm Psychol*, 80:37–42, 1972.

Johnson, R. F. Q., Maher, B. A., and Barber, T. X.: Artifact in the "essence of hypnosis;" an evaluation of trance logic. *J Abnorm Psychol*, 79:212–220, 1972.

Kirchner, J. H., and Hogan, R. A.: The therapist variable in the implosion of phobias. *Psychotherapy: Theory, Research and Practice*, 3:102–104, 1966.

Klein, M. H., Dittman, A. T., Parloff, M. B., and Gill, M. M.: Behavior therapy: Observations and reflections. *J Consult Clin Psychol*, 33:259–266, 1969.

Klinger, E.: *Structure and Functions of Fantasy*. New York, Wiley, 1971.

Lang, P. J. The mechanics of desensitization and the laboratory study of human fear. In Franks, C. M. (Ed.): *Behavior Therapy: Appraisal and Status*. New York, McGraw-Hill, 1969, pp. 160–191.

Lang, P. J., Lazovik, A. D., and Reynolds, D. J.: Desensitization, suggestibility, and pseudotherapy. *J Abnorm Psychol*, 70:395–402, 1965.

Larsen, S.: Strategies for reducing phobic behavior. *Dissertation Abstracts*, 26:6850, 1966.

Lazarus, A. A.: *Behavior Therapy and Beyond*. New York, McGraw-Hill, 1971.

Leitenberg, H., Agras, W. S., Barlow, D. H., and Oliveau, D. C.: Contribution of selective positive reinforcement and therapeutic instructions to systematic desensitization therapy. *J Abnorm Psychol*, 74:113–118, 1969.

Litvak, S. B.: Hypnosis and the desensitization behavior therapies. *Psychol Rep*, 27:787–794, 1970.

Locke, E. A.: Is "behavior therapy" behavioristic? (An analysis of Wolpe's psychotherapeutic methods.) *Psychol Bull*, 76:318–327, 1971.

Lomont, J. F., and Brock, L.: Cognitive factors in systemic desensitization. *Behav Res Ther*, 9:187–195, 1971.

Lomont, J. F., and Edwards, J. E.: The role of relaxation in systematic desensitization. *Behav Res Ther*, 5:11–25, 1967.

London, P., Cooper, L. M., and Johnson, H. J.: Subject characteristics in hypnosis research: II. Attitudes toward hypnosis, volunteer status, and hypnotic susceptibility. *Int J Clin Exp Hypn*, 10:13–21, 1962.

LoPiccolo, J.: *Effective Components of Systematic Desensitization*. Department of Psychology, University of Oregon, 1971 (Mimeo).

Marcia, J. E., Rubin, B. M., and Efran, J. S.: Systematic desensitization: expectancy change or counterconditioning? *J Abnorm Psychol*, 74:382–387, 1969.

McGlynn, F. D., Experimental desensitization following three types of instructions. *Behav Res Ther*, 9:367–369, 1971.

McGlynn, F. D.: Systematic desensitization under two conditions of induced expectancy. *Behav Res Ther*, 10:229–234, 1972.

McGlynn, F. D., and Davis, D. J.: *A Factorial Study of Cognitive Exposure and Relaxation in Experimental Desensitization*. Department of Psychology. State College, Mississippi, 1971 (Mimeo).

McGlynn, F. D., and Mapp, R. H.: Systematic desensitization of snake-avoidance following three types of suggestion. *Behav Res Ther*, 8:197–201, 1970.

McGlynn, F. D., and Mealiea, W. L., and Nawas, M. M.: Systematic desensitization of snake-avoidance under two conditions of suggestion. *Psychol Rep*, 25:220–222, 1969.

McGlynn, F. D., and Reynolds, J. E., and Lindner, L. H.: Experimental desensitization following therapeutically oriented and physiologically oriented instructions. *J Behav Ther Exp Psychiatry*, 2:13–18, 1971.

McGlynn, F. D., Reynolds, J. E., and Lindner, L. H.: Systematic desensitization with pretreatment and intra-treatment therapeutic instructions. *Behav Res Ther*, 9:57–63, 1971b.

McGlynn, F. D., and Williams, C. W.: Systematic desensitization of snake-avoidance under three conditions of suggestion. *J Behav Ther Exp Psychiatry,* 1:97–101, 1970.

McLemore, C. W.: Imagery in desensitization. *Behav Res Ther,* 10:51–57, 1972.

McPeake, J. D.: Hypnosis, suggestion, and psychosomatics. *Dis Nerv Syst,* 29:536–544, 1968.

Melei, J. P., and Hilgard, E. R.: Attitudes toward hypnosis, self-predictions, and hypnotic susceptibility. *Int J Clin Exp Hypn,* 12:99–108, 1964.

Miller, S. B.: The contribution of the therapeutic instructions to systematic desensitization. *Behav Res Ther,* 10:159–169, 1972.

Murray, E. J.: Learning theory and psychotherapy: Biotropic versus sociotropic approaches. *Journal of Counseling Psychology,* 10:250–255, 1963.

Myerhoff, L.: *Tension and Anxiety in Deconditioning.* Unpublished doctoral dissertation, University of Southern California, 1967.

Nawas, M. M., Mealiea, W. L., Jr., and S. Fishman, S. T.: Systematic desensitization as counterconditioning: A retest with adequate controls. *Behav Ther,* 2:345–356, 1971.

Oliveau, D. C., Agras, W. S., Leitenberg, H., Moore, R. C., and Wright, D. E.: Systematic desensitization, therapeutically oriented instructions and selective positive reinforcement. *Behav Res Ther,* 7:27–33, 1969.

Orne, M. T.: The nature of hypnosis: Artifact and essence. *J Abnorm Soc Psychol,* 58:277–299, 1959.

Orne, M. T.: Hypnosis, motivation and compliance. *Am J Psychiatry,* 122:721–726, 1966.

Orne, M. T.: Demand characteristics and the concept of quasi-controls. In Rosenthal, R., Rosnow, R. L. (Eds.): *Artifact In Behavioral Research.* New York, Academic Press, 1969. pp. 143–179.

Orne, M. T.: Hypnosis, motivation and the ecological validity of the psychological experiment. In Arnold, W. J., and Page, M. M. (Eds.): *Nebraska Symposium on Motivation.* Lincoln, University of Nebraska Press, 1970, pp. 187–265.

Paul, G. L.: *Insight versus Desensitization in Psychotherapy: An Experiment in Anxiety Reduction.* Stanford, California, Stanford University Press, 1966.

Pavio, A.: *Imagery and Verbal Processes.* New York, Holt, Rinehart and Winston, 1971.

Persely, G., and Leventhal, D. B.: The effects of therapeutically oriented instructions and of the pairing of anxiety imagery and relaxation in systematic desensitization. *Behav Ther,* 3:417–424, 1972.

Rachman, S.: Studies in desensitization: II. Flooding. *Behav Res Ther,* 4:1–6, 1966.

Rachman, S.: The role of muscular relaxation in desensitization therapy. *Behav Res Ther,* 6:159–166, 1968.

Ryle, G.: *The Concept of Mind.* London, Hutchinson, 1949.

Sachs, L. B.: *Modification of Hypnotic Behavior Without Hypnotic Inductions*. Unpublished study, West Virginia University, 1969.

Sachs, L. B.: Construing hypnosis as modifiable behavior. In Jacobs, A., and Sachs, L. B. (Eds): *The Psychology of Private Events*. New York, Academic Press, 1971, pp. 61–75.

Sachs, L. B., and Anderson, W. L.: Modification of hypnotic susceptibility *Int J Clin Exp Hypn*, 15:172–180, 1967.

Sarbin, T. R.: Toward a theory of imagination. *J Pers*, 38:52–76, 1970.

Sarbin, T. R., and Coe, W. C.: *Hypnosis: A Social Psychological Analysis of Influence Communication*. New York, Holt, Rinehart and Winston, 1972.

Schubot, E. D.: *The Influence of Hypnotic and Muscular Relaxation in Systematic Desensitization of Phobias*. Unpublished Ph.D. dissertation, Stanford, University, 1966.

Shor, R. E.: Expectancies of being influenced and hypnotic performance. *Int J Clin Exp Hypn*, 154–166, 1971.

Shor, R. E., Orne, M. T., and O'Connell, D. N.: Psychological correlates of plateau hypnotizability in a special volunteer sample. *J Pers Soc Psychol*, 3:80–95, 1966.

Skinner, B. F.: *Science and Human Behavior*. New York, Macmillan, 1953.

Spanos, N. P.: Barber's reconceptualization of hypnosis: An evaluation of criticisms. *Journal of Experimental Research in Personality*, 4:241–258, 1970.

Spanos, N. P.: Goal-directed fantasy and the performance of hypnotic test suggestions. *Psychiatry*, 34:86–96, 1971.

Spanos, N. P., and Barber, T. X.: "Hypnotic" experiences as inferred from subjective reports: Auditory and visual hallucinations. *J Exp Res Pers*, 3:136–150, 1968.

Spanos, N. P., and Barber, T. X.: Cognitive activity during "hypnotic" suggestibility: Goal directed fantasy and the experience of non-volition. *J Pers*, 40:510–524, 1972.

Spanos, N. P., Barber, T. X., and Lang, G.: *Cognition and Self-Control: Control of Painful Sensory Input*. Department of Sociology, Boston University, 1969 (Mimeo).

Spanos, N. P., and Chaves, J. F.: Converging operations and the "hypnotic state" construct. *Proceedings of the American Psychological Association*, 1969, pp. 905–906.

Spanos, N. P., and Chaves, J. F.: Hypnosis research: A methodological critique of experiments generated by two alternative paradigms. *Am J Clin Hypn*, 13:108–127, 1970.

Spanos, N. P., and Chaves, J. F.: Hypnotismus: Barber's empirische and theoretische Neuformulierung. In Katzenstein, A., (Ed.): *Hypnose: Aktuelle Probleme in Theorie, Experiment and Klinik*. Veb Gustav Fischer Verlag Jena, 1971, pp. 43–56.

Spanos, N. P., and Ham, H. L.: Cognitive activity in response to hypnotic suggestion: goal-directed fantasy and selective amnesia. *Am J Clin Hypn,* 15:191–198, 1973.

Spanos, N. P., Ham, M. W., and Barber, T. X.: Suggested "hypnotic" visual hallucinations: Experimental and phenomenological data. *J. Abnorm Psychol, 81*:96–106, 1973.

Spanos, N. P., Kosloff, M., and Chaves, J. F.: *Cognitive Activity During Systematic Desensitization.* Medfield, Massachusetts, Medfield Foundation, 1971.

Stampfl, T. G., and Levis, D. J.: Essentials of implosive therapy. A learning-theory-based psychodynamic behavioral therapy. *J Abnorm Psychol,* 72:496–503, 1967.

Stampfl, T. G., and Levis, D. J.: Implosive therapy: A behavioral therapy? *Behav Res Ther, 6*:31–36, 1968.

Sue, D.: The role of relaxation in systematic desensitization. *Behav Res Ther, 10*:153–158, 1972.

Valins, S., and Ray, A. A.: Effects of cognitive desensitization on avoidance behavior. *J Per Soc Psychol, 7*:345–350, 1967.

Vodde, T. W., and Gilner, F. H.: The effects of exposure to fear stimuli on fear reduction. *Behav Res Ther, 9*:169–175, 1971.

Weinberg, N. H., and Zaslove, M.: "Resistance" to systematic desensitization of phobias. *J Clin Psychol, 14*:179–181, 1963.

Weitzenhoffer, A. M., and Hilgard, E. R.: *Stanford Hypnotic Susceptibility Scale, Form C.* Palo Alto, California, Consulting Psychologists Press, 1962.

Weitzman, B.: Behavior therapy and psychotherapy. *Psychol Rev,* 74:300–317, 1967.

Wilkins, W.: Desensitization: Social and cognitive factors underlying effectiveness of Wolpe's procedure. *Psychol Bull, 76*:311–317, 1971.

Wilson, G. D.: Efficacy of "flooding" procedures in desensitization of fear: a theoretical note. *Behav Res Ther, 5*:138, 1967.

Wolpe, J.: *Psychotherapy by Reciprocal Inhibition.* Stanford, Stanford University Press, 1958.

Wolpe, J.: *The Practice of Behavior Therapy.* New York, Pergamon Press, 1969.

Wolpe, J., and Lazarus, A. A.: *Behavior Therapy Technique.* Oxford, Pergamon Press, 1966.

Wolpin, M.: *The Application of Modified Conditioning Procedures to Clinical Problems: Three case histories.* Paper presented at Camarillo State Hospital, Camarillo, California, 1966.

Wolpin, M., and Raines, J.: Visual imagery, expected roles and extinction as possible factors in reducing fear and avoidance behavior. *Behav Res Ther, 4*:25–37, 1966.

Woy, R. J., and Efran, J. S.: Systematic desensitization and expectancy in the treatment of speaking anxiety. *Behav Res Ther, 10*:43–49, 1972.

CHAPTER 12

"HYPNOSIS" AS A FACILITATOR IN BEHAVIOR THERAPY *

ARNOLD A. LAZARUS, PH.D.

Abstract: It is emphasized that people who enter therapy believing that hypnosis will facilitate their progress often possess a self-fulfilling prophecy that should be utilized in their treatment. Clients who requested hypnosis and received a standard relaxation sequence that substituted the word "hypnosis" for "relaxation" wherever possible, showed more subjective and objective improvements than those who received ordinary relaxation therapy. The main study contained twenty clients treated in a behavior therapy context. Six additional clients who had not specifically requested either hypnosis or relaxation showed no differences when treated by either or both methods. The differences in outcome are attributed to "expectancy fulfillment."

MEANINGFUL ANSWERS obviously depend upon cogent questions. Vague questions elicit nebulous answers. A decade or two ago, vigorous debates centered around questions of meaningless generality, such as whether or not psychotherapy is effective (e.g. Eysenck, 1952). Today, the focus is upon the interaction of technique and therapist variables under highly specific conditions (e.g. Strupp and Bergin, 1969). Thus, in evaluating the effectiveness of hypnotic intervention, perhaps the most useless question to ask would be "Is hypnosis effective?" Effective for whom, for what, and under which particular con-

* Reprinted from the January 1973 *International Journal of Clinical and Experimental Hypnosis*. Copyrighted by The Society for Clinical and Experimental Hypnosis, January 1973.

ditions, would be an obvious retort. A question such as "Does hypnosis enhance the effects of a particular technique such as systematic desensitization?"—to which the answer appears to be *no* (Lang, 1969)—is much more legitimate. The present paper addresses itself to the question of whether or not behavior therapy techniques are enhanced by the addition of hypnotic suggestions in clients who request to be hypnotized.

Problems concerning the exact nature of hypnosis and conflicting reports concerning the existence of hypnotic states have long occupied a large portion of experimental and clinical literature. Authorities disagree on the necessary and sufficient conditions for hypnosis, on criteria for the measurement of hypnotic depth, and so forth (Hilgard, 1965). In an endeavor to circumvent these thorny problems, the present definition of hypnosis is purely empirical. For example, the difference between a relaxation-training sequence and a hypnotic-induction sequence was that the words "hypnotic" and "hypnosis" were added to "relaxation" in the latter condition. Thus, clients being "relaxed" would be instructed to feel "calm and heavy all over as the relaxation flows through your body," while those being "hypnotized" would be instructed to feel "calm and heavy all over as the *hypnotic* relaxation flows through your body." Thus, in the present study, what differentiates hypnosis from relaxation is the use of the *word* "hypnosis" (e.g. Barber, 1964).

During my formal training in psychotherapy, I was warned by my teachers never to employ hypnosis with any patient who specifically requested it. I was not to be manipulated. Instead, I was told to interpret the patient's passive-dependent needs and/or examine his desire for a magical solution. I recall one of the first patients with whom I violated this taboo. A highly anxious woman who had repeatedly requested hypnosis was making no headway in therapy until I finally induced a fairly deep trance and simply allowed her to "sleep" for about half-an-hour. Thereafter her gains were so impressive that I thought I had stumbled upon a plausible theory and therapy for pervasive anxiety (Lazarus, 1963). In retrospect, it now seems to me that the success of hypnotic procedures is less related to factors such as suggestibility and "hypnotizability" than to the client's specific attitude toward hypnosis and his desire to be hypnotized. In essence, I am simply saying that people who enter therapy believing that hypnosis will facilitate their progress often possess a self-fulfilling prophecy that can be advantageously activated. This is not to deny that some people may indeed seek magical solutions or endeavor to express passive-dependent needs by asking to be hypnotized, but the mere request alone is insufficient data for a clinician to leap to such conclusions.

Over the years I have tended to experiment with hypnotic procedures in order to determine whether they can enhance behavioral techniques. My results were always varied and indeterminate. With some clients, hypnosis definitely seemed to deepen relaxation levels and tended to increase the vividness of imagined scenes during procedures like desensitization or emotive imagery. Others, although reporting trance-like states, vivid imagery, and profound relaxation, reported no enhancement, and with these clients, time and effort devoted to trance induction were considered wasteful. In trying to account for these differences, I turned to measures of introversion-extraversion, neuroticism, and self-sufficiency, but emerged with indefinite findings. The relevance of Goldstein's (1962) studies on therapist-patient expectancies finally led me to appreciate the fact "that people enter therapy with certain expectations, and that the effectiveness of the therapy is closely linked with these expectations [Lazarus, 1971, p. xii]."

An obvious test of this general expectancy hypothesis suggested itself. Some clients requesting hypnosis would have their wishes met, while others would be told that relaxation training is in many ways superior to hypnosis, and they would receive "relaxation training" rather than "hypnosis." As a semi-control, clients who requested neither relaxation nor hypnosis would also receive one or the other treatment condition.

CLINICAL TRIAL

The study outlined below is best called a "clinical trial" rather than an "experiment." The latter would at least require objective pre-test measures, independent raters, specific post-test criteria, and different therapists (to control for bias). However, as Lazarus and Davison (1971) point out, "many of our greatest advances in therapeutic theory and practice come through clinical experimentation and innovation, rather than through laboratory research . . . [p. 196]." The final burden of proof rests with the scientist (not the practitioner), but clinical ideas that are amenable to verification or disproof can send scientists scurrying off into laboratories to subject the claims of efficacy to controlled tests. I can but hope that some of the findings outlined below will spur the imagination of some enterprising researcher who will then subject them to proper investigation.

Hypotheses

1. Clients who request hypnosis will report "response enhancement" (e.g. deeper levels of relaxation, more vivid images) when treated by "hypnotic relaxation" rather than by ordinary relaxation.

2. Clients whose requests for "hypnosis" are granted will generally show greater therapeutic improvement than those who are treated by "relaxation" instead.

Subjects

People referred to the writer for treatment often bring up the subject of hypnosis. It was decided that the next twenty clients who asked for hypnosis would be alternately allocated to a "request granted" or a "request refused" condition. The group finally comprised eight males and twelve females. Subsequently, six additional clients who seemed neutral to both conditions (hypnosis or relaxation) received exposure to both treatment conditions.

Procedure

Relaxation training plays an integral role in many behavior therapy techniques. Apart from desensitization, where its purpose and function are well known, clients are often relaxed before, during, and after role-playing or behavior rehearsal, while using procedures like emotive imagery, time projection, anxiety relief, and many other behavioral techniques. Clients in the "request granted" group were first asked why they wanted to be hypno-

TABLE 17–I

TREATMENT OUTCOMES

Initial Request for Hypnosis	Reported Subjective Improvement	Evidence of Behavioral Change
Granted ($N = 10$)	9	8
Refused ($N = 10$)	4	3
Exact p [a]	.10	.20

[a] Two-tailed.

tized, what their previous experiences with hypnosis had been, and how deeply hypnotized they desired to be. Gross misconceptions were thus detected and discussed. Emphasis was placed upon the fact that "deep" trance levels are not necessary to achieve good therapeutic results—especially when "hypnosis" is employed as a therapeutic adjunct.

Clients in the "request refused" group were told that hypnotic induction was probably a waste of time, that ordinary relaxation would possibly be more effective, and that it was advantageous to become proficient at relaxation since it obviated the necessity of being dependent upon a hypnotist.

The *relaxation* clients were given the instructions outlined in Appendix C of my earlier book (Lazarus, 1971). Depending upon the exigencies of various cases, I would read the instructions aloud and/or lend the client a tape recording of the regimen.

The *hypnosis* clients were treated identically except for the addition of the words "hypnotic" and "hypnosis" where appropriate (e.g. towards the middle of the second paragraph of the relaxation instructions clients would be instructed "to feel the deepening hypnotic relaxation," "as the hypnotic relaxation now spreads very beautifully into the face," "as the hypnotic relaxation becomes more and more obvious"). In the hypnosis group, the third paragraph commenced as follows: "Now to increase the feelings of *hypnosis* at this point what I want you to do is just keep on relaxing . . . Just think the work *hypnotism* as you breathe out."

As stated above, opportunities for "hypnotism" or "relaxation" frequently occur during behavior therapy. A client mentions that he is feeling tense. A role-playing sequence makes him feel agitated. He is encouraged to picture himself performing an assertive act without anxiety. Regression or time projection techniques are being employed.

At the end of the sequence, clients would be asked questions such as: "How did that go?" "Do you feel less tense now?" "Were the scenes vivid?" "How relaxed did you feel?"

During the course of therapy, six additional clients who seemed neutral toward hypnosis and relaxation were treated by both methods. Three were first given "hypnotic relaxation" and subsequently changed to "ordinary relaxation." The order was reversed for the other three clients. They too were asked to rate and compare the effects of "hypnotic relaxation" and "ordinary relaxation."

RESULTS AND DISCUSSION

In general, the people who requested hypnosis and received "hypnotic relaxation" were noticeably more enthusiastic about the procedure and reported deeper levels of relaxation, more vivid images, and greater anxiety relief than their counterparts treated by regular relaxation. Clients in the combined hypnosis and relaxation conditions who had not asked for either procedure reported no differences. The outcome seemed to confirm the first hypothesis, viz., that fulfilling clients' expectancies will tend to enhance their responses to therapy.

Regarding the second hypothesis, that expectancy fulfillment will augment therapeutic outcomes, the clinical findings also showed that this was usually the case. Specifically, two tension-headache sufferers in the "request granted" group reported a noticeable decrease in frequency and intensity after four sessions of hypnotic relaxation, whereas a client (after ten non-hypnotic relaxation sessions) reported no diminution in the frequency or intensity of his headaches. Interestingly, he then received the "hypnotic relaxation" sequence and reported a significant improvement after two sessions. Similarly, two impotent men showed the same improvement pattern—the man receiving "ordinary relaxation" (in addition to other behavior therapy techniques) showed significant improvements after receiving "hypnotic relaxation."

It must be emphasized that I am not presenting these findings or impressions as experimental evidence but purely as clinical impressions. In the light of these clinical findings, however, I would now consider it unethical for me to withhold hypnotic relaxation from clients who specifically request it (unless I have independent reasons and information to the contrary).

The differential results may be a function of my bias (I may have inadvertently influenced the clients with covert expectancies of my own), but I can argue fairly convincingly that the clients' needs and expectancies were probably more influential in determining the final outcomes. For instance, verbal reports from clients who had requested "hypnosis" but were given "relaxation" instead, tended to be as follows: "I feel something is lacking." "It seems sort of superficial." "I'm just not very good at relaxing." When subsequently given relaxation training defined as hypnosis, they reported: "Wow! I got a good spaced-out feeling." "I felt as if I was wrapped in cotton." "I could really feel the relaxation this time." "It made me warm and I tingled."

While a controlled experiment concerning the precise active ingredients underlying these clinical findings is lacking, as a clinician I am satisfied with our present understanding of these factors. This seems to be a special case of a more general notion that "If the therapist's attitude and approach differ markedly from the patient's 'ideal picture' of a psychology practitioner, positive results are unlikely to ensue [Lazarus, 1971, p. xii]."

REFERENCES

Barber, T. X.: Hypnotizability, suggestibility, and personality: V. A critical review of research findings. *Psychol Rep, 14:*1964. (Monogr. Suppl. 3).

Eysenck, H. J.: The effects of psychotherapy: An evaluation. *J Consult Psychol, 16:*319–324, 1952.

Goldstein, A. P.: *Therapist-Patient Expectancies in Psychotherapy.* New York, Pergamon, 1962.

Hilgard, E. R.: *Hypnotic Susceptibility.* New York: Harcourt, Brace and World, 1965.

Lang, P. J.: The mechanics of desensitization and the laboratory study of human fear. In Franks, C. M. (Ed.): *Behavior Therapy: Appraisal and Status.* New York, McGraw-Hill, 1969, pp. 160–191.

Lazarus, A. A.: Sensory deprivation under hypnosis in the treatment of pervasive ('free-floating') anxiety: A preliminary impression. *S Afr Med J*, 37:136–139, 1963.

Lazarus, A. A.: *Behavior Therapy and Beyond.* New York: McGraw-Hill, 1971.

Lazarus, A. A., and Davidson, G. C.: Clinical innovation in research and practice. In Bergin, A. E., and Garfield, S. L. (Ed.): *Handbook of Psychotherapy and Behavior Change: An Empirical Analysis.* New York, Wiley, 1971, pp. 196–213.

Strupp, H. H., and Bergin, A. E.: Some empirical and conceptual bases for co-ordinated research in psychotherapy: A critical review of issues, trends, and evidence. *Int J Psychiatry*, 7:18–90, 1969.

CHAPTER 13

THE USE OF COVERT CONDITIONING IN HYPNOTHERAPY*

Joseph R. Cautela, Ph.D.

Abstract. Covert conditioning involves the manipulation of imagery to modify behaviors such as phobias, alcoholism, over-eating, and sexual deviations. A rationale and description of covert conditioning procedures are described. Covert conditioning and hypnotic induction procedures employing imagery are compared. The advantages and disadvantages of combining covert conditioning and hypnosis are discussed. It is concluded that some of the issues raised in this paper can only be resolved by controlled research.

COVERT CONDITIONING is a term used to describe conditioning procedures in which the stimuli and responses are presented in imagination *via* instructions.

In 1966, while treating a patient with a serious alcohol problem and searching for some relevant experiments, I became interested in some literature on the application of aversive stimuli (in the form of electric shock) to reduce homosexual responses. I conjectured that, if overt punishment was successful in inhibiting positive responses to males, perhaps aversive stimuli presented in imagination only would have a similar effect. There were a number of reasons for favoring this latter treatment. It would: (1) decrease patient attrition rate, (2) make for a better therapist-client relationship, (3) be easier to apply, since no external apparatus was needed, (4) not be limited to a clinical setting,

* Reprinted from the *International Journal of Clinical and Experimental Hypnosis*, 1975 (in press). Copyrighted by the Society for Clinical and Experimental Hypnosis.

188

and, most important, (5) better enable the patient to bring his behavior under his own control, by giving him a technique for use whenever needed.

The main assumption underlying the covert conditioning procedures is that stimuli presented in imagination via instructions affect covert and overt behavior in a manner similar to stimuli presented externally, i.e. if an individual is asked to imagine a noxious stimulus just after he has imagined a response, probability of the response occurring will decrease. A response decrement involves both covert and overt behavior (given all the conditions that produce response suppression when stimuli are presented externally). Also, if a pleasant or reinforcing stimulus is presented to a S just after he has imagined a particular response, then we can expect the probability of that response occurring to increase in a manner similar to external reinforcement.

Imagery has been used by hypnotherapists both to facilitate hypnotic induction and to treat maladaptive behaviors.

The purpose of this paper is to propose that hypnotherapists' successful treatment results may be in part due to covert conditioning. I will further speculate on the possibility that the utilization of covert conditioning procedures by hypnotherapists will increase the probability of successful treatment results. And, finally, I will speculate as to the possibility that the hypnotic induction procedure can facilitate covert conditioning.

Four widely-used procedures to change response probability are: punishment, positive reinforcement, negative reinforcement, and extinction. These procedures involve the manipulation of the functional relationship between responses and stimuli. I have modified these procedures in clinical situations by asking the client to imagine that he is making particular responses and receiving various kinds of stimulation.

COVERT SENSITIZATION (PUNISHMENT)

In 1966 and 1967 I published a description of a procedure which I labeled Covert Sensitization (CS) (Cautela, 1966, 1967). The procedure was labeled thus because the client is asked to imagine himself as he is performing an ordinary act such as walking along a street, and then imagine that he decides to perform some aspect of the maladaptive behavior for which he is being treated. Thus, if the person is very overweight, he could imagine himself walking past a bakeshop window and salivating in response to the goods he sees there. (The client has been asked beforehand about the particular circumstances under which he usually overeats, what is likely to give rise to this response, and what maintains his overeating. If the external stimulus of delicious food usually leads to a response of buying it and eating it, no matter what the time of day or state of the person's hunger, that scene would be a good one for the therapist to use. In other words, a good behavior analysis would have made apparent the stimuli eliciting the maladaptive response, as well as the consequences.)

Using a scene typical in the client's response repertoire, then, the therapist has the patient imagine that the events mentioned above are really going on at the exact moment of therapy. He is told, e.g. not just to *see* himself walking down the street and stopping at the bakeshop, but really to *be* there. He is to try to use all his senses—he can really feel the sidewalk beneath his feet, really smell the delicious aroma of baking bread and cakes, really hear the cash register ringing up another sale, really see other people buying desserts. Now he imagines that he decides to go in and buy some of his favorite pastries. As he steps into the store, he gets a faint queasy feeling in the pit of his stomach, but he ignores it, thinking of the taste of his coveted food. As he tells the proprietor what he wants, he feels clammy and a little nauseous, but again he ignores these physical symptoms. As he pays for the pastry, he really begins to feel sick, food particles coming up into his throat and the insistent, choking feeling of imminent vomiting. Still, ignoring this, he opens the bag of desserts he has just bought, and reaches in for one to munch on his way home. At the door of the store, just as he puts a pastry into his mouth, he cannot suppress the vomit any longer, and he pukes all over the pastry, himself, the floor. Other customers begin to stare at him in horror. He is terribly embarrassed. As he looks down into the bag full of vomit, he gets sick once more, and people start moving away from him and leaving the store. The salesperson is rushing around nervously, and the client wishes he could just disappear. He throws down the bag of pastries and rushes out of the store. As soon as he gets away, he feels better. He goes home and washes up, and sits down to a well-balanced meal with other people. He feels fine in this adaptive situation.

After the scene is run through, the therapist asks the client about the clarity of his imagery, and about the effect it had on him. More scenes are then practiced. The client is then given homework and asked to practice covert sensitization on himself ten times per day. The next week, his fidelity to homework practice is checked, his overt behavior discussed (e.g. how much overeating was done given a lot of practice of covert sensitization) and more office work is done in needed areas.

Experimental and anecdotal evidence indicates that covert sensitization is effective in reducing maladaptive approach behaviors such as smoking (Viernstein, 1968); alcoholism (Ashem and Donner, 1968); and sexual deviations (Barlow, Leitenberg and Agras, 1969; Davison, 1968; Cautela and Wisocki, 1971).

A search of the literature reveals that hypnotherapists have commonly employed covert sensitization-like procedures in treating maladaptive approach behaviors. Feamster and Brown asked alcoholic patients to imagine the worst hangover they had ever experienced after they had come in contact with alcoholic beverages (1963). Hollander gave post hypnotic suggestions in which the patients were to think of the word "scar" each time they picked their faces (1959). Secter had patients imagine revolting scenes every time they bit their nails or performed some other maladaptive behavior (1960). In describing his treatment of alcoholics, Wolberg states that he had his patients imagine that they were getting nauseous when they took a drink. Also, they were told to imagine alcohol as poison if they were about to drink it (1948, p. 333).

COVERT POSITIVE REINFORCEMENT

The operant framework explains response increase or decrease by the different consequences following that response. In this paradigm, a punishing event following a response will result in the response's decrease. Conversely, a reinforcing or rewarding event following a response will result in the response's increase.

The therapist's task is to punish inappropriate responses and to reinforce appropriate ones.

As seen above, the punishing events administered in imagination only had been effective in reducing maladaptive responses. It seemed logical to argue that reinforcing events administered in imagination only could also be used effectively. In this manner, I developed a technique called Covert Positive Reinforcement (COR) (Cautela, 1970).

The patient is first asked to fill out a Reinforcement Survey Schedule (Cautela and Kastenbaum, 1967; Cautela, 1972), to determine what events or things are highly reinforcing for him. This written report is later checked by the therapist, who then circles those items the patient has indicated as highly reinforcing. The therapist then has the patient imagine these items, and finally settles upon the few for which the patient reports high clarity of imagery and high feelings of reinforcement. After the patient practices imagining his reinforcing scenes, the therapist tells him that when he says the word "Reinforcement" the patient is to go through that pleasant scene in his mind. He does some more practice just saying the word, "Reinforcement," and getting the client used to imagining the pleasant scene upon hearing that word.

The actual pattern for office sessions using the Covert Reinforcement technique is the following: the patient is asked to imagine himself performing some adaptive response that is diametrically opposed to his customary maladaptive one, e.g. the obese patient used in the example above imagines that he is walking down the street and that he sees the bakeshop window full of delicious treats. Instead of going in, however, he thinks to himself, "Those will taste good, but they will add more fat to my body and will perpetuate my problem. Besides, I just had lunch." Or, he might say, "It's almost time for supper and I don't have to eat everything I see just because it looks good. A thin person would just walk by here and never think of stopping to buy something unless to save it for a proper eating time, or to give it to guests. I'm not going in there." After one of these thoughts, or a combination of them, he raises his finger. The therapist then says, "Reinforcement," and the patient imagines a pleasant scene. After many office trials of this kind, and home practice, the client begins to associate appropriate responses with pleasant consequences. This, combined with the overt reinforcement of losing weight and looking and feeling good are effective means of treating the problem. The reinforcing scene introduces a relaxed and pleasant feeling after a patient's making an adaptive response, when the patient could ordinarily be feeling still tempted, or anxious at being deprived of what formerly was giving him pleasure, albeit at great cost to himself.

Besides being used to reinforce responses antagonistic to maladaptive behavior, COR has been effectively used to treat phobias, and is easier to apply than systematic desensitization. In systematic desensitization, the therapist must use the formal relaxation technique (Jacobson, 1938) to get a client to feel relaxed at each step of the way in the move toward the feared object. Also, it is necessary to build a hierarchy to ferret out the different fear components of the total experience of the phobia. This is not necessary when employing COR. Since a person cannot really feel very pleasant and reinforced by an event and remain tense, relaxation is not necessary. Thus, if reinforcement is delivered at each successive step on the way to adaptive behavior, this behavior can be shaped without employing relaxation.

Like the other covert conditioning procedures, COR is a self-control procedure, which, once learned by the client, may be used by him whenever necessary. He can employ it for other problems, or if he feels that the problem he was treated for is again appearing in his life.

COR has also received experimental confirmation. It appears effective in reducing phobic responses (Flannery, 1972); reducing test anxiety (Wisocki, 1970); changing perception of circle-size in college students (Cautela, Steffan, and Wish, in press) and in schizophrenic subjects (Steffan, 1971). COR has been used to change attitudes toward the mentally retarded (Cautela, Wish, and Walsh, 1971). Also, Krop, Calhoon and Verrier used this technique to modify self-concepts in children (1971).

There are also some examples of COR in the literature concerned with hypnotherapy. Secter had patients imagine a pleasant scene after they performed appropriate behavior (1960). Shibata had patients with dietary problems imagine pleasant feelings after they had eaten disliked food (1967). Krippner asked children with reading problems to imagine that they were happy and proud after they read a sentence (1966). Wolberg treated phobias by having patients imagine pleasant images as they approached the feared object (1948, p. 235).

COVERT NEGATIVE REINFORCEMENT

As effective as COR has been, it cannot be used with some few patients who claim that there is nothing at all reinforcing in their lives. When pressed to search for at least one thing, even hypothetical, that could be reinforcing, they cannot even imagine anything pleasant. For these patients, I developed the technique of Covert Negative Reinforcement (CNR) (Cautela, 1970), a procedure based on the escape-conditioning paradigm. In this method, the therapist discovers what scenes or objects are particularly aversive to the client by administering the Aversive Scene Survey Schedule (Cautela, 1969) and the Covert Conditioning Survey Schedule (Cautela and Ascher, 1972). With this knowledge, he has the patient imagine an aversive scene or event, trying to evoke in him the actual emotions associated with the corresponding overt situation. When the patient can vividly imagine the stressful situation, and indicates this to the therapist by raising his index finger, he is told to "shift" and imagine the adaptive behavior the therapist is trying to increase. Thus, the adaptive behavior becomes an aversion-relief from the unpleasant scene. A typical example follows: A patient suffering from agoraphobia is asked to imagine that she is bound, hand and foot, to a chair, whereupon a rat enters the room and slowly advances toward her. She is unable to escape and focuses, horrified, on the advancing rodent. Just as the rat is about to leap, she is told to "shift" and imagine herself walking briskly down the street on a bright, pleasant day. Leaving her house thus becomes a behavior associated with terminating a very unpleasant situation, whereas, before, it was in itself a fearful event.

It is important that the patient be able to shift *completely* from one scene to another so that the properties of the aversive scene are not carried over to the imagined desirable behavior. A common error in conceptualizing the technique of CNR is that it is the same as covert punishment. Unlike CS, CNR does not punish a maladaptive response, but reinforces an adaptive one. It can be used by itself or in conjunction with other techniques for almost any behavior disorder.

In a recent experiment, Ascher and Cautela (1972) have some experimental data to indicate that CNR can increase response probability.

Abraham (1968) provides a good example of the use of CNR by a hypnotherapist. He treated a case of hysterical paralysis of the legs. He had his patient imagine (while hypnotized) that he was sitting on a beach in uncomfortably cold water, and that he could only escape the cold water (noxious stimulation) by lifting his legs out of it.

COVERT EXTINCTION

There are times when a patient's undesirable behavior is being maintained by high reinforcement from individuals and situations not under the therapist's control. In certain circumstances, e.g. while treating disruptive classroom behavior, perhaps the therapist would ask the teacher and other students to ignore the patient, if he jumps out of his seat, or "clowns around." Sometimes, however, when a response is subjected to "extinction" (i.e. evokes no change at all, positive or negative, in the environment) it first increases sharply, levels off, then drops gradually. So, when the teacher and students ignore disruptive behavior it initially becomes much worse and these very agents find it difficult to keep ignoring it. In these circumstances, it is impossible to get cooperation from the reinforcing agents to discontinue their reinforcing responses. For these situations, I developed another technique termed Covert Extinction (CE) (Cautela, 1971). As in the other Covert Conditioning procedures, the therapist outlines a scene to be imagined by the S, making it as vivid as possible. When the patient can imagine himself performing the undesirable behavior, the therapist makes it clear that there is absolutely no reaction from other people to his behavior, e.g. if a woman's headaches occur every time her husband goes out of the house, and the husband feels it cruel (no matter what the therapist says) to leave her in pain, the therapist can have the patient imagine this scene: "You are reading when you realize that your husband is dressing to go out bowling. You try to concentrate on the book, but a headache is beginning to bother you. Thinking of his leaving you makes it seem worse. You tell him how sick you feel, but he just says, 'Why don't you lie down to rest. I am going bowling'." In such a case, the therapist has to be careful that the patient doesn't begin to resent her husband for what has taken place in imagination.

There are many other problems which seem to be maintained by social reinforcement and which can be treated effectively by CE, e.g. a stutterer imagines he calls a girl up for a date and he stutters frequently, but there isn't the slightest indication from the girl's voice that she notices it.

Once a behavior has been extinguished, it is well to go through some trials to get the behavior below extinction level to guard against spontaneous remission.

Recent studies (Ascher, 1970) also indicate that CE is effective in reducing response probability.

A number of hypnotherapists employ a sort of latent extinction procedure by having the patients imagine that they are confronted with an anxiety-provoking stimulus without any anxiety (Summo, 1960; Logsdon, 1960; Verson, 1961; Erickson, 1965).

In all of the covert conditioning procedures, as many as possible different reinforcing and aversive stimuli are used to avoid satiation or adaptation. Before clients are discharged, they are thoroughly familiar with the rationale and application of covert conditioning procedures. They are taught how to use the procedures as self-control methods for the rest of their lives.

It becomes evident upon close examination of the literature of hypnotherapy that I am not the only one who has used covert conditioning-like procedures. After all, there is hardly any psychological procedure or concept that has not been used by others one way or another; e.g. Wolpe's desensitization procedure (1958); Freud's concept of the unconscious. I believe my contribution has been in explicitly labeling the procedures as specific conditioning procedures that can best be conceptualized within an operant framework. Besides labeling the procedures, I have systematized their use and extrapolated from learning studies to utilize them in an effective manner. This labeling of the covert conditioning procedures and the systematization of their use has enabled investigators to attempt controlled experimental verification. Also, investigators are in the process of determining the variables within the procedures that contribute to therapeutic effectiveness.

Hynotherapists might increase the effectiveness of their treatment by systematically employing covert conditioning procedures. The explicit use of covert conditioning has the advantage of providing guidelines for treatment strategy, since these procedures have as their base a body of empirical knowledge developed from experimental studies of learning. By way of example, after 100 percent reinforcement, a therapist could switch to partial reinforcement (Lewis, 1960)—this should increase resistance to extinction or decrease the probability of relapse. In other words, all the parameters known to affect learning could be taken into consideration in treatment.

Conversely, covert conditioning could be made more effective by employing hypnotic induction procedures. What variables in the hypnotic induction procedure could contribute to covert conditioning's effectiveness? Some investigators claim that hypnotic induction can be used to produce clearer imagery (Todd and Kelley, 1970). Clarity of imagery is an important variable in the effectiveness of covert conditioning and intensity of stimulation is a relevant variable both in overt and covert conditioning. In general, the stronger the stimulation, the more effective the conditioning. Also, the clarity of imagery will affect generalization. As of yet, though, there is no experimental evidence that hypnotic induction is more effective than other procedures in producing clarity of imagery. We, of course, have developed methods for increasing vividness of imagery. Thus far I have been able to employ covert conditioning procedures with all my clients. Generally a client is able to obtain clear imagery in one or more sense modalities. If a client appears to have poor imagery in one sense modality than in our scenes we emphasize the other senses, e.g. with a client who has a plane phobia but has poor visual imagery, I emphasize the sound of the motor, the voice of the stewardess, and the kinesthetic sensations involved while the plane is taking off, in flight and descending. If it is necessary to use a particular sense modality (e.g. visual modality involving a male nude), then the scenes are made shorter in duration and described in greater detail. Also, the client is asked to practice obtaining visual imagery by looking at a picture or an object, examine the details, then close his eyes and try to reproduce the sensation in imagery. He is asked to practice this not only to the stimuli involved in therapy but to the many stimuli he encounters daily.

Some investigators also claim that hypnotic induction facilitates rapport (Abrams, 1964). If this is true, then perhaps covert conditioning can indeed be more effective with the use of hypnosis, since the therapist will be a stronger reinforcer. Our own procedures also allow us to become powerful reinforcers. Since we have to be aware of the clients' reinforcing menu to employ covert conditioning procedures, then we can manipulate the reinforcers to increase our own reinforcing value. The therapist will thus be more apt to elicit cooperation from the S. However, thus far, investigations have indicated that neither the hypnotic induction procedure (Lang, Lazovik and Reynolds, 1965; Paul, 1969) nor degree of suggestibility (Paul, 1966) increases the effectiveness of procedures which involve the manipulation of imagery such as desensitization. It is necessary to note that these studies did not involve the covert conditioning studies discussed in this paper.

DISADVANTAGES OF USING HYPNOSIS

It seems reasonable to ask—Why not use hypnosis when you are employing covert conditioning procedures? What do you have to lose? Well, for one thing, some clients will not cooperate when told that a hypnotic induction procedure is going to be used (Taylor, 1964). Also, some clients do not seem to meet the criteria for hypnotic Ss. Then why not use hypnosis with the clients who respond favorably to the procedure? I feel that, unless there is some substantial evidence that hypnotic induction procedures would facilitate covert conditioning, it is more parsimonious not to use them. This assumption needs testing both anecdotally and experimentally. I, myself, have not combined the procedures; though some of my colleagues have told me that they are beginning to do so.

RESEARCH

Answers to some of the questions raised in this paper can only come from controlled research. Studies comparing the effectiveness of covert conditioning procedures with and without the use of hypnotic induction are necessary. Also, a comparison of the hypnotic treatment of behavior disorders with a covert conditioning treatment of the same disorders is important. I hope that I have alerted hypnotherapists as to the possibility of systematically employing covert conditioning procedures. I also hope that I have stimulated behavior therapists to inquire as to the possibility of making their treatment approaches more effective by employing hypnotic induction procedures.

REFERENCES

Abraham, H. A.: Hypnosis used in the treatment of somatic manifestations of a psychiatric disorder. *Am J Clin Hypn, 10:*304–309, 1968.

Abrams, S.: Implications of learning theory in treating depression by employing hypnosis. *Am J Clin Hypn, 6:*313–321, 1964.

Ascher, L. M.: Covert extinction: An experimental test. Unpublished data, State University of New York, 1970.

Ascher, L. M., and Cautela, J. R.: Covert negative reinforcement: An experimental test. *Behav Ther Exp Psychiatry, 1:*1–5, 1972.

Ashem, B., and Donner, L.: Covert sensitization with alcoholics: A controlled replication. *Behav Res Ther, 6:*7–12, 1968.

Barlow, D. H., Leitenberg, H., and Agras, W. S.: Experimental control of sexual deviation through manipulation of the noxious scene in covert sensitization. *J Abnorm Psychol, 5:*596–601, 1969.

Cautela, J. R.: Aversive scene survey schedule for use in covert sensitization and covert negative reinforcement. Paper presented at Boston College, 1969.

Cautela, J. R., and Ascher, L. M.: Covert conditioning survey schedule. Unpublished questionnaire, Boston College, 1972.

Cautela, J. R.: Covert extinction. Behav Ther, 2:192–200, 1971.

Cautela, J. R.: Covert negative reinforcement. *Behav Ther Exp Psychiatry, 1:*273–278, 1970.

Cautela, J. R.: Covert reinforcement. *Behav Ther, 1:*33–50, 1970.

Cautela, J. R., Steffan, J., and Wish, P.: Covert reinforcement: An experimental test. *J. Clin Consult Psychol,* in press.

Cautela, J. R.: Covert sensitization. *Psychol Rep, 20:*459–468, 1967.

Cautela, J. R., and Wisocki, P. A.: Covert sensitization for the treatment of sexual deviations. *Psychol Rec, 21:*37–48, 1971.

Cautela, J. R.: Reinforcement survey schedule: Evaluation and current applications. *Psychol Rep, 30:*683–690, 1972.

Cautela, J. R., and Kastenbaum, R.: A reinforcement survey schedule for use in therapy, training, and research. *Psychol Rep, 20:*1115–1130, 1967.

Cautela, J. R.: Treatment of compulsive behavior by covert sensitization. *Psychol Rec, 16:*33–41, 1966.

Cautela, J. R., Walsh, K., and Wish, P.: The use of covert reinforcement in the modification of attitudes toward the mentally retarded. *J Psychol, 77:*257–260, 1971.

Davison, G.: Elimination of a sadistic fantasy by a client-controlled-counter-conditioning technique: A case study. *J Abnorm Psychol, 73:*84–89, 1968.

Erickson, M. H.: Hypnosis and examination panics. *Am J Clin Hypn, 8:*356–358, 1965.

Feamster, J. H., and Brown, J. E.: Hypnotic aversion to alcohol: Three-year follow-up of one patient. *Am J Clin Hypn, 6:*165–166, 1963.

Flannery, R. B., Jr.: A laboratory analogue of two covert reinforcement procedures. *J Behav Ther Exp Psychiatry, 3:*171–177, 1972.

Hollander, M. B.: Excoriated acne controlled by post-hypnotic suggestion. *Am J Clin Hypn, 1:*122–123, 1959.

Jacobson, E.: *Progressive relaxation.* Chicago, University of Chicago Press, 1938.

Krippner, S.: The use of hypnosis with elementary and secondary school children in a summer reading clinic. *Am J Clin Hypn, 8:*261–266, 1966.

Krop, H., Calhoon, B., and Verrier, R.: Modification of the "self-concept" of emotionally disturbed children by covert reinforcement. *Behav Ther, 2:*201–204, 1971.

Lang, P. J., Lazovik, A. D., and Reynolds, D. J.: Desensitization, suggestibility and pseudotherapy. *J Abnorm Psychol, 70:*395–402, 1965.

Lewis, D. J.: Partial reinforcement: A selective review of the literature since 1950. *Psychol Bull, 57:*1–28, 1960.

Logsdon, F. M.: Age-regression in diagnosis and treatment of acrophobia. *Am J Clin Hypn, 3:*108–109, 1960.

Paul, G. L.: Inhibition of physiological response to stressful imagery by relaxation training and hypnotically suggested relaxation. *Behav Res Ther, 7:*249–256, 1969.

Paul, G. L.: *Insight vs. Desensitization in Psychotherapy: An experiment in Anxiety Reduction.* Stanford, Stanford University Press, 1966.

Secter, I. I.: Tongue thrust and nail biting simultaneously treated during hypnosis. *Am J Clin Hypn, 3:*51–52, 1960.

Shibata, J.: Hypnotherapy of patients taking unbalanced diets. *Am J Clin Hypn*, 10:81–83, 1967.

Steffan, J.: Covert reinforcement with schizophrenics. Paper presented at the annual meeting of the Association for Advancement of Behavior Therapy, Washington, D. C., 1971.

Summo, A. J.: The control of inappropriate blushing. *Am J Clin Hypn*, 3:59–60, 1960.

Taylor, W.: Psycho-therapeutic methods with hypnosis. *Am J Clin Hypn*, 6:322–325, 1964.

Todd, F. J., and Kelley, R. J.: The use of hypnosis to facilitate conditioned relaxation responses. *Behav Ther Exper Psychiat*, 1:295–298, 1970.

Verson, R. D.: A technique to control hallucinatory obsessive ideas. *Am J Clin Hypn*, 4:115–116, 1961.

Viernstein, L.: Evaluation of therapeutic techniques of covert sensitization. Unpublished data, Queens College, Charlotte, North Carolina, 1968.

Wisocki, P. A.: An application of covert reinforcement to the treatment of test anxiety. Unpublished doctoral dissertation, Boston College, 1970.

Wolberg, L. R.: *Medical Hypnosis*. New York, Grune and Stratton, 2 vols., 1948.

Wolpe, J.: *Psychotherapy by Reciprocal Inhibition*. Stanford, Stanford University Press, 1958.

CHAPTER 14

AVERSIVE IMAGERY THERAPY USING HYPNOSIS*

BURTON S. GLICK, M.D.

INTRODUCTION

IN THE RELATIVELY SHORT TIME that scientifically controlled aversive conditioning has been in existence its use has expanded to include the treatment of a great variety of pathologic conditions. Among these disorders are obsessions and compulsions, sexual disturbances (fetishism, transvestism, exhibitionism, homosexuality), alcoholism, and drug addiction—and such "normal" disorders as smoking and gambling. The unconditioned (aversive, "punishing") stimulus which, by close temporal association with representations or actualities of the deviant behavior is supposed to extinguish such behavior, has been limited mainly to emetic drugs and electric shock, with occasional forays into respiratory paralysis (via succinylcholine), imagined shameful or dangerous scenes (aversive imagery), air blasts, and noxious gases. The emetics used have included apomorphine, emetine, tartar emetic, and mustard in water.

Indications in the literature point to the possible effectiveness of suggested "imaginary" nausea (without emesis) in aversive therapy. Raymond (1964) intimated that vomiting is not an essential part of the apomorphine treatment of alcoholics (nausea being sufficient), and Feldman and MacCulloch (1965) specified that the unconditioned stimulus intensity need not exceed a

* Originally published in the *American Journal of Psychotherapy*, Volume XXVI, No. 3, July 1972, pages 432–436.

certain level (since its effect is linear above that level). In 1966 Cautela (1966) originated the term "covert sensitization" to describe a treatment situation in which both the conditioned and unconditioned stimuli are covert (that is, imaginary). While in a deeply relaxed state the subject is asked first to visualize himself engaging in the behavior to be extinguished (for example, smoking, drinking, fetishism) and then is instructed to become nauseated almost to the point of vomiting. To prevent vomiting, the subject must refrain from committing the imaginary act. Using this technique Cautela successfully treated two cases of compulsive overeating and alcoholism.

Employing this same method as the first part of a three-pronged attack against smoking behavior in two subjects, Tooley and Pratt (1967) found it was "quite effective in the early stages, but accommodation to the aversive stimulus decreased its effectiveness in later stages." Others have used the term "aversive imagery" to describe essentially the same therapeutic concept that characterizes covert sensitization.

Neither Cautela, Tooley and Pratt, nor others employing the aversive imagery technique have utilized hypnosis as part of the treatment paradigm, preferring instead deep muscular relaxation à la Wolpe's (1958) systematic desensitization. To the best of the author's knowledge no one has yet paired nauseous feeling with imagined scenes depicting pathologic behavior (at times in quite extreme forms) while the patient was in the hypnotic state. In this connection, it strikes me that neither the term "aversive imagery" nor "covert sensitization" accurately describes the true state of affairs since both imply that the nausea is an imagined or simulated condition whereas I have reason to believe, based on patients' facial expressions during hypnosis and verbal reports after it, that hypnotically induced nausea is akin, if not identical, to the real thing. I would also venture to assert that the nausea experienced under hypnosis is more extreme and realistic, and the imagined scenes more vivid, than that to be obtained with mere relaxation.

The following is an account of a case of severe, chronic fetishism treated with what may loosely be termed the aversive imagery technique.

The patient is a twenty-seven-year-old single, white male social worker who has been a clothing fetishist since the age of three or four years, at which period he would rub his penis against his mother's laundry. Prior to seeing me he had received three years of "freudian" psychotherapy once to three times weekly which he felt had "exaggerated the symptom."

He was particularly attracted to feminine underwear, slips, panties, garter belts, and dark stockings. He would frequently rummage through garbage pails searching for the desired garments and would masturbate two or three times a day using direct fetish-genital contact. In his frequent heterosexual relations he had no special desire for penetration, wishing merely to "undulate" his genitals against his partner's undergarments. It occasioned no thrill for him to view a nude female: "The clothing is the sexual object."

Whenever he saw an attractively clothed woman, he experienced a strong urge to return home to masturbate. He dated only mature women in their thirties and forties, fearing rejection from younger girls. A quite specific affective constellation overwhelmed him when he saw a seductively clad woman; an acute sensation of anguished loneliness which "devastated" him. This feeling would bring him to a near-panic state, to avoid which he often preferred not to leave the house.

The patient believed that were he to masturbate on his mother's underclothes, or were she to "just sit and show me the clothing or handle it," this would, by its very repulsiveness, turn him away from his symptoms. He was becoming quite desperate about his plight and maintained that he "must get relief" or else commit suicide. He expressed the strong belief that some type of aversive therapy would be beneficial to him.

Accordingly, aversive conditioning was started with the patient in the hypnotic state. He was given the following instructions under hypnosis: "When I clap my hands like this [clap, clap clap] you will become nauseated. As I continue to clap you will become increasingly and extremely nauseated, but you will not vomit [protection for my chair, rug, and the patient's clothes]. Throughout the entire hypnotic period, even when I am not clapping, you will feel a constant low level of nausea which will increase when I start clapping. I am also going to present to your imagination a series of scenes and situations which you will visualize as clearly and vividly as possible."

Most of the scenes used were suggested by the patient prior to the sessions. A few were of my own devising. Some of them were truly calculated to produce nausea and disgust (even without hypnosis) in all but the most strongly stomached individuals. Among the most offensive were the following:

"Visualize a pair of panties and a pair of black stockings stained with urine and covered with feces."

"Visualize your mother's panties in the sink, all covered with feces."

"Visualize your mother sitting across from you in the living room where you used to live. She is holding up and handling her panties while leering at you in an evil, provocative way."

I would not advise using this procedure with a psychotic patient.

The timing between the presentation of unconditioned and conditioned stimulus was at best a crude affair. Not knowing how long it would take to elicit nausea in response to clapping, I clapped just before introducing each scene and just before uttering such key-words as "panties," "stockings," "feces," "urine," "mother," and so forth. At times I interjected, with dramatic intensity, reinforcing remarks such as, "Ugh; how disgusting, nauseating, vile, filthy." At other times I had the patient repeat the key-words over and over while I clapped vigorously and steadily. If one could judge from the patient's facial expressions and oral contortions his gorge often rose to a considerable extent, but he did not vomit.

After the first aversive conditioning treatment the patient claimed to notice some benefit in that he panicked less. A total of six sessions in six weeks was devoted to the clothing fetish. These visits gave rise chronologically to the following statements by the patient: "For two days after the last session it was beautiful; there was no fetish at all. I was normal but it didn't hold. The garbage pail business is some-what modified. I still get intense loneliness when I see an attractively dressed girl. . . . I don't flip out completely. The bad, lonely feeling is less intense. . . . The clothing thing is definitely lessened. I don't feel as bad when I look at women. I threw out half the clothing and masturbate much less on them. . . . The fetish is markedly reduced. I tune into the nausea whenever I want to. . . . The painful feeling has subsided. . . . I'm not particularly attracted to women wearing dark stockings. I'm less distracted by women's clothing in the street. . . . I wouldn't now ask a woman to wear dark stockings. I don't have the clothing fetish very much any more."

FOLLOW-UP

Up to the time of this writing, nine months after the last of the six aversive conditioning sessions, the patient's marked improvement has been maintained. He is currently receiving supportive and direc-tive therapy in other areas of his life.

DISCUSSION

Raymond (1956) has described fetishism as the "tendency to be sexually attracted by some special part or peculiarity of the body or by some inanimate object." While mildly fetishistic be-havior undoubtedly occurs in many normal males, Yates (1970) feels that in its "perverse" form it is relatively rare and, further, that classical aversive conditioning with electric shock has "proved remarkably successful in dealing with a sexual disorder which has proved in the past to be exceptionally refractory to treatment" (p. 236).

Classical aversive conditioning with nausea-inducing and emetic drugs has been largely replaced by aversive shock conditioning, mainly because the former is "unpleasant and even traumatic in the extreme to the patient" (p. 228). However, aversive shock conditioning is not without its disadvantages. In the first place, it hurts, and may occasion interfering anxiety. Secondly, the administration of an enormous number of individual shocks is apparently necessary to produce significant results; grand totals of 400, 450, and even 675 are not uncommon. Thirdly, it requires the use of special instrumentation not readily available to, nor desired by, most therapists.

The aversive imagery technique using hypnotically induced nausea as the unconditioned stimulus offered a possible way out of the dilemma in that, while unpleasant, it is not "traumatic in the extreme" (the hypnotized patient may "escape" by refusing to become nauseated or by rousing himself from hypnosis); it is painless and probably not as anxiety-provoking as electric shock; it seems to necessitate fewer applications to produce significant clinical change than does shock; and finally, it is noninstrumental, demanding no special equipment, drugs, or personnel.

Considering the usual intractability of such severe and chronic fetishism as my patient exhibited, the marked improvement obtained with only six conditioning treatments is to be reckoned something of value. Certainly the clinical result should offer encouragement to essay this particular technique in the treatment of all those disturbances for which aversive conditioning has been employed.

SUMMARY

A severe, chronic male fetishist was treated with a variant of the aversive imagery technique. While he was in the hypnotized state suggested nausea was paired with imaginary scenes depicting his pathologic behavior. Six treatment sessions over a six-week period resulted in a definite abatement of the symptom. Because aversive conditioning using hypnotically-induced nausea does not require the employment of emetic drugs or electric shock it may prove to be a very simple and convenient therapeutic approach in appropriate cases.

REFERENCES

Cautela, J. R.: Treatment of compulsive behavior by covert sensitization. *Psychol Rec*, 16:33, 1966.

Feldman, M. P., and MacCulloch, M. J.: The application of anticipatory avoidance learning to the treatment of homosexuality. *Behav Res Ther*, 2:165, 1965.

Raymond, M. J.: Case of fetishism treated by aversion therapy. *Br Med J*. 2:854, 1956.

Raymond, M. J.: The treatment of addiction by aversive conditioning with apomorphine. *Behav Res Ther*, 1:287, 1964.

Tooley, J. T., and Pratt, S.: An experimental procedure for the extinction of smoking behavior. *Psychol Rec*, 17:209, 1967.

Wolpe, J.: *Psychotherapy by Reciprocal Inhibition*. Stanford, Stanford University Press, 1958.

Yates, A. J.: *Behavior Therapy*. New York, John Wiley, 1970.

CHAPTER **15**

VERBALLY SUGGESTED RESPONSES FOR RECIPROCAL INHIBITION OF ANXIETY*

MORTON RUBIN, D.O.

INTRODUCTION

A new and rapid technique for effecting change on the reciprocal inhibition principle is described. The patient after a detailed explanation of the learned character of his unadaptive anxiety habit, is forcefully told that through being juxtaposed with a different response, the stimuli concerned will come to evoke the latter in place of the anxiety. The counter-anxiety response is then induced in the patient by direct suggestion. Next, anxiety-evoking stimuli are presented in imagination while the counter-anxiety response is verbally sustained. The anxiety-evoking stimuli are not presented in hierarchial order, but a weaker scene will be used if the chosen one is found to evoke more anxiety than the suggested response can inhibit. The manner of introducing scenes departs from standard practice in that the patient is told not to imagine the scene while it is being described, but only at the presentation of a signal to be given shortly thereafter.

THIS PAPER PRESENTS a new technique which appears to be unusually effective in treating a wide variety of neurotic behaviors. It is based on the reciprocal inhibition principle (Wolpe, 1958), which bears repeating: "If a response antagonistic to anxiety can be made to occur in the presence of anxiety-evoking stimuli so that it is accompanied by a complete or partial sup-

* Reprinted with permission from Morton Rubin, D.O., in J. Behav Ther Exp Psychiat, Volume 3, pages 273–277, 1972, Pergamon Press. Copyright 1972. The discussion has been rewritten for this book.

pression of the anxiety responses, the bond between these stimuli and the anxiety responses will be weakened."

Behavior therapy practice has made use of numerous methods of eliciting responses antagonistic to anxiety. However, there is one readily available source of responses that has been remarkably neglected, and that is verbal suggestion. The only report of the regular use of hypnosis and suggestion in a reciprocal inhibition framework appears to be that of Hussain (1964), although as Barrios (1966, 1970) has pointed out, some well-known hypnotists (e.g. Erikson, 1948; Van Pelt, 1958) seem to carry out similar procedures without an explicit conditioning formulation.

I have used the method to be described for about five years. It consists of a constant series of steps, each of which, I believe, contributes to its efficacy, although, of course, only experimental testing can really decide this.

METHOD

A brief history is taken, paying particular attention to the circumstances of the onset of the patient's neurotic responses. The history should identify the original precipitating stimuli (S1) to the anxiety responses (R1), and take account of later events that may have modified the responses or conditioned them to second order stimuli. A diagram (Fig. 15–1) is drawn to illustrate the essential conditioning history, including stimuli that have been secondarily conditioned. The present unadaptiveness of anxiety responses to these stimuli is pointed out. The figure shown here relates to a case of claustrophobia.

A second diagram (Fig. 15–2) is now drawn to illustrate that alternative responses (R2) are available that could compete with the anxiety (R1). It is pointed out that these are adaptive responses, and if evoked strongly enough in the presence of the stimuli conditioned to anxiety, will inhibit the latter. The bond between the various stimuli and the anxiety will then be weakened. These figures seem to enhance the patient's participation in the steps that follow.

The therapist now carefully seeks out elements of pleasurable response that may be evokable by other aspects of the fearful situations. When some of these have been identified, the patient

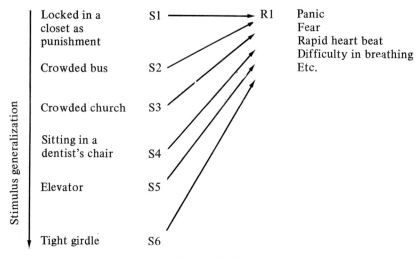

Figure 15–1

is hypnotized and told to relax as completely as possible. (A scene that might be relaxing may be suggested to augment this.) If it seems that the patient can visualize scenes satisfactorily, the central therapeutic procedure is begun. He is told that he will be expected to imagine a scene incorporating a stated anxiety-provoking stimulus at the count of three. Thereupon, the previously identified counter-anxiety responses are very strongly suggested, usually together with further suggestions of calm and relaxation. The alternative responses are suggested in varied de-

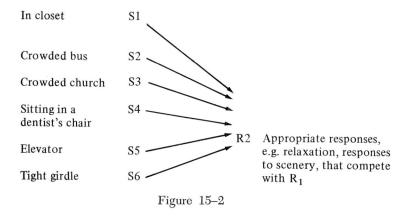

Figure 15–2

tail, drawing on the fact that every situation, no matter how simple, is a source of complex multi-faceted reactions. For example, in riding as a passenger in a car the normal reaction includes thoughts directed towards the destination and the ramifications of this, reactions to the radio broadcast, the driver, other cars, buildings, and scenery. In contradistinction, the individual who is anxious riding in a car is scarcely aware of these other stimuli.

Having ascertained that the patient comprehends what is required, the count of three is given to signal the start of visualization. The patient is directed to indicate by a finger signal when visualization takes place. Then suggestions are continued that he feel relaxed and respond in pleasurable ways to the scene. If the patient visualizes the scene without anxiety, he is rewarded by the enthusiastic approval of the therapist. Before being brought out of the hypnotic state he is told to practice the scenes at home, relaxing and eliciting the alternative mode of responding now available to him. If anxiety should ever develop, either during a practice session or during a real life exposure to a stimulus to neurotic anxiety, he is to make every effort to evoke the alternative responses.

To exemplify the foregoing, we may consider a young man with extreme anxiety whenever he took a shower or even washed his face, dating from an early age when he had been thrown into deep water by his brother in an attempt to force him to swim. (He also recalled his mother making repeated statements to the effect that an individual could drown in a tablespoon of water.) After the induction of the hypnotic state, he was asked to visualize himself taking a walk in the rain (which, he had revealed, he enjoyed) and feeling the pleasure of the water trickling down his face. While maintaining the pleasurable response, the rain was changed to a shower bath. The similarity between walking in *the rain* and standing in the shower was now stressed, while pointing to the greater control he had in the shower—regulating the temperature, stepping out of the stream or even turning it off. The delights of a feeling of cleanliness were also suggested together with calm and relaxation. Seven sessions were required to rid the patient of his phobia.

CASE ILLUSTRATION OF TECHNICAL DETAILS

A thirty-seven-year old married woman gave the history that two years earlier at a restaurant, in lifting a cup of coffee to her lips, her hand began to tremble. When she attempted to steady it with her other hand, both hands trembled and she experienced an extreme attack of anxiety. She also felt a spasm in the posterior cervical region and some occipital pain. She remained seated for about an hour, too distressed to leave. Two days later, in another restaurant with her husband, as the food was being served, she experienced a similar but even more intense attack. The anxiety was so severe that she felt compelled to leave immediately.

The next two years were a nightmare. The stimuli capable of precipitating an attack of anxiety had generalized to sitting at her own table, applying cosmetics, sitting down at work, going to the beauty shop and numerous similar situations. Consequently, she had stopped working, would eat standing, and could not visit the beauty shop or apply cosmetics. Because of the neck and head pain, she had consulted two neurosurgeons, the second of whom had performed a cervical laminectomy. This did not resolve her problem, but added discomfort and limitation of motion. With the passage of time, she became increasingly depressed and eventually came under the care of a psychiatrist who gave her twelve electro-shock treatments and then continued interviews for six months until she came to see me.

Her earlier history revealed one especially pertinent fact. About five years previously, her mother had been rendered aphasic by a stroke. This was especially distressing because she had been a vibrant, active person. The patient agreed with my suggestion that the cervical spasm and occipital pain had implications to her of an impending stroke.

By means of Figs. 15–1 and 15–2, the facts of her conditioning were made clear to her. She was made especially aware of the part played by interoceptive stimuli.

The following are excerpts from a transcript of the third treatment session:

> I would like to repeat some of the reasons for the attacks you have had. First, there was the incident of your mother's stroke fixed in

your mind. Certainly, it was a horrible experience for a woman who previously had led a very active life to become a semi-invalid. When you developed your head and neck pain, you instinctively had fears of also suffering a stroke; so that every time you felt pain there afterwards, you automatically became frightened. Your heart would beat rapidly; you would experience difficulty in breathing, and you would have a feeling of impending doom.

To complicate the situation further, the fact that your very first attack occurred while you were seated in a restaurant and had something in your hand that you tried to bring up to your mouth, provided you with signals that would come into play each time you were seated in a restaurant. Similar situations also became signals so that attacks would also occur when you were seated at other places, including your own kitchen, and at work, and when bringing other objects to your lips, such as lipstick.

We realize that there was no real threat to your health or your well being, or any danger of a stroke. Nevertheless, your brain had become conditioned to respond to these stimuli as if to the development of a stroke, and you came to respond instinctively in this anxious manner.

Your problem will be solved when you are able to relax, to feel calm and unafraid even when you are sitting down with discomfort in the back of your head or neck, doing such things as applying cosmetics. And so we will rehearse these activities in the manner of a calm, relaxed person. When you are able to rehearse and experience these events in this manner, which I will describe to you, you will find that these responses transfer to the real life situation. I want you to understand and accept this completely with no doubt in your mind whatever.

Now I am going to describe a series of scenes to you. Please listen carefully while I describe a scene, but do not attempt to visualize it until I have given you the signal by counting to three. Then visualize the scene as I have described it. Indicate that visualization is taking place by raising your index finger and drop it only when the visualization has ended. It is important that you visualize each scene exactly as I describe it, but free of any fear or anxiety and in a calm, relaxed state.

First I would like you to visualize that you are sitting down to eat in your own kitchen. You have prepared a delicious-looking filet mignon and you are quite hungry. As you sit eating the meat, you feel quite comfortable and relaxed, and it is such a wonderful feeling to enjoy the food and feel relaxed. You are really not worried or concerned. You do have a feeling of some pain and discomfort at the back of your head and neck, but in spite of this you feel good. It is such a wonderful feeling to sit there feeling relaxed and enjoying the

food. When I count to three, you may begin to visualize the scene
and indicate this to me by raising the index finger of your left hand
and keep it elevated until visualization is completed . . . One, two,
three.

As long as the patient indicated satisfactory visualization, the
description was periodically augmented. Additional scenes were
then offered—applying cosmetics, being seated while at work, eating at other people's homes, eating in restaurants, and other situations which would ordinarily provoke anxiety. The manner in
which the patient was "prepared" to accept the therapist's suggestions is indicated by the following excerpt dealing with visiting
the beauty shop.

> "You are at the hairdresser's. You are familiar with the place and
> you enter feeling very comfortable and relaxed. I know that when I
> go to the barber shop, it is an opportunity for me to relax, and fre-
> quently I almost doze off. Sometimes, because of the position I am
> in, I develop some pain and discomfort in my head and neck. How-
> ever, it doesn't disturb or frighten me. I am relaxed, and that is ex-
> actly the way I want you to feel. So when I give you the signal, I
> want you to picture yourself in the beauty shop feeling very com-
> fortable and relaxed. You have some discomfort in the back of your
> head and neck, but it doesn't worry you. You realize that it has no
> significance. It certainly does not indicate that you are going to have
> a stroke, and so when I count to three, please start to visualize the
> situation, remaining calm and relaxed."

In a total of four sessions, the patient improved so markedly
that she was able to return to work. The other situations that
provoked anxiety were also less disturbing. A follow-up nine
months later revealed that the improvement had been maintained.

RESULTS

Table 15–I summarizes the results of treatment of forty patients during the past eighteen months. A few cases that could
not be followed up are excluded. The results are given on a four
point scale based on the reports of the patients and my own observations:

1) Complete relief from maladaptive responding.
2) Marked improvement with only occasional maladaptive
responding.

3) Some improvement but with a moderate amount of mal-adaptive responding.

4) No change.

Relatively few therapeutic sessions were required as a rule. This was especially true of the sexual dysfunctions. In most cases where marked improvement was obtained, treatment was terminated by mutual agreement of the patient and therapist when the patient could function with little or no distress, and it was felt that life itself would afford further improvement.

The number of sessions required ranged from one to fifty. The mean was 7.5 and the median 4. Twenty-six of the forty cases had five or less sessions. Fourteen cases were phobic, fourteen had interpersonal anxieties, nine suffered from sexual dysfunction, and three others had diagnoses of depression, hysteria and obsessional neurosis.

DISCUSSION

If we isolate the factors involved in the technique, we find it includes relaxation, manipulation of imagery, role enactment, directly suggested changes in affect, and changes in attention or inattention.

The strategy involved in applying these factors to the method requires strict adherence to the principle of "Reciprocal Inhibition." The scenes suggested for imagery and role playing must be designed to pair previously anxiety-provoking stimuli with non-

TABLE 15–I

RESULTS FROM THERAPY ON A SCALE OF 1–4

	N	Complete relief from maladaptive responding	Marked improvement	Some improvement	No change
Phobias	14		12	1	1
Interpersonal anxieties	14	1	10	3	
Sexual dysfunction	9	4	2	3	
Depression	1				1
Conversion Hysteria	1	1			
Obsessive-Compulsive	1		1		

anxious responses. The use of hypnosis appears to facilitate all of these factors so as to effect behavioral change more readily. Hilgard (1965) lists seven characteristics shown by subjects demonstrating a high degree of susceptibility to hypnosis. Included among these are six characteristics whose relationship to the technique is readily apparent; subsidence of the planning function, redistribution of attention, heightened ability for fantasy production, increased suggestibility, increased role behavior, and a tolerance for reality distortion.

Subsidence of the planning function permits the patient to turn this function over to the hypnotist willingly and comfortably. Redistribution of attention allows greater attention to be directed towards stimuli apt to result in adaptive responses and inattention to those stimuli which elicit anxious responses. In commenting on the effect of hypnosis on imagery and fantasy, Hilgard states "the arousal of visual memories and the play of visual imagination appear to be more vivid than in the usual waking state." An example of reality distortion might be the suggestion to a patient with a public speaking phobia that he feels relaxed while speaking, and his audience is markedly impressed by his speech. Increased suggestibility is probably the most widely accepted characteristic of hypnosis. There appears to be a continuum between the acceptance of suggestions in the induction process and their acceptance in the hypnotic state. The characteristic of increased role behavior enables the patient to become so deeply involved in enacting the suggested roles that he behaves as if he were actually living it.

Sheehan (1972) speaks of imagined events serving an "as if" function. Under the direction of the hypnotist, they enable the subject to react to suggestions as if they were literally true. Bowers and Bowers (1972) assembled extensive evidence pointing to the conclusion that hypnosis leads to a rise in fantasy or suggestibility. Other studies which have demonstrated that imagery is more vivid in hypnosis than under non-hypnotic conditions include those of Rossi, Sturrock, and Solomen (1963), and Stross and Shevrin (1962). Blum (1972) has shown on the basis of extensive experimentation that subjects can be trained to experience various degrees of pleasure and anxiety while in a hypnotic state.

Personal experience has shown that attention must be paid to several factors if the technique is to be utilized most beneficially. First, the behavioral analysis must be thoroughly and skillfully developed so that the specific stimuli concerned are dealt with. Second, extraneous stimuli may be added to the scene if it increases the likelihood of inhibiting the anxiety responses. Third, anxiety must be prevented during visualization by direct interdiction. Some diminution in anxiety seems to be accomplished by asking the patient to delay any visualization during the verbal description until the pairing of anxiety-provoking stimuli with non-anxious responses has been completed. As Bendura (1969) has pointed out, "In the extinction of avoidance behavior, absence of expected adverse consequences provides a powerful source of reinforcement for completing responses." Fourth, inhibitory and calming suggestions must be directed against autonomic responses which have the ability to elicit further anxiety responses. Reinforcement of new responses is probably brought about by the therapist's enthusiastic display of approval whenever the patient shows evidence of performing as suggested.

REFERENCES

Bandura, A.: *Principles of Behavior Modification.* New York, Holt, Rinehart and Winston, 1969.

Barrios, A. A.: *A Theory of Hypnosis: An Explanation of Hypnotic Induction, Hypnotic Phenomena and Post-Hypnotic Suggestion.* (Mimeograph), Los Angeles, University of California, 1966.

Barrios, A. A.: Hypnotherapy: A reappraisal. *Psychotherapy,* 7:2–7, 1970.

Bridger, W. H., and Mandel, I. J.: A comparison of GSR fear responses produced by threat and electric shock, *J. Psychiat Res,* 2:31–40, 1964.

Cautela, J. R.: Covert reinforcement. *Behav Ther,* 1:33–50, 1970.

Erickson, M. H.: *Hypnotic Psychotherapy.* New York Number. Med. Clin. North America, May, 1948, pp. 571.

Guthrie, E. R.: *The Psychology of Human Learning.* New York, Harper Brothers, 1965.

Hilgard, E. R.: *Hypnotic Susceptibility.* New York, Harcourt Brace and World, 1965.

Hussain, A.: *Behavior Therapy Using Hypnosis.* The Conditioning Therapies. New York, Holt, Rinehart, and Winston, 1966.

Paul, G. L.: Psychological effects of relaxation training and hypnotic suggestion. *J Abnorm Psychol,* 74:425–437, 1969.

Van Pelt, S. J.: *Secrets of Hypnotism.* Los Angeles, Wilshire, 1958.

Wolpe, J.: *Psychotherapy by Reciprocal Inhibition.* California, Stanford University Press, 1958.

Wolpe, J.: *The Practice of Behavior Therapy.* New York, Pergamon Press, 1969.

CHAPTER **16**

THE USE OF HYPNOSIS TO FACILITATE CONDITIONED RELAXATION RESPONSES: A REPORT OF THREE CASES*

FREDERICK J. TODD, PH.D.
ROBERT J. KELLY, PH.D.

INTRODUCTION

Three cases are presented in which hypnotic procedure was used to facilitate the substitution of relaxation for tension responses which had led to headaches in one case, drug taking in another, and insomnia in a third. The procedure provides conditions for vivid rehearsal along with strong suggestion for the initiation of the new response pattern.

HYPNOSIS HAS BEEN CONSIDERED a useful procedure in behavior therapy ever since Wolpe's use of it in his early application of systematic desensitization (Wolpe, 1958). Eysenck (1964, p. 285) has suggested that the integration of hypnosis with behavior therapy might be a most worthwhile development. Nevertheless, this potentially valuable aid has been overlooked in situations where it might have been of service. Although we do not use hypnosis routinely in behavior therapy, we have encountered several cases in which it seems that hypnosis has facilitated the application and increased the effectiveness of the therapeutic procedures.

* Reprinted with permission from Frederick J. Todd, Ph.D. and Robert J Kelley, Ph.D., in J Behav Ther and Exp Psychiat, Volume 1, pages 295–298, 1970, Pergamon Press. Copyright 1970.

In the three cases presented briefly below, hypnosis was employed on the assumptions that (1) in the "trance" state the experimental aspects of the responses to be conditioned (e.g. relaxation, early tension signs, preparation for retiring) could be more vividly experienced and more intently focused on by the patient and (2) by means of post-hypnotic suggestion, the behaviors rehearsed in the office would acquire increased probability of occurrence when tried by the patient at home.

CASE HISTORIES

Case One

Mrs. K., a thirty-five-year-old housewife, had been troubled over a period of about four years with almost daily headaches which had become progressively more severe in the three months preceding treatment. She sought help from behavior therapy after a thorough medical check-up which resulted in the diagnosis of "tension headache." In the initial interview it was explained to her how deep muscle relaxation was to be used in an attempt to alleviate the headaches. She was instructed to keep a record of the times of occurrence of the headaches, the situations in which they occurred, and the physiological or psychological sensations which preceded them. Training in deep muscle relaxation was then begun, using a modified Jacobson technique.

For the next four weeks Mrs. K was seen twice a week during which time she learned to relax profoundly and experienced some success aborting headaches by lying down and relaxing at the first signs of their approach. She complained, however, that it was sometimes inconvenient for her to lie down, and she was not always able to intercept the beginning headache soon enough. Since it appeared that Mrs. K could abort some headaches by relaxing deeply, it was planned to attempt, in a series of steps, to condition relaxation to the covert command "Relax" in a manner similar to that described by Cautela (1966) and, if possible, to bring about the condition in which relaxation rather than headache became a response to the early sensations preceding headache. At this point the hypnotic procedure was called upon.

A fairly deep "trance" was induced by the eye-fixation method, and Mrs. K was directed to relax and to focus her attention on the sensations she associated with relaxation, e.g. heaviness, warmth, calmness. While attending to these sensations she was instructed to think to herself "I am relaxed." After the procedure was repeated several times, she was directed to "experience" herself walking into a room, sitting down in a chair, taking a deep breath, then exhaling while thinking "relax," letting all the muscles go limp and noting the positive sensations accompanying relaxation. This sequence was suggested seven times. While deeply relaxed Mrs. K was told, "After you wake from the trance we will have you practice relaxing to your own command 'relax.' You will take a deep breath, and when I say 'relax' you will think 'relax,' exhale, and relax *just as you are now, just as you are now.*" Carrying out this procedure put Mrs. K in a "trance" again. Once more the sensations accompanying relaxation were pointed out and it was suggested to Mrs. K that whenever she told herself to relax in the manner we had just practiced she would relax very well. She was brought out of the "trance" and told to practice the routine five times a day. She was advised that if she found she could relax quite well during her practice trials she could attempt to prevent a headache from developing by employing the procedure at the very first signs of a headache. If she could not abort a headache by this means she was to continue practicing the procedure but was not to make further attempts to use it for headache. Her usual method of lying down and relaxing completely was to be continued instead.

At her appointment four days later Mrs. K happily reported that she had had but two beginning headaches both of which she had stopped by sitting down, exhaling, and thinking "relax." She was hypnotized again and asked to focus on the sensations accompanying relaxation. Then it was suggested that she was experiencing the early signs of headache onset, e.g. tension in stomach, tightness in shoulders and neck, tightness in eyes. When she began to experience them clearly she was asked to raise her forefinger. At that moment she was instructed to think "relax," let her body go limp, let tension fade away, and notice the feeling of calm. She indicated when she felt completely relaxed by again raising her forefinger. This procedure was repeated eight times with the patient experiencing herself sitting, standing, and reclining in a number of different settings. She was given the suggestion that when she stopped whatever she was doing for a moment and thought "relax" she would feel the easing of tension and would experience a feeling of calm.

Following her emergence from the trance she was instructed to practice thinking "relax" and letting herself go limp for a moment in so far as possible while sitting, standing or reclining. She was told she might also try out the procedure at the beginning signs of headache, but to make a second attempt only if the first was successful. Otherwise she was to return to the procedure of sitting down, exhaling and going limp while thinking "relax."

When she returned in three days Mrs. K claimed she could relax by stopping what she was doing for a moment and thinking "relax." She was not certain whether she had aborted a headache this way or not although she thought she had detected early signs of headache onset once prior to relaxing in the prescribed manner. She was seen two more times at weekly intervals at which times the procedure described for the last session above was essentially repeated. She reported on the final occasion that she could successfully abort headaches in that manner.

On follow-up one month after her last appointment, Mrs. K said she could still abort headaches by stopping and thinking "relax" if she caught them soon enough. However, she said she had had only three actual headaches during that period, and they were not severe compared with her almost daily headaches before treatment. At a three-month follow-up she said she no longer considered headache a problem. She had them infrequently, perhaps once or twice a month, and they were easily aborted. Her reports at six months and a year were the same.

It is worth noting that not only did the patient become able to abort headaches, but the headaches themselves became much less frequent. This result would be expected if some component of relaxation had been substituted for the responses subserving headache.

Subsequently, the authors treated a second headache case in a similar manner with similar results.

Case Two

Mrs. R, a forty-nine-year-old physician's wife, had suffered for six years from intractible stomach pains for which no organic basis could be found. For relief from the pain she gave herself injections of Demerol®. As a result of treatment by deep muscle relaxation and systematic desensitization the pains diminished greatly both in frequency and intensity; the infrequent mild attacks which did occur were easily aborted. Nevertheless, she discovered that she could not get to sleep at night without her usual injection of Demerol. For treatment of this problem the authors carried out the following program in which the hypnotic procedure was used.

From Mrs. R a detailed account was obtained of her activities from the moment she decided to go to bed until she actually lay down. An appointment was made for her at 7:00 in the evening, at which time she was hypnotized and instructed to relax. It was then suggested that she was preparing to go to bed. Each step of her bedtime routine was described to her along with the suggestion that she was becoming more and more relaxed, drowsier and drowsier, until she lay down and fell asleep, sleeping through the night until awakened by the alarm. In this sequence of events, however, the step of taking the Demerol was omitted. The routine of preparing for bed was repeated eight times with the step of taking the drug omitted each time. Then Mrs. R was given the suggestion that when she did prepare for bed that night she would experience the relaxation and drowsiness and would fall asleep just as she had in the trance, sleeping until awakened by the alarm. When awakened from the trance, Mrs. R was instructed to imagine becoming progressively more relaxed and drowsy as she prepared for bed that night and to omit taking the drug. Telephoning the next day, as she had been requested to do, she reported she had fallen asleep with no difficulty and had slept through the night without taking the Demerol.

The hypnotic procedure was repeated again the next evening,

and when Mrs. R called and again reported success for this second attempt, she was instructed to try it on her own, imagining increasing drowsiness and relaxation as she prepared for bed. The next day she reported success without the hypnotic procedure. She was advised to continue the program and to report back in a week unless she experienced some difficulty before then. When seen a week later, she reported continued success. Follow-up of 3 months, 6 months and a year revealed no return to the Demerol and no particular difficulty in sleeping.

The focus here was on having the patient alter her previous response pattern at bedtime by substituting relaxation for the previous Demerol-taking response. The hypnotic procedure was used to raise the probability of the new response by rehearsing the new pattern in a vivid and intense way and having the patient experience the relaxation. It was hypothesized that relaxation might serve as a reinforcer for the new pattern as well as a response which would compete with the Demerol-taking for producing sleep.

Case Three

Two months after beginning behavior therapy for a number of problems which were treated by systematic desensitization, assertive training and operant self-control procedures, Mrs. B, a thirty-two-year-old graduate student, gave birth to her third child. This event added to the already large number of situational pressures which had developed over the past six months. Feeling exhausted most of the time, Mrs. B had little difficulty in falling asleep at night; but once having awakened for her new child's three o'clock feeding, she found it impossible to get back to sleep even though she tried to relax. Sleeping pills, she said, made her feel groggy the next morning and unable to function efficiently during her morning classes. On the other hand, she feared her lack of sleep was leading to a collapse.

Details of the three o'clock feeding were obtained from Mrs. B and then in a "hypnotic trance" she was asked to imagine putting the baby in its crib and going back to bed. Simultaneously with her experiencing the return to bed, it was suggested that she was becoming progressively more relaxed and sleepy, falling asleep as her head sank into the pillow and she thought "relax." This sequence was repeated eight times while Mrs. B was hypnotized, and she was given the post-hypnotic suggestion that she would that night perform the behaviors as rehearsed. She called the next morning with the information that she had immediately fallen asleep after returning to bed following the early morning feeding and had slept until the alarm went off at 6:30. She was told over the telephone to repeat the procedure of imagining getting sleepier and more relaxed following the three o'clock feeding on this and subsequent nights. At her regular appointment a week later she claimed she was experiencing no difficulty with sleeping nor did she have any sleeping problem during the following 3 months she continued in behavior therapy.

DISCUSSION

In each of the cases presented, the therapeutic task was seen as being to condition the cues which were initially associated with tension (resulting in headache or insomnia) to responses associated with relaxation. The hypnotic procedure was employed only after the patient had been trained in relaxation. (For each of the three patients presented, formal training in relaxation took up part of at least eight sessions with daily practice between appointments.) However, the patients reported that the experiences of relaxation, e.g. heaviness, warmth, calmness, were more vivid in the "trance" state than in the usual non-trance relaxed state. Other experiences such as headache onset, preparing to retire, and drowsiness were likewise described as being more vivid in the trance state than when simply imagined. These effects of the hypnotic procedure recommended it to the authors who reasoned that the more vivid the experiences were in the conditioning procedure, the greater the likelihood that the corresponding stimuli and responses of the actual situation would be conditioned. Also the more intensely the patients could focus on the stimuli and responses the more efficient conditioning would be. In addition, the device of post-hypnotic suggestion appealed to the authors as a possible means of increasing the likelihood that success would attend the patient's first attempts to apply the hypnotically rehearsed procedures in the life situation.

In the cases presented, the consequences of the combined relaxation-hypnosis procedure were highly gratifying. Nevertheless, the question remains whether the hypnotic suggestion would have been as effective without the prior training in relaxation. Having used hypnosis and relaxation separately, the authors believe that the combination enhanced the results. However, controlled studies are needed on the model advanced by Paul (1969).

REFERENCES

Cautela, J. R.: A behavior therapy approach to pervasive anxiety. *Behav Res Ther*, 4:99–109, 1966.

Eysenck, H. J.: *Experiment in Behavior Therapy*. New York, Pergamon Press, 1964.

Paul, G. L.: Physiological effects of relaxation training and hypnotic suggestion. *J Abnorm Psychol*, 4:425–437, 1969.

Wolpe, J.: *Psychotherapy by Reciprocal Inhibition*. Stanford, Stanford University Press, 1959.

CHAPTER 17

TREATMENT OF A SEVERE PHOBIA FOR BIRDS BY HYPNOSIS*

DAVID L. SCOTT, M.R.C.S., L.R.C.P., D.A., F.F.A.R.C.S.I.

INTRODUCTION

A case of a severe phobia for birds is presented together with a progress report one year after the commencement of treatment. The method of treatment is discussed in detail and conclusions are drawn from mistakes made by the author. The advantages of using hypnosis in such cases as well as points of general advice are summarised.

P HOBIAS ARE probably more prevalent and varied in their nature than many doctors imagine. The New Gould Medical Dictionary defines some 275 phobias by name, and even that extensive list does not include a phobia for birds.

Many of these only affect the patient slightly and are under adequate control. In other instances, as in the case to be described, the phobia has become a real disability, affecting not only the patient but also her immediate relatives and close friends. Many such patients are informed by their doctors that nothing can be done and that they will just have to "live with it." Other advice may include the suggestion to "pull yourself together;" but no amount of willpower will diminish an established phobia.

The general features of phobias are as follows:

* Originally published in *The American Journal of Clinical Hypnosis*, Volume 12, Number 3, January 1970, pages 146–149. Copyright 1970 by the American Society of Clinical Hypnosis.

1. They generally occur in otherwise well-integrated individuals.
2. Some degree of anxiety is usually present.
3. There may be an obvious aetiological event(s), but sometimes there is nothing to account for the phobia.
4. The phobia can finally become a "way of life," **not** only for the sufferer, but also for his or her next of kin.

Case History

A married hospital theatre sister,* aged twenty-seven (born November 1942). She has no family, and is quite happy both in her home and at work. She gave a history of extreme fear of birds all her known life, which had extended to include other flying things (insects, moths), and especially fluttering wings. Even feathers lying on the ground caused fear and she was unable to walk past them. She was more afraid when her arms were bare.

She had no memory of the cause, but her mother had told her that when she was four or five years old, a hen pinned her against the wall in her back garden. Prior to treatment her *only memory* was seeing a hen with its wings flapping (post mortem) under the stairs in her home.

This fear was so great that she could not walk down the street, if there was a single sparrow on the other side. She used to scan the sky for birds whenever she left a building. It once took her over an hour to cover the short six to seven minute journey home from the hospital, owing to the presence of small birds in the road; this followed a long day's work with overtime and in the rain!

Outline of the Method of Treatment

Treatment was commenced during July, 1968. The patient was rapidly conditioned and became a deep trance subject. When age regressed she exhibited total amnesia for all events subsequent to the regressed period (i.e. "true" age regression.). The following methods of treatment were used:

1. General relaxation and relief of anxiety.

* Not at Whiston Hospital, where the author works.

2. Ego strengthening—originally advocated by Emil Coué (1857–1926) and now advocated by Dr. John Hartland.
3. Age regression in order to:
   a. Check details of her past history.
   b. Abreact the different situations revealed.
4. Psychic desensitization under hypnosis, using a hierarchy of situations.
5. Auto-hypnosis, which she used for general relaxation.

Age regression confirmed her mother's story. The patient's grandfather kept a few hens in the back garden (regressed patient says: "There were hundreds."). When she was five years old, a white hen flew up at her and pinned her against the wall. She recalls that it was on a Wednesday (early closing day in Liverpool), that she had a short-sleeved blue dress on, and that she screamed for her mother. Her grandfather maintained that she had teased this hen; her uncle killed it and hung it up in the cupboard under the stairs, but unfortunately the grandfather asked her to put a penny in the gas meter, which was situated in the same cupboard. The fright of seeing this white hen hanging there in a pitch dark cupboard with its wings flapping was the one and only memory she had. This story agreed with that given to her by her mother and seemed to the author to be adequate as a cause for her phobia. The scene was abreacted at each session, her anxiety for this gradually diminished. Her conscious mind recalled each item, one at a time. A "block" was created so that conscious memory of events would not occur until she was ready.

The patient did not, however, improve adequately and the story seemed too much like a textbook description. I decided, therefore, to regress her to an age *prior* to the hen incident and ask her what she thought of birds (then). "Don't like them," came the reply. It was thus obvious that at least one other event had occurred, and this was traced in one session as follows:

1. Exit speedometer technique gave the number 1945. She was three years old in November, 1945.
2. Theatre visualization showed an old lady in a long dress and a large white bird on a stage.
3. The jigsaw puzzle technique revealed a similar picture to theatre visualization, with the addition of a large yellow egg.

This was Mother Goose and the Golden Egg. The patient was then regressed to the Christmas, 1945 period, and there she was at the pantomine, sitting hemmed in on the front row of the dress circle staring at this huge bird which was "going to fly at her." When regressed to this age and scene, she can never believe that this "bird" was a man dressed up as a bird ("He couldn't be a man—he was flapping his wings."). No amount of "sensible" talk at this age level will convince her otherwise; this is indeed "true" age regression.

It was felt that this was still not the full story, so a more careful and detailed history was taken. The history revealed that when the patient was very small her mother had been ill off and on and her elder sister had played a big part in her up-bringing. This sister, thirteen years her senior, has today a mild fear of birds which is now quite under control. It is highly probable that over twenty-five years ago this fear was greater and that it was imparted, probably non-verbally, to the patient at a very early age.

Hierarchy

The patient originally wrote out the following fear hierarchy:
1. Can tolerate a sparrow out in the open from a distance.
2. Just tolerate small birds in a secure cage (in practice, this was at a distance).
3. Not too bad with a bird on the outside of a closed window, myself being in the room.
4. Could not tolerate a larger bird on the sill outside a closed window—with me on the inside.
5. Apprehensive with the window open and a small bird on the sill.
6. Bird bigger than a sparrow on edge of pavement (would cross the road).
7. Moth flying in room (would leave the room).
8. Birds at Pier Head, Liverpool; e.g., seagulls.
9. Beach with seagulls and pigeons.
10. Could not tolerate any bird free in a room.

It soon became clear that even this hierarchy would have to be subdivided and detailed; e.g., the size of the room defined, as well as the patient's position relative to the bird cage. She was able to try out situations at her sister's home where there were two budgies in a cage. Later on positive feelings towards birds were incorporated, such as feeding them through the cage, changing the water.

Whenever stress was noted (by ideomotor finger signalling) a peaceful scene to which she had been conditioned was reverted to (in this case, one of being in a wood).

Progress of Treatment

The author felt that she had improved enough by the end of last year (1969) to discontinue actual hypnotic treatment. Since then she has been left to improve herself at her own pace. "Bird situations," of course, happen, rather than are planned. The author feels that the progress of treatment can have a modern simile—it seems rather like a moon rocket. Initial hypnosis and conditioning are like the big first stage; desensitization and ego-strengthening like the second stage, and then a very slight "puff" seems all that is required for the rocket to continue its preset course. This patient is now slowly improving herself over the months without any additional help from me.

Present Status (July 1969, i.e., one year after commencing treatment)

She is now not worried at all by any birds in cages; she no longer crosses the road to avoid them; and if one gets too close, she can scare it away. She would not leave a room when a moth flew in, but could not be in a room with a bird flying about (she feels that lots of people not normally worried by birds feel this way, and the author concurs with this view).

Positive thinking and action are seen in the fact that she now uses a feather duster at home, that she puts crumbs out in her back garden for the birds, and that she has fed ducks in the open as well as her sister's budgies (but she would not open the cage). She is still more afraid when her arms are bare.

Her phobia is no longer a disability, and she feels that she is no longer making a fool of herself. This is as far as I have aimed treatment to progress.

Incidental Other Uses

When she informed me that she had an appointment for conservative dental work, I taught her how to produce dental analgesia. She has now used this as the sole means of analgesia for eight fillings, some of which have been deep re-fillings. The dentist concerned has had no experience with hypnosis.

Early during treatment, she spontaneously stopped biting her nails, but this has recurred. I have not tried to stop this as it seems a safety valve to her emotional make-up, and staff shortages have made theatre work hectic in recent months.

Summary of Advantages of Using Hypnosis in Treating Phobias

1. It is probably the quickest method.
2. The situations created are far more vivid and realistic under hypnosis than when the patient just uses his or her imagination.
3. Relaxation is superior.
4. Reassurance can be more readily accepted.
5. By using auto-hypnosis the patient can learn to relax completely at home and thus gain much more self confidence.
6. There is the opportunity to make a fresh psychotherapeutic reassessment under hypnosis, if this is indicated.

Points to be Learned from This Case History

1. One should never decide in advance the cause of any illness. The author unfortunately jumped to the conclusion that the patient's mother's story was the only one, as it tallied so well with the details obtained by age regression and the case history.
2. The original case history should be constantly referred to during treatment, and may have to be re-checked for completeness at any stage.
3. A severe persistent phobia is probably the result of more than one traumatic episode. Check this by:
4. Age regression to a period prior to this episode, and determine the patient's reaction at this regressed age.

5. Abreactions should be repeated until their details are known to and accepted by the conscious mind without causing any mental trauma (the conscious mind should be "blocked" to protect it). After this stage has been reached, there is no point in continuing these abreactions.
6. The patient's original written hierarchy will probably have to be subdivided and modified to obtain an adequate gradation of traumatic situations. It may be advantageous later on to incorporate situations that the patient had not originally thought of; for example, in the case described the positive thought of feeding birds. Prior to this, the patient had always felt and said: "They could all die from starvation as far as I was concerned."
7. Let the patient set the pace of progress. A phobia of many years duration can take many months to diminish.

Follow-up status October 1974

The printing of this book has given the author the opportunity to assess this patient's progress after the cessation of hypnotherapy, which has not been given for over five years. She feels that this "levelled out" some two years ago. Feather pillows and dusters no longer worry her, but "bird situations" still can. These she divides into two categories:

1. Situations in which she has a choice of action.
2. Situations in which there is no choice of action.

In the former, she now usually takes what she calls "the easy way out." In this respect she feels that she has slipped back a little. Three to four years ago she would have tried to overcome such a challenge.

In the second group, where she has no choice, the effects of treatment still remain with her. She gave the following example from the day before my 'phone call to her from which this report is taken.

She had to walk down a one-way street to meet her husband who was in the family car at the "wrong" end of the street. Her way was "blocked" by some 8–10 pigeons. Under such circumstances she is still able to overcome her fear and she passed the pigeons. She still uses Calvert Stein's hand clenching technique to give her increased confidence; it is interesting that over the years the effect of this has not waned.

She can now go to a zoo, where caged birds no longer cause her anxiety. She would not, however, enter an enclosed area with free flying birds (e.g. humming birds), nor would she pass a chained bird on a perch, such as a falcon or parrot. This she regards as a reasonably normal response.

The sister who had the two budgies in a cage has unfortunately died. This patient took over looking after her deceased sister's children and has now adopted them. She gave the budgies away, however.

The writer's opinion is that the original object in treatment of restoring a reasonably normal manner of living for this individual, of elimination of the more serious elements in her severe phobia, and of creating a self-dependence which would last over the years, has been achieved. Maybe continued hypnotherapy would have secured a far more dramatic result; maybe it would have resulted in increasing dependence upon the therapist! The final conclusion to be drawn is for the doctor to be content with a reasonable result and not be overambitious. Hypnotherapeutic aims should never become stunts.

REFERENCES

Coué, E.: *Better and Better Every Day*. London, George Allen and Unwin, 1960.

Hartland, J.: The value of "ego-strengthening" procedures prior to direct symptom removal under hypnosis. *Am J Clin Hypn*, 8:89, 1965.

Stein, C.: The clenched fist technique as a hypnotic procedure in clinical hypnotherapy. *Am J Clin Hypn*, 6:113, 1963.

CHAPTER 18

HYPNOSIS AS VERBAL PRO-GRAMMING IN EDUCATIONAL THERAPY*

Stanley Krippner, Ph.D.

INTRODUCTION

THE HYPNOTIC TRANCE is generally defined as a state of con-sciousness that is characterized by a heightened responsive-ness to direct suggestion. Because suggestion is a frequent con-comitant of the teaching process, it is likely that many educators have, without knowing it, used some form of hypnosis in many of their most successful pedagogical efforts. Classroom teachers use hypnotic principles when they attempt to relax their pupils before embarking on a difficult assignment. High school athletic coaches who motivate their teams by delivering "pep talks" are capitalizing on another form of hypnosis. College instructors who capture their students' attention by the use of colorful language and visual aids are utilizing another hypnotic tech-nique. Hypnosis, in one form or another, has long been used as an educational tool.

However, during the past decade, hypnosis has become more widely used in such professional fields as surgery, dentistry, ob-stetrics, and psychotherapy. In these areas, hypnosis has been more deliberately implemented than it has in education. It is possible that hypnosis could be put to wider use by trained pro-fessionals in educational settings as well.

Over the past fifteen years, my work with elementary school pupils, secondary school students, and college students has dem-

* Originally published in *Academic Therapy*, Volume VII, No. 1, Fall 1971, pages 5–12.

onstrated three areas in which hypnosis has potential for aiding education: in the improvement of study habits, the reformation of test-taking behavior, and the strengthening of academic motivation. Bernard Aaronson has described hypnosis as a form of "programing" (1969) and I believe that this perspective has pertinent implications to education. Thus, I have designed a verbal programing approach for use in educational therapy. Following my initial work with hypnosis, I noted that only a light hypnotic trance needs to be induced for positive change to take place in these three academic areas; present evidence indicates that most of the student population is able to enter a trance of this depth.

After determining whether it is wise to use hypnosis with a particular student, and after deciding what areas of academic behavior can be helped by hypnosis, I assist the student in entering a hypnotic trance. The most effective screening procedures in my experience have been the *Minnesota Multiphasic Personality Inventory* and the *Brown-Holtzman Survey of Study Habits and Attitudes* (see References). Similar procedures are also followed by a number of my colleagues, among whom are Leo Wollman, Cecelia Pollack, and Leslie LeCron, who have utilized hypnosis for educational purposes for a number of years.

The student is first asked to fix his attention upon a specific stimulus such as the hypnotist's right eye, the stone in the center of a ring, or a colored spot attached to the ceiling of the room. The hypnotist makes several comments to encourage relaxation on the part of the student. Hypnotic induction then proceeds according to one of several possible methods. The student often is asked to indicate, by some ideomotor response (raising a finger, for example), when he feels ready to receive a suggestion.

If the student is able to perform a simple posthypnotic suggestion, it is assumed that he can be given another suggestion that might in some way improve his reading and studying behavior. Sometimes only one session is needed to help the student attain a trance that is profound enough for the performance of a post-hypnotic suggestion (such as becoming glued to the chair whenever the hypnotist pronounces the student's name). Sometimes two or more sessions are needed to enable a student to react in this manner.

Some students will not react to a posthypnotic suggestion, even after several sessions. In these instances, no work should be done to alleviate the student's study problems by hypnotic suggestion. For those students who do respond favorably, a number of positive results often take place.

STUDY HABITS

Robert is an example of a student whose concentration while studying was consistently blocked by a number of distractions. After studying for a few minutes, he would feel the need to open the window, to get a drink of water, or to visit the candy-vending machine. He would turn on the radio, turn on the record player, or remember that he had to make an urgent phone call. He claimed that it was impossible for him to concentrate on his studies for more than ten minutes before his thoughts would wander to other matters.

Robert was hypnotized several times in the course of a few weeks. One by one, the bad habits were replaced with other patterns of behavior. During posthypnotic suggestion he was told that he would ignore the room temperature while studying, that he would ignore his own sensations of thirst and hunger, that he would ignore the appeal of the radio, record player, and telephone. He was further told that his attention span would continuously increase. So successful were the suggestions that, by the end of three weeks, Robert was spending several consecutive hours on his studies each night without interruption.

Lee had a problem regarding classroom lectures. He had difficulty paying attention to the speaker and in concentrating on the material that was being presented. Lee wore a large ring, and he was told that, whenever his mind wandered, he merely had to rub the front of the ring to refocus his attention on the lecturer. This suggestion worked very well, and within a few weeks the new habit was so firmly installed that the ring-rubbing technique no longer had to be utilized.

When working with young children who have poor study habits, I often use the following statement:

> When you open your eyes, you and your clinician will select a story in a book that interests you. After looking it over for a few minutes to make certain that it is really interesting, you will start to

read the story. You will find that you are able to pay very close attention to the story. You will pay close attention for many, many minutes. It will be just as if your eyes are glued to the page. In fact, you will not want to take your eyes away from the story until you have read several pages. Perhaps you will even finish the whole story. When you have trouble with a word, your clinician will help you out. But this will not affect your attention, which will be very, very strong. At the same time, your concentration will be better than it has been for a long, long time. You will think about nothing but the characters in the story and what is happening to them. You will understand what you are reading. You might even see the characters in your mind's eye. You will enjoy what you are reading. Your concentration and attention will be so good today that you will find it even easier to concentrate and to pay attention tomorrow.

TEST-TAKING BEHAVIOR

Test anxiety is a phenomenon that frequently afflicts college students. Many individuals claim to be well prepared when they enter the examination situation, and then they find that they forget essential data, make minor errors, and allow nervous reactions to depress their test score. Hypnotic suggestions can be given to students to increase accuracy, reduce nervous tension, and improve recall.

I have often used hypnosis in an attempt to relax youngsters while they are studying for a test. For example, I often use this suggestion with elementary school pupils:

As you relax, you begin to stop worrying. You stop worrying about reading. You begin to think how much you would like to read better. You begin to think how much you would like to improve your reading ability. You know that you can read better if all the muscles of your body are relaxed. If all your muscles are relaxed, you will be able to pay closer attention to what you read. You want very much to relax all the little muscles in your eyes while you read. This will help you to read with your eyes wide open so that you will not miss any of the letters. If your eyes are wide open, you will not miss any of the words. If your eyes are wide open, you will read much, much better.

The references to vision reflect the finding that many disabled readers have poor visual skills and that in many of these cases, acute anxiety lies behind the blurred perception. In one remarkable case, a client attempted to recite the words on a basic word list and made seventeen errors out of twenty words. Under hypnosis, he was told that his second reading would be more successful because the eye muscles would relax. With his eye muscles relaxed, he would be able to read with his eyes "wide open" and would be able to see "all the letters in each word." The second reading produced only five errors, and a first reading of a different word list produced only seven errors out of twenty words.

College students who request therapy under hypnosis to improve their test-taking behavior are warned that several sessions are required. A student cannot report for hypnosis one night and realistically expect that it will help him on an examination the following day. Instead, suggestions are presented and developed over a period of several days or several weeks. Hypnotic suggestions are made regarding the interest a student will find in the subject matter. He is told to think of his long-range goals and to realize how important his academic record will be in the attainment of these goals. As might be suspected, those students without vocational goals or with little concern for the future have the most difficulty in benefiting from this type of hypnotic suggestion. Hypnosis, after all, does not implant new ideas into one's thought processes; it merely reinforces ideas that have been there all along. Hypnosis, therefore, is ineffective if there is nothing to reinforce.

Suggestions are also made that improve the student's ability to concentrate on crucial examination items. The student is told that no outside stimuli will distract him, that he will be paying such close attention to the test that nothing else will be of interest to him, unless an emergency situation arises, such as illness, or a fire. The hypnotist tries to keep the student from developing nervous symptoms and feelings of undue anxiety. A modicum of anxiety often helps to sharpen one's reactions during a test; more than that, however, hampers the effectiveness of the student. Therefore, he is told that his self-confidence will be very high as a result of his thorough preparation for the examination. Because his self-confidence is high, there will be no reason for him to develop fear reactions toward the test situation. He is told that he will approach the examination with an alert, but not anxious, attitude; he will be attentive, but not tense, while answering the examination questions.

At times, suggestions are also given to enable the student to sleep soundly the night before the test. He is discouraged from spending all night studying and is instructed to begin preparing for the examination well in advance so that the gambit of "all-night cramming" will not be necessary.

Harry, an engineering student, had an IQ of 138, but he was concerned because he was only receiving *B* grades. He felt that "examination panic" prevented him from doing well in a test situation. He also claimed that he made careless errors and that this depressed his grades. During the academic quarter, Harry was put in a hypnotic trance before he took several of his examinations. He was given suggestions designed to decrease his anxiety and fears, and other suggestions were given to improve his recall and memory in specific academic areas. For example, he was told that he could easily "revisualize" material that appeared in texts and "reauditorize" material from classroom lectures. For comparative purposes, he took alternate examinations without having previously entered a hypnotic trance. On the latter examinations, Harry made a *B* average during the quarter. On those examinations that he took following hypnosis, he received, without exception, *A* grades. He was later taught self-hypnosis, which enabled him to achieve the same effect without the aid of a hypnotist.

Carl claimed that he needed a high grade in a Spanish examination in order to pass the course. He was so anxious about the test that he had been unable to concentrate on the subject matter and had difficulty getting to sleep. Hypnotic sessions began one week before the scheduled test. The night before the examination, Carl was put into a light hypnotic trance and informed that he would spend the next several hours studying, that he would be studying so intently that he would not worry about the test itself, he would not talk to his roommate, and he would not leave his desk except to answer the telephone or go to the washroom. Furthermore, he was told that at midnight he would become very tired, would have a pleasant night's sleep, and would awaken at 7:30 A.M. He was told that he would feel that he was in excellent condition in the morning and that he would do well on his Spanish examination.

So well did the suggestions take effect that Carl refused to speak to anyone who entered his room that evening. He left his desk only once, and on his way to the washroom he was heard to mumble, "I must get back to that Spanish book." He later reported that he had adequately covered the material by 11:45. However, he said he was unable to close his book and reviewed the material again until 12:00. At this point, he felt very drowsy and went to bed. After a sound night's sleep he awoke refreshed, took the Spanish examination, and received a B. This was the highest grade he had ever received on a test in that subject.

ACADEMIC MOTIVATION

The difference between an excellent student and a poor student is often as much a matter of interest as it is of intelligence. A student with high persistence and strong motivation generally does well in his work. He prepares his assignments. He follows a schedule for study. He applies himself energetically. Often, what he lacks in mental ability he compensates for in his purposefulness. On the other hand, many bright students do poorly in college because they have little interest in the learning process and no strong motivation to succeed academically.

An interview with the student will often reveal that, in spite of his poor motivation, he has several reasons why he feels impelled to attend college. He will often state his vocational ambitions, his academic intentions, and his life-long goals. He knows why he is pursuing his education, but he is not acting with purpose. Under hypnosis, his motivation can be strengthened and reinforced so that he commits himself to his goals, feels strongly about them, and acts upon them.

Rosie is a student who seemed to be burdened with motivational problems. Although her high school record was excellent and her IQ was 125, she was having difficulties with her college work. She claimed that she could do well academically only if she liked a professor, enjoyed a course, and was "in the right mood" for studying. Rosie proved to be an adept student in learning self-hypnosis. Eventually, she was able to put herself in a light trance and tell herself that she would take a keen interest in an assignment. Using this method, she was able to follow her assignments through to completion; as a result, her academic record showed a marked improvement.

Walter felt little motivation toward the learning process. He knew that a college education was necessary for the attainment of his vocational objectives, but could not develop an interest in his coursework, even in business subjects, his major field. Walter's exact words regarding his long-range goals were repeated to him under hypnosis. Eventually, he was permitted to state these goals himself while in the hypnotic trance. Finally, he discussed his goals with the hypnotist while in hypnosis. The positive statements about career objectives were reinforced in this manner and gradually began to bring about a change in his academic performance. It can be seen in this and other cases that the student is encouraged to take an active part in the hypnotic process: success in hypnotic suggestion depends more on the student than on the hypnotist.

Guy had problems in motivation and in maintaining his academic persistence. He often fell asleep during class and while doing his homework. On several occasions he was able to enter the hypnotic trance, but he fell asleep while in the trance and no suggestions could effectively be introduced. In other words, he went from a *hypnotic sleep,* in which the individual is actually very much conscious of what is going on, to an *actual sleep,* in which he is not aware of what the hypnotist is attempting. During the few sessions in which Guy remained awake, he did not go into the trance deep enough for posthypnotic suggestions to be effective. Some months later, Guy's college career was terminated when he was found to be the producer of counterfeit drivers' licenses and falsified student identification cards.

Guy's case demonstrates that deep-seated drives toward college failure cannot be treated effectively by hypnotic suggestion unless they are preceded by personality change. In most cases, extensive psychotherapy would be required to bring about these changes. Although Guy's consciously-stated attitudes regarding college were positive, his unconscious motives toward failure and self-defeat were too strong to be easily contramanded. Hypnosis can be an efficient reinforcer of drives that are already present; however, it cannot reinforce a drive that is absent or that is considerably weaker than motives that oppose it within the personality.

What special qualifications must a professional person have to successfully utilize hypnosis in an educational setting? This is a crucial point because it is likely that the lack of trained personnel rather than the lack of student interest is a major factor among those that inhibit the development of this field. A sound knowledge of educational psychology as well as a solid background in hypnosis is necessary. The hypnotist must understand the psychological and physiological concomitants of such educational concerns as the improvement of reading skills and study habits. In addition, he should be a member of either the American Society of Clinical Hypnosis or the Society of Clinical and Experimental Hypnosis, which are national professional organizations for psychologists, psychiatrists, physicians, and dentists who use hypnosis in their work.

The use of hypnosis in education deserves wider application. For those students who are able to enter at least a light hypnotic trance, improvement may occur in such areas as studying course material, taking examinations, and committing oneself to long-range educational and vocational goals. Hypnosis is not a panacea. Further, it must be used in collaboration with other methods and techniques. However, it demands greater attention and utilization as the nation continues its task of developing to the maximum extent the talents and skills of all its young citizens.

REFERENCES

Aaronson, B. S.: The subject as programmer. *Am J Clin Hypn*, 11:245–252, 1969.

Brown, W. F., and Holtzman, W. H.: *Brown-Holtzman Survey of Study Habits And Attitudes.* New York, N. Y., The Psychological Corporation, 1956 (revised).

Hathaway, S. R., and McKinley, J. C.: *Minnesota Multiphasic Personality Inventory.* New York, N. Y., The Psychological Corporation, 1951 (revised).

CHAPTER **19**

HOMEWORK AND SELF-HYPNOSIS: THE CONDITION-ING THERAPIES IN CLINICAL PRACTICE*

Irwin Rothman, V.M.D., DO
M. Lynn Carroll, B.A., and
Frances D. Rothman, Ed.D

A GENERAL PROBLEM

MANY PSYCHOTHERAPISTS feel that there is insufficient time in one therapeutic session per week to produce and establish lasting attitudinal, emotional, and behavioral changes desired and needed by patients. Patients, too, can be discouraged and their resistance enhanced by their feelings of regression into unhealthy behavior patterns over the time between appointments. The lack of measurable or readily perceptible progress also tends to discourage them.

American psychiatrists and psychologists may hesitate to utilize behavior modification which involves classical and/or operant conditioning. This may be due to unfamiliarity with the extensive literature on conditioning, its seeming complexity, and a lack of awareness of the practical applications of the methods. Some reluctance may be due to the presentation of conditioning as a total therapy, exclusive of other techniques already being used by the therapist.

Familiarity with the literature on conditioning is, of course, advisable; and there are many sources available to clarify the

---

* Original manuscript.

principles to be used. (Consult the references following this paper as well as the voluminous literature now available.)

A COMBINED METHOD

Once an understanding of the basic principles of conditioning is established, the therapist becomes increasingly aware of the feasibility of using conditioning in conjunction with other therapeutic methods.

One combined approach encompasses hypnosis, self-hypnosis (or relaxation), and conditioning supported by "homework" steps suggested to the patient. This involves daily efforts on the part of the patient to achieve certain changes and provides a record for both patient and therapist to evaluate.

Advantages to the Therapist

The first advantage to the therapist in having a patient follow a daily homework program is that it is time-saving. Once the program is established, the therapist need not consume session time with details of what the patient needs to do. Instead, he can focus on those areas where are particularly difficult for the patient and so work towards faster progress.

Second, homework tends to increase a patient's motivation in therapy since there is considerable positive reinforcement for efforts made by seeing actual steps in progress. The patient's progress is also gratifying and reinforcing to the therapist.

Third, the use of homework frequently increases the insights often cognitively gained by the patient, who may develop self-insights outside of the therapeutic sessions. Homework also becomes an excellent tool for spotlighting and clearly delineating areas of resistance.

Fourth, the method is widely applicable and can be used in a variety of cases including stuttering, phobias, obesity, tics and torticollis, impotence and frigidity, and certain other types of obsessive, depressive, and anxiety symptoms.

Advantages to the Patient

Besides the therapeutic values previously discussed, there are additional benefits to the patient. First, the use of homework increases the amount of time spent in constructive effort. It is, therefore, an adjunct to office sessions and provides some tangible measurement of progress or indication of negative transference and resistance (in the analytic sense).

Second, homework can be substituted for self-destructive rumination by the patient about his problems.

Third, homework in easy successful steps increases patient participation in therapy; and progress made often bolsters self-confidence since the patient becomes more active and tends to feel less helpless.

Possible Disadvantages

There are relatively few disadvantages to the use of homework. One contraindication may be in the case of some schizoid patients whose imaginary visualization might constitute a danger. If the therapist feels that the self-hypnotic part of the homework might be threatening to such a patient, or would result in further withdrawal or dissociation, the time spent on this part of the routine can be strictly limited or even omitted altogether.

Second, a homework program may elicit strong resistances. This is particularly possible with those patients whose symptoms bring them strong secondary gains like attention, sympathy, or freedom from responsibility. In such cases, the patient may terminate treatment before improvement can reinforce the method.

Finally, the method may not be easy or initially effective with passive aggressive individuals who tend to fight direction. However, even with such patients, homework can be useful in helping them to become aware of their negativism and allowing them more constructive ways of working through their problems. With such patients the failure to do self-monitored homework is not criticized in treatment sessions; rather, it is explained in learning terms that the teacher (therapist) gave too much of an assignment, so an easier and more rewarding one is desirable.

OUTLINE OF THE METHOD

The first step is the induction of light to deep hypnosis, depending on the individual circumstances. The goals are improved relaxation and imagery. Next, the patient learns self-relaxation or hypnotic procedures. This is demonstrated, and rapidity of learning is enhanced by having the therapist induce the hypnotic state. Then a stepladder (hierarchy) of items suitable for desensitization (gradual exposure to and constructive handling of steps without fear or anxiety) is established. Next, a specific homework program including self-relaxation, visualization of the stepladder or hierarchy, and additional *in vivo* practices is described and demonstrated, preferably with simultaneous cassette tape recording, which the patient then utilizes at home for further reinforcement. Finally, positive rewards or reinforcements are established and recommended for use following each successful homework session.

REVIEW OF REFERENCES

The use of relaxation in psychotherapy will be familiar to those who use hypnotherapy. This author (1956) treated a group of stammerers with such a technique. Wolberg (1948) described a similar method. Kline (1955) mentioned the facilitation of conditioning through hypnotism. Kroger also quotes Platonov and Patterson's research indicating the greater durability of conditioned reflexes (desired behavior is taught and rewarded) established under hypnosis.

In some cases, particularly when a patient is too anxious to relax sufficiently to face his fears, an intravenous injection of a relaxant such as amobarbital is useful in inducing the hypnotic state and in helping the patient to make constructive *in vivo* efforts. This practice was described by the author in 1957. Wolpe (1958) also discussed the use of amphetamines and other medications in conjunction with conditioning.

AMPLIFICATION OF THE HOMEWORK METHOD

Self-hypnotic procedures can be taught to the patient by combining the method used in therapeutic sessions along with simple muscle relaxation and visualization exercises. The method chosen should be one which is quick and easy for the patient. Arm gravitation or eye-rollback are frequently used. The patient, once familiarized with the hypnotic method, is instructed to practice this technique for ten to fifteen minutes at least once daily and more often if necessary until he or she can attain a state of at least light hypnosis fairly quickly and with minimum effort.

Some individuals, although excellent hypnotic subjects, have great difficulty with, or resistance to learning, self-hypnosis. In many such cases, a simple alternative is for the therapist to make a tape recording of the hypnotic induction. Some or all of the steps of the hierarchy may also be included if deemed helpful. The patient is then instructed to play the tape daily in accordance with his homework program.

A hierarchy of steps is formulated with the patient relating to his problems. The steps start with a neutral or non-threatening scene and *gradually* lead up to those situations in which the person experiences severe anxiety. The individual is instructed to use the stepladder daily—to visualize, under hypnosis, successfully completing several steps. Actual *in vivo* efforts to try the steps are strongly encouraged.

The patient is usually advised to use self-hypnosis and positive self-imagery and visualization in increasing steps in place of self-defeating, negative rumination. Whenever possible, constructive action is encouraged.

A homework sheet is given to the patient to keep a daily record. This includes the date, number of self-hypnotic visualization practices, time spent on homework, how far the patient has been able to go successfully on the stepladder, and what constructive *in vivo* efforts he has made. All of this serves to provide daily continuation of the therapeutic process.

Positive reward (reinforcement) *must* be closely connected with the homework steps. All constructive efforts are warmly encouraged in office sessions. Along with verbal reinforcement, the importance of the individual crediting himself for positive action is stressed. Each patient is asked to rate preferred activities on a modified reward schedule based on the work of Cautela and Kastenbaum (1967). Ellis (1965) has also written on the utilization of reward and homework methods.

Once the reward schedule or schedules have been completed, a variety of reinforcing steps can be chosen. The patient is to follow up each constructive bit of effort with some enjoyed activity or fantasy. Rewards can vary and may include items such as watching a favorite television show, having a snack, seeing a movie, calling a friend or visualizing a two-minute pleasant scene. (See operant covert reinforcement list in Appendix.)

When the conditioning program of effort and reward is firmly established, further operant conditioning may be applied. For example, as progress is made, the patient may then reward himself only for constructive *in vivo* moves. Another variation is the use of a point system. In such a program, therapist and patient rate constructive moves to be made with a point value. Specified rewards are also given a point rating, and the patient is asked to compile the required number of points before giving himself that reward.

Aversive stimulation may also be used to extinguish undesirable and self-defeating behavior. *Self*-aversive conditioning may be done by the patient with the use of an inexpensive plastic card pack shocker or a shocking fountain pen operated by flashlight batteries. These readily available items give a mild but effective buzzing shock. The patient in such a case is to administer the shock to himself each time he acts or visualizes acting in a self-defeating way. Positive and desirable behavior is of course to be followed by reward, either real or fantasy. This is described by the senior author in Wolberg (1948).

SUPPLEMENTARY HOMEWORK

Additional homework is based on the individual and his problem. In cases of obesity, for example, homework includes a daily record of weighing in, all foods and beverages consumed, and when they are taken.

In these cases, aversive stimulation may be initiated by the covert association under hypnosis of something unpleasant such as castor oil with the foods the patient overeats. It is our own experience that these aversive methods are the last resort because, for difficult cases, the patient is often "aversed" out of treatment altogether! (Samples of reward schedules, homework sheets and specific hierarchies are included at the end of this chapter in the Appendix.)

CASE STUDIES

Case One: After undergoing ten years of intensive orthodox analysis, the wife of a surgeon feared going anywhere alone and was limited in range even when she was with someone else.

Hypnosis was used in office sessions and a hierarchy of phobic situations was established. The patient learned self-hypnosis and used it to reduce general anxiety and for desensitization with the hierarchy. These were incorporated with her daily homework program. After twelve office visits and use of daily homework, she was able to travel considerable distances with a companion.

The homework program was continued and, after approximately twelve visits, the patient was able to take a long train trip with someone meeting her at the terminal. This was particularly significant since the initial phobic reaction was precipitated on a train. Eventually, she was able to travel to Florida by plane, and therapy was gradually discontinued.

Case Two: A man troubled by heterosexual impotence was referred by a urologist. He was not strongly motivated to change but was concerned by his wife's intention to terminate the marriage. His early life history and castration fears were readily available to provide insight. However, this man's ego weakness, limited intellectual range, time limitations, and financial circumstances precluded insight therapy. Since he was able to achieve and maintain an erection only in homosexual activity or fantasy, aversive stimulation was used initially. The plastic card pack shocker was used whenever the patient visualized homosexual activities and fantasies. His own use of the aversive stimulus was continued daily in the homework program until he was unable to visualize homosexual scenes clearly and until such fantasies finally disappeared.

The next phase involved Wolpe's method of sexual desensitization *in vivo*, and the conditioning techniques based on Masters and Johnson's work (1970) were included. These steps encompassed a gradual range from pleasurable, non-sexual touching up to actual heterosexual intercourse. Homework for this patient was to try each of the steps until successful.

Although his wife was very inhibited and initially uncooperative, she agreed to try the homework program with him after she had seen a female psychologist working with us for a few sessions. Her participation in the homework was (a) to avoid critical or demanding behavior with her husband; and (b) to respond affectionately to his positive efforts and (c) to participate with him on the step-ladder process.

After relatively few visits, the man was able to have an erection and shortly afterwards the couple was able to engage in intercourse.

Case Three: One young woman was treated for severe, suicidal depression and more than borderline obsessive fears. She had had a history of therapeutic failure, including hospitalization with at least twelve electroconvulsive treatments and 1000 mgms of Thorazine® a day, and had been told that her case was "hopeless." Of her many phobias, the strongest was a fear of driving because she felt and believed that she was killing people. This woman was extremely non-assertive probably because of an over-protective and dominant mother. The single exception to her submissiveness was with her over-indulgent husband with whom she would fly into a rage. Conditioning to free her from her fears, realistic assertive training, and learning a non-destructive means of ventilating conscious and unconscious hostilities were needed.

The homework program included self-hypnosis for relaxation and visualization, a hierarchy of assertive moves including independence from the mother, and an additional hierarchy of steps in driving (e.g. looking at the car, sitting in it, starting it up, etc.) Aversive stimulation with a shocker was to be used initially to stop obsessive thoughts of killing.

One of the most important steps was to find a means of ventilation for this patient's considerable anger. Any expression of hostility resulted in severe feelings of guilt. To circumvent this process, each person the patient felt anger toward was described to her as having two sides—good and bad. She was to direct her anger only toward the "bad" side of the individual. During the therapeutic sessions the patient was directed to express anger fully, both verbally and with her body by kicking and hitting a couch or mattress in a kind of "temper tantrum" mode. This release of anger was instrumental in relieving her symptoms. A tape recording of one of her office sessions using this method is available through the American Academy of Psychotherapists Tape Library (1972).

The patient was initially reluctant to cooperate with the homework program since she obtained much secondary reinforcement of her symptoms from her family. The family was also drawn into the homework program and helped by beginning to reward her only for constructive behavior. Symptom relief also prompted her to gradually do more in the homework procedure.

By the time this young woman terminated treatment, she had achieved much more independence from her mother, was more active with her husband, children, and friends, was more assertive, drove more frequently, and had learned to cope with most of her phobic fears. She has functioned as a happy and successful housewife over at least a two-year followup period.

GROUP ASSERTIVE TRAINING HOMEWORK

Assertive training in groups and self or group assignment-homework for the following week's assertive step has proven to be more effective in measurable results than any other form of group therapy; open-ended groups of this type have shown more rapid and tangible practical results after two years of evaluation than insight groups or encounter groups.

Tapes are also used a half hour before bedtime for those who passive-aggressively resist using them during the day. Even if the patient falls asleep (a positive reinforcement for using the tape), there seems to be clinical evidence that, at least during this first half hour, some "sleep learning" takes place. After the first half hour we do not believe that further "sleep learning" occurs.

SUMMARY

A method is offered whereby the time between office visits may be utilized by the client for the practice of self-reinforced, positive, and progressively motivating behavior modification techniques assigned as daily homework by the therapist. A combination of self-relaxation and conditioning, with a hierarchy designed as a collaborative project between therapist and client, is widely applicable to a variety of obsessive-compulsive, depressive, and anxiety symptoms. Examples are given of sample hierarchies, reward schedules, and homework record sheets.

REFERENCES

Agras, C., and Marshall, C.: The application of negative practice to spasmodic torticollis. *Am J Psychiatry 122:*579, 1965.

Astrup, C.: *Pavlovian Psychiatry.* Springfield, Thomas, 1965.

Ban, T.: *Conditioning and Psychiatry.* Chicago, Aldine, 1964.

Case, H. W.: Therapeutic methods in stuttering and speech blocking. In Eysenck, H. J. (Ed.): *Behaviour Therapy and the Neuroses.* Oxford, Pergamon, 1960.

Cautela, J. R., and Kastenbaum, R.: A reinforcement survey schedule for use in therapy, training and research. *Psychol Rep, 20:*1115, 1967.

Dunlap, K.: *Habits, Their Making and Unmaking.* New York, Liveright, 1932.

Dunlap, K.: cited by Walton, D., in Experimental psychology and the treatment of a ticquer. *J Child Psychol,* 2:148, 1961.

Ellis, A.: Some uses of the printed, written, and recorded word in psychotherapy. In Pearson, L. (Ed.): *The Use of Written Communications in Psychotherapy.* Springfield, Thomas, 1965.

Franks, C. M. (Ed.): *Conditioning Techniques in Clinical Practice and Research.* New York, Springer, 1964.

Hendry, D.: *Conditioned Reinforcement.* Homewood, Dorsey, 1969.

Hilgard, E., and Marquis, D.: *Conditioning and Learning.* Revised by Kimble, G. A. New York, Appleton-Century-Crofts, 1961.

Jones, H. G.: Continuation of Yates treatment of a ticquer. In Eysenck, H. J. (Ed.): *Behaviour Therapy and the Neuroses.* Oxford, Pergamon, 1960.

Kline, M. V.: *Hypnodynamic Psychology: An Integrative Approach to the Behavior Sciences.* New York, Julian, 1955.

Krasner, L., and Ullmann, L. (Ed.): *Research in Behavior Modification.* New York, Holt, Rinehart and Winston, 1966.

Masters, W. H., and Johnson, V. E.: *Human Sexual Inadequacy.* Boston, Little, Brown, 1970.

Rafi, A. A.: Learning theory and the treatment of tics. In Eysenck, H. J. (Ed.): *Experiments in Behaviour Therapy.* Oxford, Pergamon, 1960.

Rothman, I.: Psychiatry and anesthesiology (including hypnosis and anesthesiology). *Internat J Anesth,* 2:186, 1955.

Rothman, I.: Hypnotherapy and narcotherapy. *J Am Osteopath Assoc,* 55:306, 1956.

Rothman, I.: Clinical use of drugs in induction and termination of the hypnotic state. *Int J Clin and Exp Hypn.* 5:25, 1957.

Rothman, I.: Biodramatic conditioning. *Tape #66.* Orlando, Fla., American Academy of Psychotherapists Tape Library, 1972.

Salter, A.: *Conditioned Reflex Therapy.* New York, Creative Age Press, 1949.

Skinner, B. F.: *Science and Human Behavior.* New York, Free Press, 1953.

Wells, H. K.: *Pavlov.* New York, International, 1956.

Wolberg, L. R.: *Medical Hypnosis.* Vol 1. New York, Grune and Stratton, 1948.

Wolpe, J.: *Psychotherapy by Reciprocal Inhibition.* Stanford, Stanford Univ. Press, 1958.

Wolpe, J., and Lazarus, A. A.: *Behavior Therapy Techniques.* Oxford, Pergamon, 1966.

Yates, A. J. Cited in Eysenck, H. J. (Ed.): *Experiments in Behaviour Therapy.* Oxford, Pergmon, 1964.

APPENDIX*

1. DAILY HOMEWORK SHEET—Irwin Rothman
2. SELF-DESENSITIZATION OR ANXIETY REDUCTION TECHNIQUES IN MAN—Irwin Rothman and M. L. Carroll
3. SELF-HELP RELAXATION METHODS—Irwin Rothman
4. REWARD SCHEDULE—L. M. Carroll and Irwin Rothman
5. IMPROVING HUMAN SELF IMAGES RAPIDLY—Irwin Rothman
6. HUMAN AVOIDANCE OR AVERSIVE CONDITIONING HOMEWORK

1. DAILY HOMEWORK SHEET

Change for the better, a learning or growth experience, usually just as school requires "homework" or practice in life *outside of* office sessions. This should include *at least one period* of practice daily—sometimes more. When the good changes become habits, then less frequent review or practice is needed. Breaking the harmful habit usually by ignoring it is most important. *You* must really make *real* effort to motivate and reward yourself to gain the changes you want sometimes. Pushing yourself into useful activity against moderate fear even or *especially* if you *"don't feel* like it," can lead to a happier life.

You may have already made up a desensitization list, or decided on some other homework. On this homework sheet, you are to list each day's date, how many practices you were able to do and how long they lasted, list the last step on your list you were able to reach successfully through visualization, (without over-whelming anxiety) and *also list any positive accomplishments for the day.* (This is to include any real accomplishments, *no matter how slight or insignificant you think you are* (even a

* The Homework Sheets in this Appendix supplied through the courtesy of Allied Psychological-Psychiatric Services, 6420 City Line Avenue, Philadelphia, Pa. 19151.

255

fraction of second's worth). Set a regular time or times in advance *by the clock for self-improvement.*

Don't be discouraged if you are only able to take a step at a time—regular practice is important and will gradually help you to go further. If any step seems too difficult, try to break it down into several smaller steps.

Let yourself make some notation each day and bring this sheet with you to each visit. Use the back of this sheet or additional paper when necessary.

"HE HAS NOT LEARNT THE LESSON OF LIFE WHO DOES NOT EVERY DAY SURMOUNT A FEAR." (Emerson)

Date	No. of Practices	Length of Practice	Positive Accomplishments

2. SELF-DESENSITIZATION OR ANXIETY REDUCTION TECHNIQUES IN MAN

A. Frequently you will be given a choice of self-relaxation or self-hypnotic techniques described in a booklet or in instructions given to you by the doctor. Practice the method you choose. Other types of training for self help may also be shown you.

B. Make a written stepladder of situations which disturb you or are problems to you. Arrange these in order from the *most disturbing* to the *least,* or from *least* to *most* if you prefer. Please provide a clear copy of your stepladder for the doctor.

C. During your 70 percent successful relaxation periods, visualize dramatically (get a vivid mental picture of) yourself successfully handling the situations (going up your stepladder) from the least to slightly disturbing until you feel slightly tense, then stop. Relax until you are again at ease. This procedure should be done daily, usually for not more than ten minutes at bedtime, or some other convenient time. This visualization should be about things you actually want and intend to do and not just daydreaming. Make it a practice to *try* the things you have successfully pictured yourself doing whenever possible. After a few days, longer or more frequent practice periods or several separate stepladders may be prescribed.

D. Try to record where you are on the list daily. The faithfulness with which you practice daily visualization is an indication of how much your healthy self is willing to cooperate in the treatment against your self-destructive side. If your mind wanders from successful picturing, repeat the last successful picture. Remember that the mind can only concentrate on one thing at a time, although it may skip quickly. Bring back the thought you wish to work with for at least two to three seconds at a time. Your visualization will improve with practice. Stop when you feel anxiety at the same step on the stepladder more than three times, go back to a comfortable relaxation, and later add extra smaller steps between the worrisome ones.

E. The situations listed below are merely suggestions of areas which *may* be problems to you and how to handle them with this method. If any of the examples *do* apply to you, include them in your own stepladder(s), along with any other problem areas *not* listed here. Each area can be divided into *as many as twenty or more gradual steps to visualize* and to conquer in actuality. If you do not experience any anxiety while first visualizing situations which you find much too difficult to accomplish in real daily life, consult the doctor or his associates concerning this.

EXAMPLES

(The first example is broken down to give you an idea of how to place situations on your own list.)

I. Assertion Examples

Asserting yourself with other people without guilt, listing different types of people in order of decreasing difficulty from the boss (possible #1) to the office boy (possible #9) to the janitor, (possible #15). This is a most important category for people with depression, strong self-damaging tendencies and anxieties in dealing with other people.

Picture yourself: (a) expressing affection openly for (1) pets; (2) children; (3) immediate family; (4) more distant relatives; (5) friends; (6) acquaintances—possibly in that order of difficulty for you: (b) being assertive with your family, clerks, waitresses, policemen, and authority figures in the degree and order of difficulty fitting you.

(c) Discussing topics which are of interest to you with your family, other relatives and close friends.

(d) Making an effort and succeeding in discussing their interests.

(e) Stating your wishes without guilt to family, relatives and close friends.

(f) Expressing disagreement without guilt to family, friends, other relatives.

(g) Following the same steps with casual friends and acquaintances.

(h) Requesting firmly that clerks, janitors, or any subordinates do their jobs promptly and properly.

(i) Expressing disagreement or your feeling of annoyance with those who do not fulfill their duties correctly.

(j) Talking about your job with fellow workers or firmly requesting that they do their share of any mutual job.

(k) Giving a report and expressing disagreement if necessary with your immediate superior in a tactful way.

(l) Giving a report and expressing disagreement if necessary to the highest superior with whom you must deal in a tactful way.

II. Fear of Criticism, Rejection, Disapproval or Healthy Disagreement

(a) Successfully facing sarcasm from family, friends or associates

(b) Successfully facing direct disapproval or criticism from family, friends, or associates

(c) Successfully arguing and being unafraid of arguments

(d) Successfully facing feelings of being excluded by others

(e) Successfully facing being ignored or reprimanded
(f) Successfully dealing with persons you feel dislike you.

III. Symptoms You Have Been Told Have No Medical Importance

Getting busy with activities and ignoring symptoms such as rapid heartbeat, buzzing in ears, constant or intermittent pain from rheumatism or similar symptoms if you know that they are not medically important. Arrange a stepladder of increasing time for enduring them and carrying on despite them.

IV. Stage Fright

Successfully speaking to a group. Perhaps start with an empty room and gradually increase the number of people present to 100.

V. Social Fright

Enjoying entertaining and parties of increasing size from one friendly couple to any number of relative strangers.

VI. At Ease in Crowds of Increasing Size

Elevators, trains, cramped quarters, open spaces, etc.

VII. Being at Ease in Applying for a Job

Starting with an interview you do not really want. Actually having several interviews before taking a job.

VIII. Being at Ease with Members of the Opposite Sex

Starting with someone unimportant to you and increasing periods of time and difficulty.

IX. Being at Ease in Making Your Own Decisions

Making decisions without regrets and afterthought. Start with small decisions and increase importance.

3. SELF HELP RELAXATION METHODS

I. Letting Go

For most, it is a mistake to "try to relax." Just tense the muscle group and then visualize and verbalize to the muscle group "let go and keep on letting go."

II. Breathing

A Yogic style of deep slow breathing (6000 years old). Filling up from the lower belly (abdomen and diaphragm) toward the chest—like filling a glass of water, and *exhale slowly* thru the nostrils. Can first tense, or suck in the belly and feel tension in these muscles and then say "I will allow these muscles to let go" and visualize letting go on exhalation. Can place hand below belly button and feel area move up on inhalation and down on exhalation. Relaxed breathing should continue throughout other exercises.

III. Forearm

Many people can most quickly be aware of tensing the forearm and relaxing it on exhalation. Making fist is one way of tensing and visualizing.

IV. Face and Forehead

Wrinkle forehead as tightly as possible and then say to muscles "let go and keep on letting go." Practice this often. Furrow between the brows often and "let go and continue to let go."

Clench teeth, feel jaw muscles and let go with lips and teeth slightly parted. Show teeth and relax these muscles. *Push* tongue against upper palate (top of mouth) and let it relax between lower teeth (just almost touching bottom teeth). Close eyelids tightly and let go slowly. IMPORTANT—Look as far to left as possible with eyes closed, lids relaxed, and then let go and let eyes go and drift. Same to right and up and down. (Rolling eyeballs up with Yogic breathing and keeping them up is one way to be helpful for inducing self hypnotism and later sleep in insomniacs). Visualize and let the entire face smooth out as though you are smoothing it with both hands and let it stay smooth. (*Relaxation of eyes and tongue often controls unwanted thoughts and helps with insomnia*).

V. If Mind Wanders, Get it Back to Thinking of Breathing and Muscle Group Pictures as Best You Can—Tighten on Inhalation and let go on Exhalation.

VI. Repetition

Do not become discouraged as tension patterns have existed all of your life—practice whenever possible. Soon shortcuts such as deep breathing and word "calm" or "let go," or "relax," or words or pictures of your choosing may help form a habit. You may find for you, certain muscle groups such as face, shoulders, breathing muscles allows you to relax adequately.

VII. Neck Practice

The same procedures of breathing and tensing muscle groups apply to all parts of body you can, especially in the beginning. Bend head back, relax. Head to the left and right.

VIII. Shoulders

Hunch up as far as possible and let go. Backward and forward also.

IX. Lower Extremities

Pinch buttocks together—feel tension and let go. Let go to toes.

GENERAL: Practice at every available moment to do things in a relaxed fashion, then let yourself consciously breathe deeply and relax in situations ordinarily causing tension. If possible, condition or habituate the relaxation of entire musculature, or letting go to deep breathing and the same key words or words that seem to suit you.

TIME: Persistence and review are worthwhile since everyone agrees on the desirability and harmlessness of relaxation.

4. REWARD SCHEDULE

The purpose of this self-survey is to help you to decide on specific rewards which you can give yourself each time you complete a given step on your stepladder of progress. It is most important that you attempt a pleasurable thought or act as a reward each time (or almost each time later on) as you reach a specific goal in your treatment.

NOTE: The sections on eating and alcoholic beverages should be skipped if these are problem areas for you.

In filling out the survey, circle the number which best describes how much enjoyment you get from the specific activity.

0 means: "Not at all"
1 means: "A little"
2 means: "A fair amount"
3 means: "Much"
4 means: "Very much"

The best activities to use as rewards are those which you give ratings of 3 or 4. In broad categories, specify and rate as many things you like as possible.

I. INDIVIDUAL

1. *Eating*
   a. Sweets 0 1 2 3 4
   b. Meat   0 1 2 3 4
   c. Vegetables 0 1 2 3 4
   d. Low caloric snacks (carrots, celery, cottage cheese, etc.) 0 1 2 3 4
2. *Beverages*
   a. Water 0 1 2 3 4
   b. Milk   0 1 2 3 4
   c. Soft drinks 0 1 2 3 4
   d. Tea   0 1 2 3 4
   e. Coffee 0 1 2 3 4
3. *Alcoholic Beverages*
   a. Beer   0 1 2 3 4
   b. Wine 0 1 2 3 4
   c. Hard liquor 0 1 2 3 4
4. Television (Comedy, Drama, News, Sports, etc.) 0 1 2 3 4
5. Movies   ("   "   "   "   ") 0 1 2 3 4
6. Plays   ("   "   "   "   ") 0 1 2 3 4
7. Concerts   (Classical, Jazz, Folk, Popular, Rock) 0 1 2 3 4
8. Listening to Records 0 1 2 3 4

9. Radio 0 1 2 3 4
10. Reading 0 1 2 3 4
11. Solving Problems (Puzzles, mathematical problems, do-it-yourself projects, etc.) 0 1 2 3 4
12. Hobbies—(Painting, sketching, building, photography, collecting, sewing, singing, playing a musical instrument, alone or with others) 0 1 2 3 4
13. Attending Church 0 1 2 3 4
14. Religious thought, or prayers 0 1 2 3 4
15. Bath 0 1 2 3 4
16. Household chores 0 1 2 3 4
17. Relaxing—Deep breathing, relaxation exercises 0 1 2 3 4
18. Working 0 1 2 3 4
19. Attending lectures or discussions 0 1 2 3 4
20. Exercising, jogging, walking or hiking 0 1 2 3 4
21. Writing letters, stories, essays, poems 0 1 2 3 4

II. INDIVIDUAL OR SOCIAL ACTIVITIES— MORE ACTION ORIENTED

1. Sightseeing (Museums, scenery, famous buildings, etc.) 0 1 2 3 4
2. Traveling—Bus, train, car, plane 0 1 2 3 4
3. Driving 0 1 2 3 4
4. Dancing 0 1 2 3 4
5. *Attending or participating in sports*
   a. Football 0 1 2 3 4
   b. Baseball 0 1 2 3 4
   c. Basketball 0 1 2 3 4
   d. Track 0 1 2 3 4
   e. Golf 0 1 2 3 4
   f. Swimming 0 1 2 3 4
   g. Running 0 1 2 3 4
   h. Tennis 0 1 2 3 4
   i. Pool 0 1 2 3 4
   j. Other 0 1 2 3 4
6. Attending classes in some subject you have an interest in 0 1 2 3 4
7. Playing cards or other games 0 1 2 3 4

8. Shopping—for clothes, food, furniture, etc. 0 1 2 3 4
9. Having, training or playing with a pet 0 1 2 3 4

III. SOCIAL REWARDS

1. Joining a club 0 1 2 3 4
2. Visiting friends or relatives 0 1 2 3 4
3. Going to parties 0 1 2 3 4
4. Going to dances 0 1 2 3 4
5. Going to small social gatherings 0 1 2 3 4
6. Talking to other people whom you enjoy 0 1 2 3 4
7. Flirting 0 1 2 3 4
8. Doing things for others 0 1 2 3 4
9. Caring for or playing with children 0 1 2 3 4
10. Volunteer work 0 1 2 3 4
11. Talking to friends on the phone 0 1 2 3 4
12. Meeting new people 0 1 2 3 4
13. Competing with others
    a) For fun 0 1 2 3 4
    b) For money 0 1 2 3 4
    c) For attention 0 1 2 3 4
    d) For a job 0 1 2 3 4
    e) Other goals 0 1 2 3 4
14. Teaching others how to do something you can do well!
    0 1 2 3 4

IV. SEXUAL REWARDS

1. Attractive Women
    a) Looking at pictures of 1) Clothed 0 1 2 3 4
       2) Nude 0 1 2 3 4
    b) Observing 1) Clothed 0 1 2 3 4 2) Nude 0 1
       2 3 4
    c) Being with 0 1 2 3 4
    d) Talking to 0 1 2 3 4
    e) Dating 0 1 2 3 4
2. Attractive Men
    a) Looking at pictures of 1) Clothed 0 1 2 3 4 2) Nude
       0 1 2 3 4
    b) Observing 1) Clothed 0 1 2 3 4 2) Nude 0 1 2 3 4

c) Being with 0 1 2 3 4
d) Talking to 0 1 2 3 4
e) Dating   0 1 2 3 4

3. Making love
   a) Physical closeness 1) Clothed 0 1 2 3 4 2) Nude 0 1 2 3 4
   b) Petting (Light) 1) Clothed 0 1 2 3 4 2) Nude 0 1 2 3 4
   c) Foreplay 0 1 2 3 4
   d) Intercourse 0 1 2 3 4

4. Talking about sex 0 1 2 3 4
5. Reading about sex 0 1 2 3 4

V. SOCIAL APPROVAL AND/OR POSITIVE FEEDBACK

Note: This section is particularly useful in evaluating self worth and increasing confidence. Rate the importance of the items in your viewpoint. They are partially dependent on the way people respond to you and your behavior. It is helpful in increasing your confidence, if you learn to identify these pieces of positive feedback daily and utilize them in building a better self concept.

1) Being with happy people 0 1 2 3 4
2) Making others happy   0 1 2 3 4
3) Doing things to make yourself happy 0 1 2 3 4
4) Others smiling at you 0 1 2 3 4
5) Being accepted by another person or a group 0 1 2 3 4
6) Being included by another person or a group 0 1 2 3 4
7) Being sought out by others
   a) For advice 0 1 2 3 4
   b) For help   0 1 2 3 4
   c) For company 0 1 2 3 4
   d) For understanding and sympathy 0 1 2 3 4
8) Being right
   a) In work 0 1 2 3 4
   b) In arguments 0 1 2 3 4
   c) In decisions   0 1 2 3 4
   d) In evaluating others 0 1 2 3 4
9) Being complimented
   a) On your appearance   0 1 2 3 4

b) On your intelligence 0 1 2 3 4
c) About your work 0 1 2 3 4
d) About hobbies 0 1 2 3 4
e) On physical strength 0 1 2 3 4
f) On your personality 0 1 2 3 4
g) About your beliefs and convictions 0 1 2 3 4
h) About your understanding of others 0 1 2 3 4
i) About your judgement 0 1 2 3 4
j) About your possessions 0 1 2 3 4
k) About your taste (choosing clothes, activities, friends, etc.) 0 1 2 3 4
l) On your cooperation with others 0 1 2 3 4
m) On your ability to achieve goals 0 1 2 3 4
n) About your ability to influence others 0 1 2 3 4
10) Direct approval of you having someone
    a) Say they like you 0 1 2 3 4
    b) Having someone say they wish to spend more time with you 0 1 2 3 4
    c) Say they value your help, opinions, or advice 0 1 2 3 4
11) Physical feedback from others
    a) Handshake 0 1 2 3 4
    b) Pat on the back or similar motion 0 1 2 3 4
    c) Casual hug 0 1 2 3 4
    d) Warm embrace 0 1 2 3 4

SECTION VI: OTHER (CONFIDENTIAL)

List things which you enjoy or would enjoy doing or thinking about, and estimate how many times daily you do or think about them.

5	10	15	20 times/day
_____	_____	_____	_____
_____	_____	_____	_____
_____	_____	_____	_____
_____	_____	_____	_____

SECTION VIII: ACTUAL THOUGHTS OR ACTIVITIES

List things which you spend time (thinking or doing) daily even if you don't like them, or are not proud of them (e.g. nibbling, watching TV, lying in bed, sitting). List the number of times a day you do this.

10	20	30	40 times/day

5. IMPROVING HUMAN SELF IMAGES RAPIDLY

INTRODUCTION

You and the doctor or his associates have agreed that a less self-critical self-image of yourself is desirable; or a self-concept in which you feel less inferior and more self-confident, or less childlike, more active at finding a new job—remedying a situation—doing more housework—getting more exercise—or more comfortable physical and social activity—or some other changes in your innermost self-concept are necessary or desirable.

METHOD I

Under self-hypnosis or relaxation leave yourself with the self-image of pleasant feelings and times in your life you, and possibly others, thought you were at least somewhat successful. Tell yourself, "I promise to act in accordance with this image."

METHOD II

A gradual stepladder of improved self-images can be used under self-hypnosis or relaxation, and you can move up this imaginary ladder of improved self-images until you feel a tinge of anxiety. Step down to the last comfortable self-image you could get. As soon as possible act in daily like according to this improved image—as if it is now you.

METHOD III

Visualize your "lazy" or passive self-image as perhaps you have looked after avoiding some important work—a picture that we have agreed should be changed. After imagining this picture for two to three seconds, give yourself a buzz usually until the image stops. Repeat as prescribed, usually for about 20 pictures at a sitting, with at least daily repetition. Substitute an image of a time when you were slightly more pleased with yourself each time you relax from the buzz.

METHOD IV

This can be used if you have been taught self-hypnosis with body imagery changes. (a) Hypnotize yourself to picture how some of your character (expressed as face and body) looks to you. Usually the doctor or his associates will have agreed with you on a given signal or word for this unconscious image to appear clearly. If you find difficulty in separating "bad mother or bad father" (or other image previously discussed with the therapist) from *your* image, i.e. they stick, then try using the buzzer to break up the fusion and leave you with an *independent self-image*, or with "good" Mother and Father's love. (b) Then you may attempt to modify by fusing your image with someone who has, as you and your therapist have agreed, some desirable traits you'd gradually like to work toward in a *realistic* fashion. (c) If the old image is stubborn in leaving, or fusing with the image you and your therapist have agreed upon, use the buzzer as described in Method III and #1 under AVERSIVE CONDITIONING to modify the old image by bussing it and thereby speeding up the desired fused image. Report changes to your therapist and keep your goals *practical* and within easy steps forward.

NOTE: It is most important that you keep careful records of frequency of use, and just what happens with the images, and discuss this with the therapist. These methods are not the same as daydreaming. Homework time is limited to approved and improved images as prescribed and should be tried out in reality.

6. HUMAN AVOIDANCE OR AVERSIVE CONDITIONING (HOMEWORK)

You can help yourself to get rid of undesirable, torturesome thoughts and habits after you and the doctor or his associates have agreed that these thoughts, or habits are damaging to you. Repeated practice is necessary for most people at least one or more times per day in the beginning and then at gradually decreasing intervals until the thought or habit is gone. The doctor or his associates may help prescribe the intervals and amount of time most helpful to you as well as other helpful ideas.

I. REPETITIVE, SELF-DAMAGING THOUGHTS (THOUGHT-STOPPING, MODIFIED BY ROTHMAN, I. AFTER WOLPE, J.)

a. Close your eyes, hypnotize, or *relax yourself* and force the repetitive thought or the picture of the undesirable habit to be *visualized* in your mind for at least two to three seconds.

b. Almost immediately, shout *STOP* or if this is not possible, *think* STOP or if this is not possible, *think* STOP emphatically and promptly give yourself an unpleasant buzz with the buzzer at the same moment. Holding your breath can be used with the buzzer, or something unobtrusive for you, e.g. a clenched fist can be used at the same time in place of "STOP." (*It is important that during the pleasant and restful time after you have stopped the shock, visualize a successful, positive, helpful image or valuable substitute activity.*) As soon as these secondary things (breath holding, fist, etc.) work, use buzzer less and less frequently.

Repeat this entire procedure at the same sitting until you can no longer get the thought at that time or until at least twenty satisfactory repetitions have occurred. The entire procedure is to be repeated up to six times per day for one to fifteen weeks. This will be prescribed in accordance with the severity of your problem and the length of time you have had it. Make a note each day on the back of an appointment card or some other record such as a homework sheet of how frequently and for what number of repetitions you have been using the buzzer, or the word "STOP" breath holding, fist, etc. A list of possible pleasant thoughts, activities, assets should be available.

II. MODIFICATION

In addition, you can carry the buzzer, or special pen if you prefer, with you and use it whenever you find yourself thinking repetitively or continuing your undesirable habit. If circumstances are such that it is impossible for you to use the buzzer during the larger part of the day, think the word STOP and imagine the uncomfortable buzz when you find yourself going back to the thought or habit. This will gradually become more successful after actual practice when practice is possible. Unless good success is being maintained with the STOP, breath holding, or other simultaneous gesture, and the pleasant thought or activity substitution report to doctor.

III. NOTE

The buzzer terminals (the two shiny metal discs at the end) should be held firmly with two fingers, one on each disc, and the buzz should *not* be too pleasant or too painful. If it seems too much to endure, even though it contains only a single pen-light type battery, a single thickness of kleenex placed under the fingers will modify the buzz sufficiently. The pinhead-sized piece of metal one-half inch in from the metallic disc is compressed by the thumb of the hand that is not being shocked. Pressing the thumb down on this "pinhead" stops the shock. Raising it delivers the shock. If your model buzzer also has an outside dial (rheostat) this can be adjusted so that the buzz is not *too* unpleasant.

AVAILABILITY: 1) A pocket pen for hidden self-buzzing will also be available soon. 2) All of the above self-help devices in addition to a stuttering desensitizer called Pacemaker, are available from Dr. Libby, Associated Auditory Instruments, 6796 Market Street, Upper Darby, Penna. 19082 upon professional prescription.

CHAPTER 20

CLINICAL HYPNOSIS: WARP AND WOOF OF PSYCHOTHERAPIES*

Gus K. Bell, Ph.D

B EHAVIORISM, as applied through behavior therapy techniques such as Wolpe's systematic desensitization, has made respectable the discussion of such forbidden topics as mental imagery, imagination and other cognitive or mentalistic functions. Wolpe (1969) has stated that he carries out desensitization under hypnosis in about 10 percent of his cases treated by reciprocal inhibition. But, in an exploratory way, he introduces hypnosis with each patient; and in those who are difficult to hypnotize, hypnosis is abandoned and instructions are given merely to close the eyes and relax according to the therapist's directions. I am sure many psychotherapists, in addition to myself, have found these relaxation instructions to be excellent hypnotic induction procedures, especially for the resistant patient.

As hypnotherapy is done today, very seldom is a symptom removed directly simply by post-hypnotic suggestion. I mention this because it seems to be what so many people expect. Nevertheless, there are more direct approaches to the removal of symptoms within the tradition of clinical hypnosis than is the case with Wolpe's systematic desensitization and its sometimes tedious hierarchies.

Recently Gibbons, Kilbourne, Saunders, and Castle (1970) reported on an investigation testing the relative merits of the methods of systematic desensitization and a "Directed Experience"

* Originally published in Psychotherapy: Theory, Research and Practice, Volume 9, No. 3, Fall, 1972, pages 276–280. This is a revised copy of the original article.

271

hypnotic technique in reducing test anxiety. Essentially, the approach was one of inducing affective states of relaxation, happiness, and tranquility directly while the client was in a hypnotic trance and then telling him he was no longer in the office but in the test-taking situation. This was brought about through the use of visual imagery but was made more realistic by administering various kinds of actual test items and allowing the subject to respond while in a deep trance. The results demonstrated that a directed experience involving hypnosis was more effective than systematic desensitization in reducing test anxiety. The essential difference in the two approaches was the Directed Experience technique induced pleasant affect directly as opposed to indirectly through deep muscle relaxation used in systematic desensitization.

One value of approaching desensitization with hypnotic procedures is that it enables one to go more directly to a maximally arousing situation. This can be done in a number of ways, but it typically involves altering the client's subjective environment so that he more vividly experiences a situation but without the usual anxiety. The approach can be quite permissive:

> For example, consider a man who had an avoidance of doing one important aspect of his job, i.e. writing reports following his week's work as a sales representative. There were other aspects of his job that gave him problems and there were other aspects of his personality which brought him to therapy with me, but I shall consider only the behavior of his sitting down and writing a report. This was a job which he often avoided until he was in trouble with his boss; and when he did approach it, it seemed to be impossible even though he knew intellectually the task was simple. While in a trance the suggestions for relaxation and confidence were given, and he was directed to carry out the "dreaded" job in fantasy. These fantasies repeated with intermittent fantasies of a very pleasant nature were a rather straight-forward way of desensitizing fear of sitting at a table and writing reports; but in order that he be able to deal with a fuller affective experience, some of the hidden feelings associated with completing a job were also elicited. The technique which I used with this man was a permissive one (Erickson, 1967). I suggested, while he was in a fairly deep trance, that he visualize a crystal ball in which he might begin to see himself in various situations at different times in his life. A particular suggestion was made that he might see himself in some way which might be related to or in some way

permit him to better understand his avoidance of report writing. He was instructed that any part of any experience which might be too disturbing for him to remember could simply be forgotten as he returned to his usual state of awareness. The gentleman in case had several flashes of imagery related to his feelings about relationship to authority. One in particular was of a high school teacher whose judgment of his work was intimidating and anger producing. Discussing his hatred of the teacher led to negative feelings about his boss whose rejection and judgment he feared. After differentiating feelings of the past and those related to the present, and after re-experiencing through trance the phobic situation several times, the newly experienced confidence and more effective coping behavior generalized to more successful week-end report writing. This illustration of hypnotic procedures is a mixture of uncovering methods of the analytic tradition and behavioral techniques, but they were applied in a relationship which was permissive and which I prefer to think of as humanistic and existential.

Another permissive approach involving induced imagery, reported by Brown (1969), takes into consideration the possibility that a patient's fear of an object or situation might be related to the idiosyncratic way he conceptualizes the phobic object. Rather than telling the patient to imagine specific scenes described to him, such as Wolpe might do, the patient is told to put his ideas and feelings about the feared object or situation into a mental image—an imagined situation, a fantasy, a caricature, a cartoon, or a representative in an animal form. The patient reveals his own peculiar distortions as he describes his conceptualizations; and as they are reimagined three or four times during the session, associated emotions decrease markedly and a psychological distancing seems to occur.

Another case which had to do with the uniqueness of one's imagery was that of a not very spry, but spunky, seventy-two-year old lady with severe rheumatoid arthritis. She needed to control pain sufficiently to be able to carry out exercises prescribed by her physician. We concerned ourselves primarily with her left knee, on which she had had surgery, to be followed by extensive physiotherapy. She had never been able, however, to raise her leg to carry out the exercises due to soreness. She was well motivated as one alternative would probably have been removal of the knee cap. My psychotherapeutic task was to help this lady to bend her knee, raising the leg straight ahead while in the sitting position. The hypnotic technique used involved the patient's picturing the pain in her knee more vividly while she closed her eyes and relaxed herself. As she relaxed deeper she was able to picture it more and more vividly and better describe it with more accuracy. It was suggested that perhaps she might also find some worthwhile associations or connections of that pain to some things quite significant and important, an open ended, permissive sort of suggestion. She was asked to describe whether the pain was more on one side of the knee than the other, attempting to focus more specifically on the location. "Is it a large pain or a small pain? Can you give some kind of description of the size of it? Is it a heavy pain or a light pain?" She described the pain as being on the left side of the knee. "Sort of a tightness, not a large area . . . sort of heavy, hard to pull against, just tight, won't loosen." And I asked, "And what color would you say the pain is?" The color associated with the pain was a rough, tan color. "I don't like that color," she stated. "And when your knee was feeling entirely normal and entirely comfortable, what color would you say it was then?" I asked. "Yellow," she replied, "I love yellow." "And how do you feel in general when you have this pleasant, yellow feeling?" Continuing to describe and compare the feelings of comfort and discomfort, the patient was led to focus on the two opposites: the rough, brown, uncomfortable, tight feeling and the yellow, relaxed, contented feeling. "Now as you relax deeper I would like you to concentrate on that brown, tense, uncomfortable feeling and I would like for you to imagine that all these feelings are present in your left forearm." After these feelings and their similarity to the pain in the left knee were acknowledged, I asked her to apply the antidote color, that nice, yellow, pleasant feeling color, and associate it to the same left forearm and notice the pain go away. It was a simple matter then to transfer the application of the antidote yellow, relaxing color to the left knee. She was then able to raise the left leg without the interfering discomfort. During our discussion of what the rough, brown color meant to her, she recalled a physician who, years earlier, had recommended surgery rather than exercise and in so doing had referred to her knee joint as being like sandpaper, "That rough, brown sandpaper must have stuck in my mind," she commented.

I am convinced that, as one fully explores the possibilities of hypnotic behavior therapy techniques, one is also likely to increasingly involve himself with intrapsychic factors or psychodynamics as well as to become more sensitive to the therapist-patient relationship.

People often come in with misconceptions about hypnosis and

its application in the clinical setting. One lady, recently referred by a surgeon because of her fear of being put to sleep by anesthesia illustrates such misconceptions. After already having experienced a trance sufficient for the therapeutic goal, she urged me to let her go "all the way under" and while she would be "asleep" she wished I would drop into her "unconscious" a list of suggestions which she had written on a slip of paper. She needed to learn more about the nature of hypnosis, particularly her own responsibility in bringing about changes.

Hypnosis is not a therapist-centered tool, but rather a patient- or client-centered one (Kroger, 1970). Fromm (1965), in clarifying the nature of a hypnotherapy relationship, has pointed out that during the nineteenth century, and until about 1940, hypnosis was used by the therapist in an authoritarian, dominating fashion: "The hypnotist would command the patient to give up his symptoms—or, as young Freud did, to bring up warded off memories. In authoritarian hypnosis defenses were not respected. The ego, therefore, often refused responsibility for material produced in a trance. Had Freud used a more permissive technique —as he soon came to do in developing free association—most likely he would not have dropped hypnosis as an investigative and therapeutic tool."

The hypnotized client remains an individual with full rights and privileges whose wishes and needs must be constantly consulted and consistently respected (Moss, 1967). For the therapist inexperienced with hypnosis, one of the most difficult realizations is that hypnotherapy can be a highly nondirective venture. Induction is the easiest part; it is the relationship which follows that is more important to consider. The individual is not asleep, not unconscious. In fact, in hypnosis one is more aware and more vigilant, since there is selective inattention to irrelevant stimuli. A person is treated in hypnosis and not by hypnosis (Kroger, 1970).

More important than the depth of a trance is the therapist's ability to establish the kind of interpersonal relationship which will allow him and the client to work successfully toward the client's goal, whether it be relief, cure or personal growth (Moss, 1967). One characteristic of the successful hypnotherapy relationship is that the therapist becomes more exquisitely aware of a responsiveness to subtle cues from the subject.

Humanistic psychology, in its concern for self, basic need gratification, love and self-actualization, has brought hypnosis into positive light by conceptualizing it as a creative act (Krippner, 1968). In this age, when more and more people are seeking freedom instead of insight, therapeutic procedures offering new and more creative experiences, and perhaps new values, may be more redemptive than a therapy which promises only to solve a problem or to teach new habits. If one accepts the hypothesis that stereotyped thinking is an inevitable result of cultural indoctrination and that hypnosis enables man to stand apart from his culture sufficient to release creative forces, there is promise for hypnosis as a tool for personal growth. Its use may be a part of the traditional psychotherapy relationship or of the many developing personal growth experiences provided by groups, workshops, or human relations laboratories.

To emphasize the relevance of hypnosis to the uniqueness of man and his personal growth, I conclude with a quote from Hilgard (1970):

> What we found out was that the hypnotizable person was capable of a deep involvement in one or more imaginative-feeling areas of experience—reading a novel, listening to music, having an aesthetic experience of nature, or engaging in absorbing adventures of body and mind. This involvement is one of the things the existentialist is talking about when he speaks of the breaking down of the distinction between the subject and the object of his experience; it is what those seeking expansion of consciousness mean by their all-embracing experiences; it is something like Maslow's (1959) peak experience.

REFERENCES

Brown, B. M.: The use of induced imagery and psychotherapy. *Psychotherapy: Theory, Research and Practice*, 6:120, 1969.

Erickson, M. H.: Pseudo-orientation in time as a hypnotherapeutic procedure. In Haley, Jay (Ed.): *Advanced Techniques of Hypnosis and Therapy, Selected Papers of Milton H. Erickson, M.D.* New York, Grune and Stratton, 1967.

Fromm, E.: Hypnoanalysis: Theory and two cases excerpts. *Psychotherapy: Theory, Research and Practice*, 2:127, 1965.

Gibbons, D. Kilbourne, L., Saunders, A., and Castle, C.: The cognitive control of behavior: A comparison of systematic desensitization and hypnotically induced "Directed Experience" techniques. *Am J Clin Hypn, 12:*141, 1970.

Hilgard, J.: *Personality and Hypnosis, A Study of Imaginative Involvement.* Chicago, University of Chicago Press, 1970.

Krippner, S.: The psychedelic state, the hypnotic trance, and the creative act. *Journal of Humanistic Psychology, 8:*49, 1968.

Kroger, W. S.: Comprehensive management of obesity. *Am J Clin Hypn, 12:*165, 1970.

Maslow, A. H.: Cognition of being in the peak experiences. *J Genet Psychol, 94:*43, 1959.

Moss, C. S.: Brief crisis oriented psychotherapy. In Gordon, Jesse E. (Ed.): *Handbook of Clinical and Experimental Hypnosis.* New York, Macmillan, 1967.

Wolpe, J.: *The Practice of Behavior Therapy.* New York, Pergamon Press, 1969.

CHAPTER 21

DISSOCIATIVE AND INTEGRATIVE PROCESSES IN HYPNOANALYSIS*

ERIKA FROMM, PH.D

In 1906 Morton Prince described for the first time a case of multiple personality, his famous patient Sally Beauchamp. She was a spontaneously dissociating personality. He treated her with hypnosis and helped her to reintegrate her opposing personalities into a single, more mature one.

We have learned since that hypnosis is a state—or a process— which easily lends itself to dissociative phenomena, even in the normal person. The dissociative phenomena that I shall discuss, and that occur in the ordinary state of trance, are not of the same dramatic quality as were those of the very sick patients of Morton Prince or of Thigpen and Cleckley who described a similar patient in "The Three Faces of Eve." (1957).

The normal dissociative phenomena that are characteristic of hypnosis can be used in exploratory, in confronting and in therapeutic ways in hypnotherapy and in hypnoanalysis.

Three major areas of dissociation are used in hypnoanalysis, namely:

1. Dissociating the observing ego from the experiencing ego.
2. De-egotizing parts of the body to express unconscious wishes, thoughts and feelings, as in automatic writing, drawing and painting in hypnosis, and hypnoplasia.
3. Dissociating various ego states, processes or functions and helping the patient to reintegrate them in a new and healthier way.

* Originally published in *The American Journal of Clinical Hypnosis*, Volume X, Number 3, January 1968, pages 174–177.

In any kind of psychotherapy, particularly in psychoanalysis, the patient must learn to observe himself while he experiences affect. In hypnosis this process occurs spontaneously—and often to the surprise of the patient who thought he would be "unconscious" or unaware of what is going on in him during trance. In hypnosis, the patient experiences strong affects, thoughts, and hypermnesia, and is aware that he does. He has thus dissociated the observing part of the ego from the experiencing or the behaving part. A patient, for instance, can be told in hypnoanalysis to watch himself making a decision—or to hallucinate a "person who looks just like him and who feels as angry as he unconsciously does, come into the room and act exactly as he wants to, without feeling fear or guilt." Similarly, a person who has to undergo surgery can be told he feels that another man who looks just like him steps out of him, walks a few steps ahead of him, is put into a wheel chair, taken up to surgery and undergoes the operation; while he himself sits over there on a chair in the corner of the surgical theatre and watches "that man" undergoing surgery. The patient's observing ego in this case retains ego cathexis, while the experiencing ego is decathexed. Because the observing ego is separated from the experiencing ego—and because the observing ego alone retains the ego cathexis ("that man —not I")—the patient does not feel any pain and can be operated on without any anesthetic. I have helped a number of women who were afraid of labor go through it in this way without experiencing pain.

Frequently in hypnoanalysis we make use of de-egotizing parts of the body, or using parts of the body to express unconscious wishes, thoughts, and feelings.

In *automatic writing* the hypnoanalyst induces glove anesthesia in a patient. The patient is then told that the anesthetized hand is separating away from his body, that it leads a life of its own . . . that it knows the patient's unconscious feelings and thoughts. The hypnoanalyst thus has separated the conscious ego from the unconscious ego, and given the unconscious a direct means of expression. When one asks such a patient a question, he may answer with "yes" or "no," according to what he consciously feels; but his hand will write the real, the unconscious answer—

often a no when he answers verbally by saying yes. The hand also will write out events, thoughts and feelings that have been repressed and are unavailable to his conscious memory.

In a way, doodling is a minor form of hypnotic automatic writing. In doodling, too, we express unconscious feelings while our conscious attention is occupied with some other task.

For the same purposes, drawing and painting are frequently used in hypnotherapy. Ainslie Meares (1958) has hypnoanalyzed a schizophrenic girl, mainly employing her hypnotic drawings and paintings.

Let me mention also the method of hypnoplasia, developed by Raginsky (1962). The patient, while in deep trance, is given colored plasticine which he kneads and models and smells, and shapes into forms and objects that satisfy his unconscious longings, or against which he expresses his hostility (e.g. many patients have in trance shaped nipples or bottles on which they began to suck, or effigies which they—mild-mannered, timid people —bashed in and smashed with abandon, often venting their hostility then also verbally.)

Borrowing Kris' (1952) expression, we can say that in trance the patient is in a state of "regression in the service of the ego" (Bellak, 1955; Gill and Brenman 1961; Fromm, 1965). Therefore the hypnotherapist will be more successful if he uses symbolic, primary-process, evocative language than when he talks to the patient in the rational, secondary process forms of speech.

For instance: A female scientist, middle-aged and unmarried, who for years devotedly had taken care of her parents, became deeply depressed and suicidal after both parents died in short succession. We analyzed her irrational guilt, and her repressed childhood anger at her father. Still, the patient felt apathetic, without much interest in life and unable to do her work.

It was in March. In hypnosis I asked the patient to raise her arms and to imagine that she was a tree, her feet being the roots which she would now sink deep into fertile soil, her body the trunk of the tree, and her arms its branches. From the Good Earth the sap would soon rise and fill the roots, the trunk, the branches . . . the whole tree with new life. Then into her dominant hand, I put a real (not an imaginary) branch of dogwood which still looked barren but the blossoms of which—I knew—would open within a few weeks. When the patient opened her eyes and looked at the branch in her hand she said: "Oh, it's real. And I felt the sap, new joy, rising in me."

She took the branch home, and improved markedly over the next few weeks as the dogwood blossoms grew and unfolded into large blooms.

Not only can various ego states or functions be dissociated easily in hypnosis, the hypnotherapist can also help the patient to integrate or reintegrate in new, more mature, healthier ways.

One such method is the Ideal-Self Technique. The hypnoanalyst asks the patient who sits at one end of the couch to imagine seeing his "ideal self" a real figure, walk into the office and sit down at the other end of the couch. He lets him describe how this "ideal self" looks and behaves. Then he suggests that the patient slowly shove over sideways on the couch . . . closer and closer to the ideal self . . . until the patient's body fully merges into that of his self-ideal . . . into every curve and plane of it. When that has occurred the hypnotherapist gently suggests that the patient fantasy the ideal self (into which he is now incorporated) go and undertake one of the tasks that ordinarily cause him anguish or difficulty.

For instance: to an acrophobia who cannot bring himself to go higher than the third floor in any building I may say: "Now you see this self take the elevator and go up to the twentieth floor. (Note that I now call it 'this self' rather than the 'ideal self'). This self steps out of the elevator and walks to a balcony from which *you* have a wide, wide view of the city and beautiful Lake Michigan; an exhilarating view that is quite different from the way in which you have looked at the city before." I encourage him to tell me what he sees from this outlook. If I sense that the patient becomes anxious, I let him grasp my hand or the "balcony's bannister." In any case, I encourage him to stay up there a little longer "inside the ideal self that is not afraid"; I may tell him also that I am right with him. A few such sessions often give the patient the impetus to ascend high locations in real life. Or they may bring to light new, valuable material for further analysis.

Another integrative method is that of assigning to the patient, in trance, ego strengthening tasks of progressive difficulty. This can be done either by means of imagery and symbolism, or through dreams. In both cases the hypnoanalyst speaks to the patient's unconscious ego.

For instance: a patient in trance can be asked to imagine vividly that he

1. walk up five flights of stairs
2. climb up a steep high sand dune without using his hands to hold on anywhere
3. walk up ten flights of stairs
4. climb up a mountain in the Rockies on a narrow road
5. scale the steep and roadless face of this same mountain in a snowstorm to rescue a friend.

Another example: A depressed patient depreciates himself, is lacking in courage, self-assertiveness and initiative. I may have him hallucinate in trance that it is a rainy, windy day and he is in a dreary landscape at the shore of a rough lake; but that in the distance, he can see the other shore of the lake bathed in warm sunshine, with relaxed people working and playing over there. This I designate as the shore of normal, healthy life. I then urge him to swim or row across that lake. Intentionally I will only mention as possibilities swimming or rowing—not, for instance, taking a ferry or a motor boat—so as to stimulate, symbolically, his own activity and coping processes. I let the patient describe how big the distance across the lake is. From time to time I will suggest that he has met with an obstacle on his way, and that he has to use his ingenuity to find means to overcome it, or a way to swim around it. I will ask him to describe the obstacle to me, and the methods he invents to deal with it. Usually I do not require the patient to "swim" the whole distance the first time. Too short a distance would symbolize an easy task. I let him rest, temporarily, on conveniently located islands. But I keep urging him on to greater and greater efforts, and wider and wider stretches to master. I attempt to develop in the patient first the hope and then the growing conviction that he can rally his coping mechanisms. Each part-success is exploited to give him renewed hope and self-confidence, as I support his efforts with the trust that eventually he can reach the other shore. I also suggest to him in trance that he can remain there when he has found out he can use his energy self-assertively and *constructively*, rather than in beating himself down, i.e. *destructively*. The imagery of the lake and swimming stand symbolically for real life obstacles and this patient's ability to master them; the other shore stands for a normal, happy life. The best therapeutic effects with this method of performing ego strengthening tasks in trance are achieved if the hypnoanalyst talks to his patient in the language of imagery and dreams, that is in primary process symbols, the language of the unconscious.

More realistic, ego supportive, encouraging hypnotic suggestion can also be used to help the patient. If the activity fantasied in trance is non-symbolic, we call it Reality-Testing-in-Fantasy. You let the patient rehearse and try to master in trance the very activity that he fears he cannot perform successfully in real life. Reality testing in fantasy—in and out of hypnosis—is another ego-strengthening, integrative process.

Why do such methods work? For two reasons: First of all, they *mobilize* the patient; they divert his emotional energies from being bound in defensive mechanisms to be channeled into productive coping activity. Secondly, research (Ruff and Korchin, 1967) has shown that the effectiveness of adaptive responses to stress is based on past experience and competence. In trance we develop a stress situation for the patient and then let him experience that, and how, he can handle it with increasing skill. Thus, in hypnosis experiential situations are created which lead to the mobilization of ego strength and the feeling of trusting oneself in real life, too.

Life is rarely without tension. We cannot "promise" our patients "a rose garden" (Green, 1964). But we can and must try to help them gain the desire and the ego strength to tackle difficulties in the paths of their lives and to deal with them to the best of their potentials.

REFERENCES

Bellak, L.: An ego psychological theory of hypnosis. *Int J Psychoanal, 36*: 1–4, 1955.

Fromm, Erika: Hypnoanalysis: theory and two case excerpts. *Psychotherapy,* 2:127–133, 1965.

Gill, M. M., and Brenman, Margaret: *Hypnosis and Related States: Psychoanalytic Studies in Regression.* New York, International Universities Press, 1961.

Green, Hannah: *I Never Promised You a Rose Garden.* New York, Signet, 1964.

Kris, Ernst: *Psychoanalytic Explorations in Art.* New York, Basic Books, 1952.

Meares, Ainslie: *The Door of Serenity.* London, Farber and Farber, 1958.

Prince, Morton: *The Dissociation of a Personality.* New York, London, Longmans Green and Company, 1906.

Raginsky, Benjamin B.: Sensory hypnoplasty with case illustrations. *Int J Clin Exp Hypn,* 3:137–147, 1962.

Ruff, G. E., and Korchin, S. F.: Adaptive stress behavior. In Appley, Mortimer H., and Trumbull, Richard (Eds): *Psychological Stress.* New York, Appleton, Century and Croft, 1967.

Thigpen, Corbett H., and Cleckley, Harvey M.: *The Three Faces of Eve.* New York, McGraw-Hill, 1957.

SECTION 4

USES OF BEHAVIOR
THERAPY IN HYPNOSIS

WHEN WOLPE, AMONG OTHERS, introduced behavior therapy, he used hypnosis as a relaxational technique; other behavior therapists continued the practice, but with lessening emphasis upon it through the years. In contrast, hypnotherapists have been using behavioral techniques with increasing interest and effectiveness. Erickson (in Beahrs, 1971) would assign tasks for the patient to do himself, thus allowing behavior modification to occur from within rather than by the imposition of external controls. Alexander (1971), Spiegel (1960; also in Dengrove, 1971), Kline (1970), and many other well-known hypnotherapists have written articles depicting their own versions of behavior therapy.

In this section, Weitzenhoffer provides a historical review of this association, detailing how hypnotherapists have long used hypnosis in conjunction with the therapeutic application of learning principles, yet without incorporating learning principles into therapy in a planned, systematic manner.

Ego-strengthening techniques are particularly suited to this association, and Hartland provides a clinically valuable, unusually effective, series of posthypnotic suggestions useful with behavioral techniques. His procedure adds an assertive quality (there is no article in the hypnosis-behavior therapy literature

285

exclusively on assertive techniques) helpful to patients who are fearful, helpless, introverted or withdrawn. Further, other suggestions specific to the patient's problems can be introduced at any point in the hypnotic procedure. Susskind describes her novel application of integration of hypnosis and cognitive conditioning principles for confidence and assertive training. The patient creates the dynamic goal of an idealized self through imagery in conjunction with hypnosis.

Hypnotherapists have commonly employed other behavior therapy-like techniques in treating maladaptive behaviors. Jabush follows with his version of ego-exhilaration, emphasizing appropriate self-assertion without anxiety by the use of hypnotic recall and intensification of a previously experienced pleasant affect. By means of two case presentations, Meyer and Tilker illustrate the use of posthypnotic suggestion and a technique very like covert positive reinforcement. Feamster and Brown employ a procedure similar to covert sensitization with aversive imagery ("worst hangover you have ever experienced") to treat alcoholism. Other authors (e.g. Smith-Moorhouse, 1969) have used similar procedures to treat the alcoholic. Schneck demonstrates the use of hypnosis incorporating a technique similar to flooding in imagination. Field describes the combined use of systematic desensitization and hypnotherapy to prevent crying.

Wickramasekera describes procedures to enhance hypnotizability through modeling, shaping, and other means. Other authors (Diamond, 1973; Kinney and Sachs, 1974), too, have used behavior modification techniques to increase hypnotic susceptibility by restructuring cognitions and attitudes, and alleviating anxiety.

Kroger concludes this section with a discussion of his combination of behavioral and hypnotherapeutic procedures to expedite therapy.

REFERENCES

Alexander, L.: Hypnotically induced hallucinations. *Dis Nerv Syst,* 32:91, 1971.

Beahrs, J. O.: The hypnotic psychotherapy of Milton H. Erickson, *Am J Clin Hypn, 14:*73, 1971.

Dengrove, E.: A single-treatment method to stop smoking using ancillary self-hypnosis: discussion. *Int J Clin Exp Hypn, XVIII:*251, 1970.

Diamond, M. J.: The modification of hypnotizability: a review. Unpublished manuscript.

Kinney, J. M., and Sachs, L. B.: Increasing hypnotic susceptibility. *J Abnorm Psychol, 83:*145, 1974.

Kline, M. H.: The use of extended group hypnotherapy sessions in controlling cigarette habituation. *Int J Clin Exp Hypn, XVIII:*276, 1970.

Smith-Moorhouse, P. M.: Hypnosis in the treatment of alcoholism. *Br J Addict, 64:*47, 1969.

Spiegel, H.: Hypnosis and the psychotherapeutic process. *Comp Psychiatry,* 3:175, 1960.

Wolpe, J.: *Psychotherapy By Reciprocal Inhibition.* Stanford, Stanford University Press, 1958.

CHAPTER *22*

BEHAVIOR THERAPEUTIC TECHNIQUES AND HYPNO- THERAPEUTIC METHODS*

ANDRE M. WEITZENHOFFER PH.D

INTRODUCTION

The literature on behavior therapy suggests that the use of hypnosis in connection with the application of learning principles is essentially limited to systematic desensitization. On the other hand, perusal of the hypnotherapeutic literature indicates that hypnotic techniques are being successfully used in conjunction with learning principles in a great many ways which clearly qualify as recognized behavior therapeutic techniques. Recognition of this fact by behavior therapists and hypnotherapists could be of considerable benefit to both groups if followed through.

A REVIEW of the behavior therapy literature published during the last five years reveals that behavior therapists hold a surprisingly limited view of the potential uses of hypnosis † (Wolpe, 1969; Franks, 1964, 1969; Schaefer and Martin, 1969). Behavioral therapists tend to discuss hypnosis only as a means of systematic desensitization for producing relaxation or enhancing imagery. ("Systematic desensitization" is not to be confused with the unqualified term "desensitization.") Wolpe (1969) does recognize the additional use of hypnosis in psychotherapy to elicit abreactions, but quite correctly states that this "is not a behavior therapy."

† The term "hypnosis" is used throughout this paper to denote "hypnosis as a state, hypnotic techniques and suggestions in general."

* Originally published in *The American Journal of Clinical Hypnosis*, Volume 15, Number 2, October 1972, pages 71–82. Copyright 1972 by the American Society of Clinical Hypnosis.

The paucity of applications of hypnosis by behavior therapists is puzzling when one considers that the hypnotherapeutic literature contains a fair number of references to the use of hypnosis in conjunction with the therapeutic application of learning principles. True, most psychotherapists who use hypnotic techniques extensively in their practice (hereafter called "hypnotherapists") never point out this fact. Not only do most hypnotherapists fail to incorporate learning principles into therapy in the planned, systematic manner of the behavior therapist, many display a barely rudimentary understanding of them. Some are even unaware of using them. Finally, whereas the behavior therapist sees hypnosis as adjunctive to the application of learning paradigms, the hypnotherapist sees this relation reversed (when he does plan his use of learning principles).

Three factors have probably helped conceal the therapeutic potential of hypnosis combined with learning principles.

1. Much relevant literature in hypnotherapy was published long before "behavior therapy" became a recognized branch of psychotherapy (Franks, 1964). For example, in 1948 Wolberg clearly discussed the use of hypnosis in systematic desensitization in his definitive work on medical hypnosis, but under the heading of "reconditioning." The expression "systematic desentization" had yet to enter the professional vocabulary.

2. Past behavior therapists have focused almost exclusively on strict Pavlovian and Skinnerian models of conditioning. Yet, other important, useful learning models exist, as described in such general texts on learning theory as that of Hilgard and Bower (1966). Wolpe (1958) did lean at one time toward the Hullian model of classical conditioning, and indications appear in the recent literature (Frank, 1969a, 1969b) that behavior therapy may be moving in a more eclectic direction in these regards.

3. Finally, behavior therapists have been inclined to work more in terms of paradigms associated with theories of learning than in terms of the many available empirically established principles of learning, such as those listed by Hilgard and Bower (1966). Such a restrictive framework has made it almost inevitable that behavior therapists would overlook certain applications of hypnosis in conjunction with learning theory.

The purpose of this article is to discuss neither the defects nor the merits of behavior modification vs. hypnotherapy. Its aim is to point out that the combination of hypnosis with learning principles has considerably more potential than the existing behavior therapeutic literature recognizes. For those readers who are prone to question the reality of hypnosis as a state, I would further add that suggestion and not hypnosis is the key concept in most modern hypnotherapy. Thus, any existing controversy regarding the existence or validity of hypnosis is not really germane to the present discussion. Even the question of whether "suggestion" is a valid concept is more or less irrelevant. The fact is that we must deal with two sets of techniques which, at least methodologically, have definite points of difference.

This article, then, will have a dual focus: (a) the extent to which behavior therapeutic techniques and the underlying principles can be used by hypnotherapists in conjunction with hypnosis and/or suggestion, and (b) how behavior therapists can use hypnosis and/or suggestion techniques in the context of behavior therapy. The evidence before us is not invariably clear-cut. Some reports in the literature written by hypnotherapists could just as easily have been written by strict behavior therapists. These pose no problems. It is the equally large (or larger) collection of reports, in which the use of learning principles is camouflaged by other therapeutic material, that raises problems of interpretation. To compound the difficulty, some behavior therapists, such as Franks (1964, 1969) and Wolpe (1969), frequently offer different interpretations regarding the principles employed in the treatment of given cases.

Finally, learning theory still contains a number of unresolved issues which inevitably affect both the design and interpretation of therapeutic techniques. Typically, no complete agreement has yet been reached concerning the existence of one-trial conditioning; the essentiality of drive-reduction continues to be controversial. Even the exact nature of reinforcement and reinforcers remains debatable. Nevertheless, it is this writer's belief that enough solid evidence exists to indicate that hypnosis has wider applicability within the framework of learning theory, and even within the stricter one of behavior therapy based on a stimulus-response (S-R) learning paradigm, than the literature reflects.

CATEGORIES OF BEHAVIOR MODIFICATION TECHNIQUES

Behavior therapy, in its broadest as well as its more limited sense, can generally be considered to consist of the systematic use of learning principles and/or theories to eliminate unadaptive behavior. It is beyond the scope of this article to explore these principles and theories in any detail. Summarily stated, they fall into two broad families: the stimulus-response (S-R) learning paradigms and the cognitive view of learning. For details the reader is referred to the excellent text of Hilgard and Bower (1966). Generally speaking, the understructure of behavior therapy has consisted of, and continues to consist of, strictly S-R theories. Accordingly, and as reviewed and discussed, for instance, by Wolpe (1969), the methods of behavior therapy fall under two main headings: classical conditioning (also known as Type I, Type S, respondent or Pavlovian conditioning), and instrumental conditioning (also known as Type II, Type R, operant conditioning, or Skinnerian conditioning).

Three basic techniques are used for classical conditioning in behavior therapy: counterconditioning, positive reconditioning, and experimental extinction (Wolpe, 1969). Counterconditioning is primarily an application of what Wolpe has called "reciprocal inhibition" (to be discussed in more detail later); he sees this as the basis of his own widely used technique of systematic desensitization, as well as of the well-known "aversion therapy." According to Wolpe, reciprocal inhibition plays some role in most of the behavior therapy techniques he discusses. Wolpe apparently uses "positive reconditioning" simply to denote the formation of a positive (adaptive) conditioned response to fill the gap left by removal of an unadaptive response. Under operant conditioning, he lists four broad techniques: positive reinforcement, extinction, punishment, and negative reinforcement. To these he adds differential reinforcement—a combination of the first two—and response-shaping, a special application of the first.

Let us now examine the various hypnotherapeutic procedures to show which of these behavior modification techniques have been used in conjunction with hypnosis.

THE USE OF LEARNING PRINCIPLES IN HYPNOTHERAPY IN THE CONTEXT OF A STRICT S-R APPROACH

Aversion Therapy and Hypnotherapy

The most striking and puzzling omission in the literature regarding the uses of hypnosis in behavior therapy is probably associated with aversive techniques. This is one of the oldest applications, dating back to the late nineteenth century or earlier. During this period nicotinism, morphinism, and especially chronic alcoholism were thus treated in Europe. Typically, the hypnotized patient was given suggestions ranging from moderate disgust to nausea and vomiting whenever he came into contact with the addictive substance (Bernheim, 1903; Tuckey, 1907; Moll, 1909; Forel, 1927; Grasset, 1904).

The practice continues to the present. For example, Abrams (1964) and Femster and Brown (1963) have recently used this method to treat alcoholics. Wolberg (1948) has outlined, under "reconditioning," a similar application of hypnosis for the control of "excessive smoking, nail-biting, eating and alcoholic indulgence." An innovation he has introduced is the association of painful and disgusting experiences from the patient's own life with the undesirable behavior. To this he has added associations with hypnotically induced, disagreeable fantasies. Others, such as Hershman (1955, 1956) and Kroger (1970), have successfully applied hypnosis to treat compulsive eaters and cigarette smokers by combining a similar aversive technique with positive reinforcement. Von Dedenroth (1964a, 1964b) has also treated smokers in this fashion with still further modifications. These modifications will be taken up in more detail in connection with operant conditioning. Finally, Erickson (1954c) has given a detailed account of the hypnotherapy of a case of enuresis which involved a subtle use of aversive therapy as part of the overall treatment. The complexity of the treatment, unfortunately, makes its complete description prohibitive in this space.

Cautela's "covert sensitization" (Wolpe, 1969, p. 214) should probably be mentioned here. Although neither he nor other behavior therapists apparently recognize any connections with hypnotherapy, covert sensitization may represent an exception to my earlier statement that behavior therapists seem to limit their use of hypnotic techniques to systematic desensitization. Cautela does not explicitly induce hypnosis, but his instructions to patients aimed at initiating aversion-evoking imagery seem otherwise indistinguishable from those used by Wolberg (1948), Hershman (1955, 1956), and Kroger (1970) for the same purpose in conjunction with hypnosis. I do not imply that Cautela's instructions owe their therapeutic potency to the fact that they are "suggestions." This remains an open question. In view of the known potency of nonhypnotic suggestions, however, the possibility cannot be excluded. Hence, covert sensitization might qualify as hypnotherapy (or perhaps, more appropriately, suggestion therapy) just as well as systematic desensitization.

General Counterconditioning Therapy, Positive Conditioning Therapy, and Hypnotherapy

Although counterconditioning is discussed in the behavior therapy literature primarily in relation to overcoming anxiety, the method is clearly not limited to this (Wolpe, 1969). "Counterconditioning" seems to be Wolpe's terms for the conditioned inhibition of certain undesirable behavior through the application of what he has called "the reciprocal inhibition principle [1958, 1959]." In its most general form, the principle states that: if a response R_1 inhibitory of another response R_2 can be elicited in the presence of a stimulus which evokes R_2, it will weaken the stimulus-response bond. This condition can be expected to be satisfied when, in particular, R_1, and R_2 are mutually exclusive and R_1 is prepotent. Wolpe (1969) makes the further point that "there are many instances of positive conditioning which *ipso facto* include the conditioned inhibition of previous habits of responses to the antecedent stimuli concerned"—a remark significant to much of the material which follows in this section.

Wolberg (1948, p. 213, 215) has given two of the earliest accounts of hypnosis applied in the context of reciprocal inhibition and systematic desensitization. These two brief accounts, which he categorizes under "reconditioning," clearly antedate Wolpe's 1958 work. In one case, a patient experienced such an unreasonably intense dislike for orange juice that it had become a very real problem. In the other instance, profound unease and discomfort in the presence of people was the problem. Both patients were treated by hypnotically inducing fantasies in which the problem stimulus (oranges, people) was experienced in the presence of hypnotically induced feelings of pleasure, happiness, relaxation, and peace.

Erickson's (1955) treatment of two patients with cosmetic problems caused by dental defects appears to be best described as involving the reciprocal inhibition of self-deprecatory behaviors. Both patients suffered from strong feelings of inadequacy focused on their dental defects, with consequent emotional repercussions. As his primary therapeutic approach, Erickson used instigated behaviors which led these patients to associate positive feelings with their dental defects, thus countering their previous totally negative feelings.

More recently, Ludwig et al. (1964) have described a procedure for treating drug addicts; it closely resembles Wolpe's description of "thought-stopping." Its uniqueness lies in the ingenious use of a complex posthypnotic suggestion to evoke hallucinations which act as automatic thought-stoppers. These hallucinations are triggered by thoughts of using drugs. Ludwig et al. mention a second technique which probably falls in this category, too. It consists in part of inducing a selective "amnesia" for the words "narcotic drugs" and the associated craving. Additionally, these authors had the patients conjointly use self-hypnotically induced relaxation within a framework of standard "desensitizing" in order to counter the drug-craving.

Another probable instance of thought- and action-stopping in hypnotherapy appears in Spiegel's recently reported method for treating smokers through hypnosis (1970). The patient is initially taught self-hypnosis and instructed under hypnosis to perform a meditative exercise in self-hypnosis throughout the day (detailed by Spiegel). The patient is instructed to do this particularly when he feels the urge to smoke. He is also given posthypnotic instructions in the ritualistic-like use of a series of acts which he can eventually substitute for the meditative exercise and perform any time he feels the need to smoke.

Clearly, this activity regimen must act as a buffer against protracted thinking about smoking and against smoking itself. Apparently, the primary function of the initial use of hypnosis is to enable the therapist to set up the above pattern of activity as posthypnotically suggested behavior. An element of aversive therapy may also enter into the technique because of the specific association which the patient is asked to make in hypnosis, and later in self-hypnosis, between smoking and bodily injury (and, indirectly, death). This is the focal theme of the prescribed meditation.

A number of the reported uses of hypnosis appear to fall best in Wolpe's class of positive conditioning simultaneously producing an associated inhibition. In these instances, a more adaptive response is substituted for a less adaptive one; the method could well be designated "direct response substitution." Baumann (1970), for instance, has shown young drug abusers how they can evoke more satisfying hallucinatory experiences with hypnosis than with drugs. This posthypnotic training is, of course, carefully accompanied by protective (limiting) instructions regarding the use of self-induced hallucinations. Mann (1961) has described similar treatment of a combined drinking-weight problem in which the patient is hypnotically induced to substitute non-alcoholic, non-caloric beverages for alcohol and excessive food—with equally satisfying results. This writer, treating an asthmatic patient who was also an inveterate smoker, used hypnotic techniques to ascertain exactly what the patient experienced when smoking. Then, by suggestion, the patient was able to substitute for actual smoking a few puffs on a nonexisting cigarette. The associated hallucination, duplicating the experience of real smoking, proved to be the key to eliminating the cigarette habit. Von Dedenroth's (1964a, 1964b) treatment of tobaccomania, to be described shortly, includes analogous procedures.

Erickson's "symptom substitution" and "symptom transformation" techniques (1954b) are probably best categorized under the above heading, too. In all of the examples discussed, hypnotic instructions were used to help the patient substitute a more adaptive form of behavior for certain incapacitating behavior, although the new behavior still contained neurotic elements. In one case, for instance, a moderate stiffness of the right wrist was substituted for a hysterical paralysis of the entire arm. In another case, anxiety elicited by the patient's enuresis was countered by suggested anxiety associated with other matters. In both cases, hypnosis was used to create a competing, prepotent, and hence inhibiting behavior.

Positive and Negative Reinforcement and Hypnotherapy

Both Hershman (1955, 1956) and Kroger (1970) have combined positive reinforcement with other techniques in the hypnotherapy of smoking and weight problems; Baumann (1970) has done this with drug abusers. For instance, both Hershman and Kroger use hypnosis to make their patients associate pleasant, positive feelings with the desired behavior (abstinence from smoking, consuming less food, and eating only the right foods). Peterson and London (1964) reported a case in which hypnotic suggestions apparently functioned in three ways; otherwise, it was a straightforward application of operant conditioning. Their patient was a young child with dyscopresis. First, a simple schedule of reinforcement was used to encourage the child to have a bowel movement which could be rewarded. Second, the act of defecation was rewarded by a (suggested) good feeling. Third, a degree of relaxation was evoked sufficient to counter the child's anxiety surrounding defecation, thus introducing an element of reciprocal inhibition and desensitization.

Von Dedenroth (1964a, 1964b) has described a treatment for tobaccomania which, from a learning standpoint, combines various techniques, the dominant one being positive reinforcement. Through hypnotic suggestions, various good feelings are associated with a particular sequence of activities in which smoking is prohibited. This is part of a response shaping program involving three sessions. Combined with this, competing prepotent activities are introduced, the subject being instructed in both the nonhypnotic and hypnotic states to perform certain activities in lieu of smoking, should he feel the urge to smoke. This step, which is probably best categorized as a use of reciprocal inhibition or positive conditioning, is also probably involved in Spiegel's treatment of smoking already discussed.

Von Dedenroth combines the above with aversive therapy. The patient is sequentially asked to use brands of cigarettes lower and lower on his preference scale. At the same time, he is repeatedly hypnotized and made to associate smoking with its various negative aspects. Later, the therapist suggests that each puff will become less enjoyable to the patient and eventually that the smoking habit will be disagreeable. Thus, smoking becomes not only less pleasurable, it is actually associated with negative affect and unpleasantness. Finally, the patient is instructed, in and out of hypnosis, to abstain from cigarettes at certain times of the day (when he is most likely to smoke), according to a schedule of progressively increasing abstention. This step represents conditioning of the abstention response to specific stimuli. Since abstention is probably self-rewarding in this situation, operant condition as well as classical (positive) conditioning is at work.

Self-reward as an active agent is not unique to this situation, of course. It is probably an important factor in many hypnotherapeutic procedures. Meyer and Tilker (1969) have used posthypnotic suggestions to induce two of their patients with character disorders to reward their own appropriate actions by strong, immediate self-approval by giving them suggestions to this effect. This writer has found a similar procedure helpful in treating habitual smokers and compulsive eaters.

Erickson (1965) used what was probably positive reinforcement in treating a patient who experienced highly distressing coldness in her buttocks. Through hypnosis he enabled her to associate directly the feeling of coldness with enjoyable feelings and experiences. The symptom was not only dealt with satisfactorily, but the patient's previously unsatisfactory sex life improved, eventuating in a happy marriage after many previous marital failures.

Finally, Erickson's "symptom substitution" technique (1954b) may also have an element of operant conditioning in the approval and disapproval which the therapist probably communicates in relation to the behavioral shift occurring or not occurring.

Other Behavioral Therapeutic Techniques and Hypnotherapy

Ludwig et al. (1964) attempted to use a "modeling" technique to cure drug addiction. Although the results were questionable, the method was interesting. Hypnotized drug addicts were repeatedly instructed to "watch" a fantasied television show in which the hero overcame his craving for drugs.

Erickson has employed techniques involving simple extinction-producing situations. For instance, his treatment of enuresis (1954c) by aversive techniques, mentioned earlier, certainly also contained elements of "negative practice," in which a repeated response vanishes due to lack of reinforcement. As also mentioned, the complexity of Erickson's *modus operandi* in this case precludes a detailed explanation here. It should be added there is some question whether hypnosis was really involved. That is, no actual, explicit induction of hypnosis was ever actually used. Erickson does, however, maintain that hypnosis was indirectly induced and employed, mainly in the posthypnotic production and enforcing of certain behaviors required by the therapy plan.

The combined use of hypnosis and extinction seems much clearer in Erickson's ingenious "pseudo-orientation-in-time" technique (1954a), whereby the hypnotized patient is projected into the future and made to experience the therapeutic goal as an actuality already achieved. As an example, he cites a patient suffering from a compulsion to visit his mother's grave daily; this severely interfered with his life. Erickson used hypnosis to project the patient's imagination two weeks into the future, at which time the patient fantasied himself to have failed to make his habitual visits to the grave. He was then reoriented to the present, brought out of hypnosis, with amnesia suggested for the hypnotic experience, and given an appointment two weeks later. During this period, the patient neither visited the grave nor gave it a thought. When this fact was brought to his attention at the next visit, he was also given the strong affirmation that now he knew he did not have to visit the grave. A follow-up ten years later showed that the compulsion remained abated. This could be considered a one-trial extinction taking place during the temporal projection and further reinforced during the next few weeks. Although a Pavlovian paradigm can be used for this, the operant model of extinction seems more appropriate. One could also view the case as a many-trial extinction, for the actual two weeks free of visits effectively amounted to fourteen trials without negative reinforcement (i.e. the unverbalized feared consequences of not going to the grave). A third possible interpretation, better suited to readers who cannot concede that extinction could take place during an imaginary situation, is simply that a posthypnotic command not to visit the grave was capable of overriding the patient's compulsion for two weeks, thus allowing him to become deconditioned. This last mechanism is not exclusive of others, and conceivably extinction could have been multi-determined in accordance with these various mechanisms.

FURTHER APPLICATIONS OF LEARNING THEORY IN HYPNOTHERAPY

Thus far we have discussed hypnotherapy mainly from the standpoint of the techniques and learning principles most often used by behavior therapists. Clearly, however, the field is open to numerous applications of learning principles such as are listed by Hilgard and Bower (1966, p. 486) which behavior therapists generally fail to consider, at least overtly.

One of the most widely recognized factors affecting learning is motivation. Proper motivation not only enhances learning, it undoubtedly contributes to the success of many forms of hypnotherapy. Motivation of the patient can be readily introduced in any hypnotherapy, through the use of appropriate hypnotic instructions and suggestions. They can be as direct as telling the patient he will want to make certain steps, or will look forward to making these shortly. The motivational instructions may, however, also be less direct, and even quite subtly built in. There is a good likelihood that some of the aversion techniques and uses of positive and negative reinforcement employed by hypnotherapists may also indirectly function as producers of added motivation. However, as Hilgard (1956) has pointed out, overly intense motivation can work against effective learning. In this writer's experience over the years, many patients seek hypnotherapy as a last resort. Their intense need to succeed now "or else" often is more of a hindrance than a help and must be reduced before learning principles can be satisfactorily used.

Little question seems to exist that appropriate and inappropriate goals can be important factors in successful learning. Appropriate therapeutic goals for the patient also are important. Many hypnotherapeutic techniques involve the creation of goals and the channeling of activities toward these goals. Not only do they reinforce the goal of attaining a cure, they often create adjunctive goals. Spiegel's hypnotic treatment of smokers (1970) may owe part of its effectiveness to the enhancing effect hypnosis seems to have on any commitment made in this state. In this case, the patient commits himself to protecting his body from the effects of smoking.

Affects and attitudes, which often have strong influences upon an individual's state of motivation, are frequently manipulated by hypnotherapists in ways which favor the application of learning principles. Most of Erickson's articles mentioned earlier contain instances of this. Apart from their influence on motivational states, affects and attitudes have other potentials for helping or hindering learning processes. Characteristically, intense affect can be highly disruptive of any ongoing learning process. It can cause breakdown of existing learned behavior and prevent new learning. While this is difficult to document specifically in the hypnotherapy literature, it is reasonable to suspect that some of the steps used by hypnotherapists have taken cognizance of this principle. My own experience with patients leaves me little doubt that my use of hypnosis specifically to decrease strong affect has made a significant contribution to otherwise nonhypnotherapeutic techniques aimed at developing more adequate behaviors through reeducation. I have also intentionally and successfully used hypnosis to bring about attitudinal changes favoring the acquisition of new, better, responses or the reinstatement of older but more adequate ones.

Perceptual factors contribute in many ways both to the learning process and to eliciting learned behaviors. Adequate stimulus discrimination is particularly important. Here, too, specific examples in the existing hypnotherapeutic literature are difficult to find, although the potentialities certainly exist. On a number of occasions, this writer has deliberately used hypnosis as an instrument to improve a patient's discrimination in dealing with outmoded, inadequate behavior which came to the surface in situations resembling earlier events. I have also used hypnosis to create a perceptual alteration to make smokers more aware of the acts of reaching for a cigarette and even smoking it, both of which are so often automatic. This has been enough to allow some patients to then acquire voluntary control over their smoking.

Transfer of learning (stimulus generalization) is another widely accepted phenomenon in learning theory. It may underlie what Wolberg (1948) has referred to as "removal of symptom with active participation by the patient." The patient is first induced to experience the production and then the removal of an artificial symptom through suggestions and other hypnotic methods. Then an artificial symptom similar to the chief complaint is produced elsewhere in his body. This is followed, in sequence, by the partial hypnotic removal of the chief complaint, enhancement of the artificial symptom, and, finally, total removal of the chief complaint. When the artificial symptom is left in lieu of the original one, the new symptom is selected so as to be minimally incapacitating. When the artificial symptom is removed, a residual form of the original symptom is allowed to remain. The basic process here appears to be a generalization (transfer) of the patient's acquired control of the artificial symptom to the control of the real symptom. The exact mechanism of the transfer remains unclear, however. Perhaps an analog of learning transfer is more valid than the actual thing. In any event, Erickson (1935) used this approach to treat a patient suffering from premature ejaculation. In his detailed discussion of the therapeutic process, he explicitly mentioned generalization as a possible mechanism effecting the cure. Posthypnotic suggestions can play a particularly important role in hypnotherapy as elicitors of specific behaviors. Both classical and operant conditioning call for the repeated production of certain responses under highly specific conditions. Posthypnotic suggestions offer an unusual degree of control over this, as in the aversion therapy situations discussed earlier.

Although many other aspects of learning actively enter into

the various forms of hypnotherapy described in the literature, we will discuss only one more here: learning capacities. This in itself is not a learning principle, but it cannot be overlooked in any treatment which involves learning processes. This aspect of a patient's makeup can be as critical to the success of therapy as his hypnotizability. Most hypnotherapists, as well as most behavior therapists, tend to ignore this factor, because, for the most part, they are unaware of making use of learning principles. Erickson, one of the few hypnotherapists who has specifically discussed and attempted to use elicited and emitted behavior within a learning framework, takes learning capacities into account. Integral to his overall philosophy as a hypnotist and therapist is the importance of using a patient's fullest learning and response-producing capacities.

SOME FINAL CONSIDERATIONS

Indirect Adjunctive Roles of Hypnosis

Thus far, we have considered rather direct uses of hypnosis to create favorable conditions for behavior therapeutic techniques. Hypnosis makes indirect contributions, as well. For example, some therapists use hypnosis to uncover important facts in the patient's past history, particularly regarding his symptoms. Although behavior therapy can certainly be successful without this, it might prove less efficient. Another element not to be regarded lightly is the apparent ease of establishing an intense rapport when one uses hypnotherapy. Moreover hypnosis imparts to patients a sense of well-being, a positive attitude toward the future, and a reduction of discomfort.

Influence of Hypnosis and Hypnotic Suggestions Upon the Learning Processes

Hypnosis and hypnotic suggestions might also be used in behavior therapy to enhance learning processes directly. Laboratory experiments have been conducted to determine whether hypnosis per se or specific hypnotic suggestions can facilitate retroactive inhibition, positive reinforcement, extinction, external inhibition, etc. This research has been reviewed by Treloar (1967), Von

Dedenroth (1964b) and Weitzenhoffer (1953, 1954, 1955). Although the results have remained generally ambiguous and, at best, offer only partial answers, there have been enough reports of positive effect in the laboratory to force one to consider the above as a strong possibility. In any case, it is debatable whether one can extrapolate laboratory data to the clinic. The difficulty lies partly in the extremely limited, circumscribed, elementary behaviors examined in the laboratory. Hypnosis experiments performed in association with behavior therapy are certainly not infeasible; they simply have not been done.

Posthypnotic and Other Hypnotic Delayed Behaviors and Learned Behavior

An intriguing aspect of hypnotic behavior is this: Whatever actual mechanism is involved, certain instructions, commands, and suggestions given to hypnotized subjects seem to be able to create more or less lasting effects which overtly look like learned behavior (if one overlooks theoretical and paradigmatical formulations). Delayed and posthypnotic suggestions operate in this manner. This feature of the elicited behaviors is especially apparent in the definition taken from Hilgard and Bower (1966); "Learning is the process by which an activity originates or is changed through reacting to an encountered situation, provided that the characteristic of the change in activity cannot be explained on the basis of native response tendencies, maturation, or temporary states of the organism (e.g. fatigue, drugs, etc.)." This definition raises the possibility that suggestions which evoke enduring change in an individual's behavior constitute learning— perhaps a form of learning as yet to be recognized as such. That unrecognized forms of learning may exist finds support in a recent review and discussion of learning categories by Melton (1964). Posthypnotic suggestions given in the course of hypnotherapy often do seem to establish responses to cues which resemble learning. Whether patients told to experience smoking as distasteful and nauseating really have this experience, the fact remains that they respond appropriately over a long-enough period for the aversion therapy to be considered successful. Frequently, such hypnotically induced associations as smoking-nausea have all of the appearances of learning in one trial, which both Guthrie and Skinner have maintained is possible (Hilgard and Bower, 1966). More often, however, and in closer parallel to the learning situation, one has to "reinforce" the posthypnotic suggestions through repeated statements to make them fully effective. One might further consider the intriguing questions of whether posthypnotic behavior instituted to occur indefinitely in response to certain cues does not eventually evolve into habitual behavior no different from other "naturally" acquired responses. Erickson (private communication) appears to believe that this does, indeed, take place.

CONCLUSIONS

Examination of the hypnotherapy literature leaves little doubt that many hypnotherapists apply a variety of learning principles in conjunction with their hypnotic techniques. In many cases, they use procedures similar enough to those employed by behavior therapists to identify their approaches as "behavior therapeutically oriented hypnotherapies," or, more simply, "behavioristic hypnotherapies," in distinction to other types of hypnotherapy (such as "hypnoanalysis," probably better termed "psychoanalytically oriented hypnotherapy"). Thus, a realistic survey of behavior therapy does not justify the limited view of the utility of hypnosis which behavior therapists seem to hold. This last can probably be explained by their professional-philosophical orientation, as well as by the historical antecedents of behavior therapy. In any event, little question seems to exist that behavior therapists could profitably make far greater use of hypnosis. On the other hand, hypnotherapists who use learning principles apparently do so on an intuitive basis most of the time, and usually not too systematically. A greater awareness on their part of the potentialities inherent in a more systematic use of learning principles would probably generate an even more effective use of hypnosis by hypnotherapists.

REFERENCES

Abrams, S.: An evaluation of hypnosis in the treatment of alcoholics. *Am J Phychiatry, 120:*1160–1165, 1964.

Baumann, F.: Hypnosis and the adolescent drug abuser. *Am J Clin Hypn,* 13:17–21, 1970.

Bernheim, H.: *Hypnotisme, Suggestion, Psychothérapie.* Paris, Octave Doin, 1903.

Erickson, M. H.: A study of an experimental neurosis hypnotically induced in a case of ejaculatio praecox. *Br J Med Psychol,* 15:34–50, 1935.

Erickson, M. H.: Pseudo-orientation in time as a hypnotherapeutic procedure. *J Clin Exp Hypn,* 2:261–283, 1954. (a)

Erickson, M. H.: Special techniques of brief hypnotherapy. *J Clin Exp Hypn,* 2:109–129, 1954. (b)

Erickson, M. H.: Undirect hypnotic therapy of an enuretic couple. *J Clin Exp Hypn,* 2:171–174, 1954. (c)

Erickson, M. H.: Hypnotherapy of two psychosomatic dental problems. *Journal of the American Society of Psychosomatic Dentistry,* 1:6–10, 1955.

Erickson, M. H.: The use of symptoms as an integral part of hypnotherapy. *Am J Clin Hypn,* 8:57–65, 1965.

Feamster, J. H., and Brown, J. E.: Hypnotic aversion to alcohol: Three-year follow-up on one patient. *Am J Clin Hypn,* 6:164–166, 1963.

Forel, A.: *Hypnotism or Suggestion and Psychotherapy.* New York, Allied Publishing Company, 1927.

Franks, C. M. (Ed.): *Conditioning Techniques in Clinical Practice and Research.* New York, Springer Publishing Company, 1964.

Franks, C. M. (Ed.): *Behavior Therapy. Appraisal and Status.* New York, McGraw-Hill, 1969. (a)

Franks, C. M.: Introduction: Behavior therapy and its Pavlovian origins: Review and perspectives. In Franks, C. M. (Ed.): *Behavior Therapy. Appraisal and Status.* New York, McGraw-Hill, 1969b.

Grasset, P.: *L'Hypnotisme et la suggestion.* Paris, Octave Doin, 1904.

Hershman, S.: Hypnosis in the treatment of obesity. *Journal of Clinical and Experimental Hypnosis,* 3:136–139, 1955.

Hershman, S.: Hypnosis and excessive smoking. *J Clin Exp Hypn,* 4:27–29, 1956.

Hilgard, E. R.: *Theories of Learning.* New York, Appleton-Century-Crofts, 1956.

Hilgard, E. R., and Bower, G. H.: *Theories of Learning.* New York, Appleton-Century-Crofts, 1966.

Kanfer, F. H., and Phillips, J. S.: A survey of current behavior therapies and a proposal for classification. In Franks, C. M. (Ed.): *Behavior Therapy. Appraisal and Status.* New York, McGraw-Hill, 1969.

Kroger, W. S.: Comprehensive management of obesity. *Am J Clin Hypn,* 12:165–176, 1970.

Ludwig, A. M., Williams, H. L., Jr., and Miller, J. S.: Group hypnotherapy techniques with drug addicts. *Int J Clin Exp Hypn,* 12:53–66, 1964.

Mann, H.: Hypnotherapy in habit disorders. *Am J Clin Hypn,* 3:123–126, 1961.

Melton, A. W.: The taxonomy of human learning: Overview. In Melton, A. W. (Ed.), *Categories of Human Learning*. New York, Academic Press, 1964.

Meyer, R. G., and Tilker, H. A.: The clinical use of direct hypnotic suggestion: A traditional technique in the light of current approaches. *International Journal of Clinical and Experimental Hypnosis, 17:*81–88, 1969.

Moll, A.: *Hypnotism*. London and New York, Walter Scott Publishing Company, 1909.

Peterson, D. R., and London, P.: Neobehavioristic psychotherapy: Quasi-hypnotic suggestion and multiple reinforcement in the treatment of a case of post-infantil dyscopresis. *The Psychological Record, 14:*469–474, 1964.

Schaefer, H. H., and Martin, P. L.: *Behavioral Therapy*. New York, Mc-Graw-Hill, 1969.

Spiegel, H.: A single-treatment method to stop smoking using ancillary self-hypnosis. *Int J Clin Exp Hypn, 18:*235–250, 1970.

Treloar, W. W.: Review of recent research on hypnotic learning. *Psychol Rep, 20:*723–732, 1967.

Tuckey, C. L.: *Treatment by Hypnotism and Suggestion*. London, Baillere, Tindal and Cox, 1970.

Von Dedenroth, T. E. A.: The use of hypnosis with "tobaccomaniacs." *Am J Clin Hypn, 6:*326–331, 1964. (a)

Von Dedenroth, T. E. A.: Further help for the "tobaccomaniacs." *Am J Clin Hypn, 6:*332–336, 1964. (b)

Weitzenhoffer, A. M.: *Hypnotism. An Objective Study in Suggestibility*. New York, John Wiley and Sons, 1953.

Weitzenhoffer, A. M.: The influence of hypnosis on the learning process. *J Clin Exp Hypn, 2:*191–200, 1954.

Weitzenhoffer, A. M.: The influence of hypnosis on the learning process. Some theoretical considerations: Recall of meaningful material. *Journal of Clinical and Experimental Hypnosis, 3:*148–165, 1955.

Wolberg, L. R.: *Medical Hypnosis. Volume I. The Principles of Hypnotherapy*. New York, Grune and Stratton, 1948.

Wolpe, J.: *Psychotherapy by Reciprocal Inhibition*. Stanford, Stanford University Press, 1958.

Wolpe J.: *The Practice of Behavior Therapy*. New York, Pergamon Press, 1969.

CHAPTER 23

THE EGO-STRENGTHENING TECHNIQUE

John Hartland, B.Sc., M.B., Ch.B., M.R.C.S., L.R.C.P.

INTRODUCTION

[The following excerpt, taken from Medical and Dental Hypnosis and Its Clinical Applications, Second Edition, Williams and Wilkins Co., 1971, provides a post-hypnotic suggestion of unusual effectiveness when added to the usual behavioral techniques. It has an assertive quality that can prove most helpful to any patient who tends to be fearful, helpless, introverted, or withdrawn. Further, other suggestions more specific to the patient and his problems can be introduced into the patter at any point.—Editor.]

THE EGO-STRENGTHENING TECHNIQUE

Psychotherapy of this kind need be neither difficult nor complicated provided that certain fundamental requirements of the patient are borne in mind. For this purpose his psychological reactions to his illness can be conveniently divided into two groups:

1. Those arising as a consequence of the illness itself, such as anxiety, fear, tension and agitation.
2. Those arising from defects in his own personality, such as nervousness, lack of confidence, dependence and maladjustment.

In planning your general psychotherapeutic suggestions to combat these, many can be adopted as standard ones which remain unchanged from case to case. Others will naturally have to be added or varied to suit each individual and his particular complaint. If once you develop the habit of using such a technique in every case that you treat under hypnosis before you proceed either with direct symptom-removal or hypno-analysis as the main object of your therapy, you will find it will pay handsome dividends. Not only will the patient obtain more rapid relief from his symptoms, but he will display obvious improvement in other ways. You will notice him becoming more self-reliant, more confident and more able to adjust to his environment, and thus much less prone to relapse. In fact, my own experience has led me to believe, and this has been confirmed by innumerable reports from professional colleagues, medical and dental both in this country and overseas, that *this combination of what I call 'ego-strengthening' suggestions and symptom-removal will enable the general practitioner to deal successfully with the majority of his cases without having to resort to hypno-analytical procedures.* Naturally, he will still encounter some cases in which a relatively simple investigation and superficial analysis of the patient's current environmental difficulties and his reactions to them will render his treatment both speedier and more effective. Even under these circumstances, I still adopt the same basic scheme in framing my therapeutic suggestions, incorporating any additions that may seem desirable as a result of analytical investigation. It has been especially interesting to hear how many dental surgeons are successfully using a specially constructed and shortened version of the standard technique in their everyday work.

In the construction of an ego-strengthening technique, quite apart from the actual suggestions themselves, it is essential that particular attention should be paid to such significant factors as *'rhythm,' 'repetition,' the interpolation of appropriate 'pauses,'* and the *'stressing of certain important words and phrases.'* The verbalization that I devised for my own use, even in psychiatric work, has been carefully constructed in accordance with these principles. In this connection, I consider certain points to be worthy of your attention. You will notice that repetition is often achieved by expressing the same fundamental idea in two or three different ways. This tends to avoid excessive monotony. Some words and phrases are stressed because of their importance and significance to the patient himself. Other words are stressed and suitable pauses included with the sole purpose of emphasizing the rhythm of the whole delivery which, in my opinion contributes considerably to its success. The manipulation of these factors should become self-evident as I describe the whole routine.

First, I must refer briefly to the question of trance depth. One of the advantages of this technique is the fact that deep trances are certainly not essential. Nevertheless, as in most hypnotherapeutic methods, the deeper the trance, the more rapidly improvement will occur and the shorter the duration of a course of treatment will be. The patient who has been conditioned to enter the hypnotic state upon a given signal, verbal or otherwise, can usually be regarded as having attained sufficient depth for treatment to be effective. Yet even this is not absolutely necessary since a satisfactory response can often be obtained in light trance states only. Under these circumstances, however, one would naturally expect treatment to be continued over a longer period and the results to manifest themselves more slowly. Methods of trance induction and deepening are of little significance and can be safely left to individual preference, although I do consider it important that the patient should be rendered as fully relaxed, mentally and physically, as possible and it is well worth while spending a little extra time to attain this objective.

In the following detailed account and analysis, I am describing in full the routine I use successfully in dealing with such cases as anxiety states, tension states, and phobias. Most of it is equally applicable as a prelude to the treatment of asthmas, migraines and various psychosomatic conditions. It lends itself admirably to shortening, adaptation and the addition of specialized suggestions in accordance with individual needs, both of the patient and of the therapist.

A TYPICAL EGO-STRENGTHENING ROUTINE

Once the patient is in a trance state and is as fully relaxed as possible, I proceed as follows:

"You have now become *so* deeply relaxed . . . *so* deeply asleep . . . that your mind has become *so* sensitive . . . *so* receptive to what I say . . . that *everything* that I put into your mind . . . will sink *so* deeply into the unconscious part of your mind . . . and will cause so deep and lasting an impression there . . . that *nothing* will eradicate it.

This tends to prepare the patient's mind to receive the suggestions that follow. Notice the stressing and repetition of the word *so* which not only adds force to the ideas presented, but also strongly emphasizes the rhythmic quality of the delivery.

> "Consequently . . . these things that I put into your unconscious mind . . . will begin to exercise a greater and greater influence over the way you think . . . over the way you feel . . . over the way you behave."

This is the first indication to the patient that he will begin to feel a gradual change in his thoughts, feelings and actions, as a result of the suggestions he is about to receive.

> "And . . . because these things *will* remain . . . firmly imbedded in the unconscious part of your mind . . . after you have left here . . . when you are no longer with me . . . they will continue to exercise that same great influence . . . over your *thoughts* . . . your *feelings* . . . and your *actions* . . . *just* as strongly *just* as surely . . . *just* as powerfully . . . when you are back home . . . or at work . . . as when you are with me in this room."

Here you will notice the introduction of the first unobtrusive post-hypnotic suggestion to the effect that the patient can expect the same changes to continue in his everyday life, after the trance state has been terminated. Note also that so far, all the suggestions have been directed towards the modification of the three fundamental psychological processes—'*thinking*,' '*feeling*,' and '*acting*.' These words have been stressed because of their importance to the patient, and the word '*just*,' in order to add to the rhythmic quality of the delivery. Repetition has been ensured by the use of three different words—'*strongly*,' '*surely*,' '*powerfully*' —all of which convey the same essential idea. Those familiar with my original descriptions of this technique will realize that these groups of suggestions are entirely new. Judging by clinical results, I am convinced that their addition has given increased force to the effectiveness of the basic routine.

> You are now so *very deeply asleep* . . . that *everything* that I tell you that is going to happen to you . . . *for your own good* . . . *will* happen . . . *exactly* as I tell you.
> And *every feeling* . . . that I tell you that you will experience . . . you *will* experience . . . *exactly* as I tell you.

And these same things *will continue to happen* to you . . . *every day* . . . and you *will continue to experience* these same feelings . . . *every day* . . . *every day* . . . *just* as strongly *just* as surely . . . *just* as powerfully . . . when you are back home . . . or at work . . . as when you are with me in this room.

Here we have repetition, not only of single words or phrases, but of the same group of expectations and ideas already expressed—'driving them home'—as it were. The patient begins to expect that he will not only experience something in the course of the trance, but that he will continue to benefit from this even when he is no longer receiving active treatment. I attach the greatest importance to this 'post-hypnotic' effect, for surely the whole success of treatment under hypnosis depends upon the simple fact that the suggestions last longer than the trance itself. The words '*will*' and '*exactly*,' together with other phrases of significance to the patient, are pronounced with increased emphasis to add force and authority to the suggestions, and although you will have noticed the continued interpolation of '*pauses*,' I have not drawn particular attention to them. Let me repeat one phrase in a slightly different manner: "*Just* as strongly . . . (pause) . . . *just* as surely . . . (pause) . . . *just* as powerfully . . . (pause)." and observe how the stressing of the word '*just*' helps to drive the idea home, almost like the blows of a hammer, and this, taken in conjunction with the pauses, establishes a rhythmical quality to the delivery similar to the beat of a metronome. In this connection, I think most of us tend to pay far too little attention to the importance of pauses in our work with hypnosis. Although this may be partly due to the limitations on our time, I am sure that this is not invariably the case. After all, when we give the patient a drug we are quite content to allow sufficient time for it to take effect, and if only we adopted the same attitude of mind when working with a patient in a hypnotic trance I am convinced that our results would become greatly enhanced.

As a result of this brief analysis of the mode of construction and delivery of these suggestive routines, you should now be able to detect these devices whenever they are used. You will find that, throughout the rest of this technique, I have strictly observed the same cardinal principles of 'repetition,' 'stressing,' and the use of 'synonymous words and phrases' intermingled with 'pauses' to secure a smooth, rhythmic delivery.

> During this deep sleep . . . *you* are going to feel physically *stronger* and *fitter* in every way.
> You will feel *more* alert . . . *more wide*-awake . . . *more* energetic.
> You will become *much* less easily tired . . . *much* less easily fatigued . . . *much* less easily discouraged . . . *much* less easily depressed.
> *Every day* . . . you will become *so deeply interested* in whatever you are doing . . . in whatever is going on around you . . . that your mind will become *completely distracted away from yourself.* You will no longer *think nearly so much about yourself* . . . you will no longer *dwell nearly so much upon yourself and your difficulties* . . . and you will become *much less conscious of yourself* . . . *much less pre-occupied with yourself* . . . *and with your own feelings.*
> *Every day* . . . your nerves will become *stronger and steadier* . . . your mind *calmer and clearer* . . . *more composed* . . . *more placid* . . . *more tranquil.* You will become *much less easily worried* . . . *much less easily agitated* . . . *much less easily fearful and apprehensive* . . . *much less easily upset.*

Here are the first group of actual 'ego-*strengthening*' suggestions, intended to improve the patient's general condition, to strengthen his weaknesses, to increase his confidence and to allay his anxieties. You will notice as we proceed how they have been designed, not only to alleviate most of the complaints made by the average neurotic, but also to improve and mitigate those defects which have contributed largely to his illness.

> You will be able to *think more clearly* . . . you will be able to *concentrate more easily.*
> You will be able to *give up your whole undivided attention to whatever you are doing* . . . *to the complete exclusion of everything else.*
> Consequently . . . *your memory will rapidly improve* . . . and you will be able to *see things in their true perspective* . . . *without magnifying your difficulties* . . . *without ever allowing them to get out of* proportion.
> *Every day* . . . you will become *emotionally much calmer* . . . *much more settled* . . . *much less easily disturbed.*
> *Every day* . . . *you* will become . . . and *you* will remain . . . *more and more completely relaxed* . . . and *less tense* each day

> *. . . both mentally and physically . . .* even when you are no longer with me.
> And *as* you become . . . and *as* you remain . . . *more relaxed . . . and less tense* each day . . . *so . . .* you will develop *much more confidence in yourself . . .* more confidence in your ability to *do . . .* not only what you *have . . .* to do each day . . . but more confidence in your ability to do whatever you *ought* to be able to do . . . *without fear of failure . . . without fear of consequences . . . without unnecessary anxiety . . . without uneasiness.* Because of this . . . *every day . . .* you will feel *more and more independent . . . more able to 'stick up for yourself' . . . to stand upon your own feet . . . to hold your own . . .* no matter how difficult or trying things may be.

You have probably noticed how much more positive and definitive the suggestions have become as the treatment proceeded.

> *Every day . . .* you will feel a *greater feeling of personal well-being . . . A greater feeling of personal safety . . . and security . . .* than you have felt for a long, long time.
> And because all these things *will* begin to happen . . . *exactly* as I tell you they will happen . . . *more and more rapidly . . . powerfully . . . and completely . . .* with every treatment I give you . . . you will feel *much happier . . . much more contented . . . much more optimistic* in every way.
> You will consequently become much more able to *rely upon . . . to depend upon . . . yourself . . . your own efforts . . . your own judgment . . . your own opinions.* You will feel *much less need . . .* to have to *rely upon . . .* or to *depend upon . . . other people.*

I have found this routine, the full and unabbreviated version of which I have just described, to be equally valuable in preceding direct symptom-removal or the more involved hypno-analytical techniques. Constant repetition at the beginning of each treatment session strengthens the 'ego-defences' to such an extent that it not only renders the symptoms more vulnerable to direct suggestion and lessens the likelihood of relapse, but will often enable a patient to co-operate eventually in an analytical investigation he was formerly ill-equipped to face.

No matter what particular branch of therapeutic activity in which you are engaged, I have always found that patients will respond much more rapidly and effectively to treatment if you will only deal with them as intelligent individuals, and explain in advance exactly what you propose to do, why you are doing it, and what they can reasonably expect to happen. Consequently, I invariably find it helpful to explain to the patient, in the waking state, why and how he can expect this method to work.

> When you first went to school, I'm sure you can remember some-times being given a short piece of poetry to learn off by heart so that you could recite it next morning without the book.
> And how did you set about this task?
> I expect that you read the poem over and over again at home, possi-bly aloud, and each time you did so, a little bit more of it became stuck in your mind until eventually you could recite the whole of it from memory, without referring to the book.
> Now this treatment acts in exactly the same way because it is also a *'learning process,'* only instead of having to do it all yourself, every time I repeat these suggestions to you, more and more of them will stick in your unconscious mind so that you will gradually notice yourself improving in your everyday life, even when you are no longer with me.
> This will happen more quickly and easily than when you are wide-awake because, whenever you enter a trance state, your memory becomes greatly improved, and your powers of concentration greatly increased.

I always begin every treatment session with this particular sequence of suggestions as soon as the induction and deepening of hypnosis have been completed. The suggestions are given slowly and deliberately, and I prefer to leave those specifically directed towards symptom-removal to the end, since this seems to render them more effective. Indeed, in certain psychosomatic cases in which symptom-removal is the principal objective, a somewhat abbreviated version may be used before proceeding with the main suggestions to that effect. In neurotic, anxiety, tension and phobic states, however, I always employ it in full, coupled at times with a relatively superficial analysis of the patient's current problems and difficulties. Used regularly in this way, its efficacy can be surprising. In my own psychiatric practice, some 70 percent of my patients recover as a result of this technique alone, usually within Wolberg's suggested limit of twenty sessions of short-term psychotherapy.

It is certainly not intended that this verbatim account should be adopted in the precise form I have described. It is the principle that I consider worthy of attention, and the sequence I have outlined should be regarded simply as a guide to the individual therapist in framing his own suggestions to conform with his own personality, method of approach, and style of delivery. It is impossible to suggest here the varying inflections of the voice, but the same cardinal rules of construction, stresses and pauses etc. should be used in order to maintain a rhythmical quality from start to finish.

The following case history, with a somewhat unexpected result, seems to illustrate the effectiveness of this technique:

> The patient was a young man, a salesman aged twenty-eight, and happily married. He had been suffering from 'claustrophobia' for about seven years and was quite incapable of remaining in confined spaces without developing acute attacks of panic and anxiety. Curiously enough, he had never sought treatment for this before I saw him. Recently, he had been moved to the top floor of an eight-storey block of flats. Since he found it impossible to use the lift (or elevator) he was compelled to climb the stairs several times a day, and this was making his life intolerable. Obviously motivation was strong. He was a highly-strung, anxious individual, lacking in confidence, but otherwise fairly well-integrated, with no gross personality defects. No significant factors emerged from routine investigation of his childhood, his family history, or his prevailing environmental circumstances.

> I concluded that only an analytical approach would be likely to solve this problem. Unfortunately, however, whilst he was easily taught to enter the hypnotic state upon a given signal, the simpler methods of analytical investigation failed to produce any clues whatsoever, and it proved impossible to deepen his hypnosis sufficiently to use the more involved hypno-analytical techniques.

> He attended for treatment once a week, and since mentioning his incapacity seemed to distress him greatly, I ceased to refer either to 'claustrophobia' or to the difficulty he was experiencing with the lift, I consequently continued with the 'ego-strengthening' technique alone, and made no attempt whatever at direct symptom-removal. I hoped that he would eventually improve sufficiently to permit this, or that it would become possible to obtain the greater depth necessary for further analysis. Certainly after a few weeks he became much calmer and less tense, and seemed to be gaining more confidence in himself. Nevertheless, I was both surprised and gratified when he attended for his eleventh session, looking extremely pleased with himself. Apparently, several days before, he was carrying home

a load of timber with which he intended to make book-cases, and while passing the lift and faced with eight flights of stairs to climb, he suddenly felt that he might be able to overcome his fears sufficiently to try to use it. This he did, on the spur of the moment, and subsequently experienced no further difficulty whatever. In view of past experiences in dealing with this kind of symptom, I can only say that such a quick and satisfactory result was entirely unexpected.

CHAPTER 24

THE IDEALIZED SELF-IMAGE
AND THE DEVELOPMENT OF
LEARNED RESOURCEFULNESS*

DOROTHY J. SUSSKIND, PH.D.

INTRODUCTION

THERE IS MUCH RESEARCH and many promising lines of endeavor in the field of cognitive-behavior psychotherapy with which the clinician, teacher, parent and community should be familiar.

The primary focus on systematic desensitization and assertive training adopted by certain behavior threapists has identified behavior therapy with a few specific techniques or a "particular bag of tricks" that can be indiscriminately applied to most behavioral problems. This is simplistic and mechanistic, almost "cultish." The important common denominator underlying advances in empirical research, theoretical analysis and clinical innovations of the behavior therapist is the adoption of the strategy and concepts of experimental-behavioral science.

It is possible to be rigorous, scientific, and yet not simplistic. Naturally, when we function as behavioral scientists in the clinical situation, we have to apply our scientific principles at a considerably lower level of abstraction than is usually found in clinical research. Of necessity, we have to cut corners and work with less than complete information. Nevertheless, as Franks has well pointed out in his important paper on the practitioner as behavioral scientist,

> It is no myth to suggest that such a conceptual unity of science and practice can exist but it is certainly in the realm of wishful thinking

* This chapter is an extension of an article previously published: "The Idealized Self-Image (ISI): A New Technique in Confidence Training, in *Behavior Therapy, Volume 1*, 538–541, 1970.

to assume that such a goal is currently being attained to any large extent in the field of traditional clinical psychology. But the reality is there and we can strive towards it. When circumstances make temporary deviations unavoidable we can do so with intellectual honesty rather than nebulous thinking and we can make concerted efforts to reduce the departure from the ways of science to the unavoidable minimum (Franks, 1969).

Another myth is that somehow behavior therapists, furtively or otherwise, control their patients. The film "Clockwork Orange" provides a typical example of the misrepresentation of behavior therapy as something that is calculating, rigid and encouraging the docility of the robot.

As is by now well documented (Franks and Susskind, 1968; Franks, Susskind, Franks, 1969), a major aim of behavior therapy is to give the individual concerned a knowledge of the principles of behavior so that he is in a position to select appropriately for himself from a multiplicity of potential behavioral options and thereby increase his command of the situation. Far from imposing his or her will on the patient, the behavior therapist takes pains to discuss the principles, practices and theory of behavior therapy with his patient, and together—it is a collaborative process—they decide on an appropriate strategy to be used.

Patients are made aware that behavior is a function of its consequences and that rewarding and punishing events serve as important determinants of behavior. Pertinent contingencies, past and present, are reviewed with the patient to make him cognizant that he may be reinforcing undesirable behavior (e.g. Mrs. B who reinforced Tommy every time he had a temper tantrum by giving

Figure 24–1

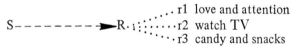

S = Mother telling Tommy to go to bed

R = Tommy's temper tantrum

him love and attention, letting him watch TV, giving him candy and snacks).

To the many so-called guardians of a free and democratic society, who profess to embrace the concept of the free man—free to make his own choice, to think his own thoughts, to become his own uniqueness—the behaviorist's response is that freedom to choose can come only from full knowledge of the choices available and the methods at hand. Unlike Freudians, behavior therapists believe that with freedom comes responsibility governed by deliberate, rational decisions and informed self-monitoring. Man is not, and should not be, at the mercy of unconscious, illogical impulses.

As behavior therapy evolves, it becomes increasingly apparent that it is not at all simplistic. It is also apparent that—at least in principle—these extensions and expansions can be accomplished without any descent into the unholy waters of mysticism, subjective thinking and psychodynamics. It is not possible here to more than touch on these many exciting developments and, for this reason, I have chosen to focus briefly upon one such area, namely self-control.

Authorities such as Kanfer (1972), Mahoney (1974), and Goldfried and Merbaum (1973) have expressed themselves most admirably with respect to the current status of self-control. It becomes clear that the concept of self-control—until recently embedded in intrapsychic personality theories, and banished from strict behavioral accounts of human activities—can be repatriated with full honors. Self-control or self-management has nothing to do with mysterious psychic processes and phenomenological inner entities. For the behavior therapist, self-control means, among other things, principles and techniques whereby the individual can learn to manipulate his environment, to monitor and regulate his behavior in the direction he desires. Here, the term environment is enlarged to include those private events more commonly subsumed under the rubric of imagery. This is legitimate because, after all, the images we build up are environmentally determined. For example, an individual cannot imagine himself obese from overeating without reference to some form of environmental cue.

Figure 24–2

MONITORING YOUR IDEALIZED SELF-IMAGE WEEK BY WEEK *

DESCRIPTION OF YOUR ISI: that you see yourself attaining after one week (please give at least two or three)

1. _____
2. _____
3. _____
4. _____
5. _____

WEEKLY MONITORING OF ISI:

1. To counter-condition negative behavior (thinking, feeling, acting).
2. Try to improve your record each day.

DATE	RELAXATION	ISI

There are many ways of developing self-control and here I would like to focus upon a technique which I have found helpful not only in this respect, but also in the development of self-esteem and learned resourcefulness (Susskind, 1970).

THE IDEALIZED SELF-IMAGE (ISI): A NEW TECHNIQUE IN CONFIDENCE TRAINING

Cognitive principles and techniques are of value only to the extent that they are part of such a broad spectrum approach. For example, one problem common to many patients seeking therapy is a lack of self-confidence, together with poor self-esteem. It would appear that their diverse life experiences have uniformly served to reinforce an expectation toward failure and rejection. Focusing upon their mistakes, inadequacies, and rejections, this continued application of the "self-fulfilling prophecy" serves merely to perpetuate and reinforce the imbalance. As a result, they withdraw from the challenges of life and "cop out." It is, therefore, necessary to train these patients to become aware of reinforcement contingencies and their concomitant effects upon the self-fulfilling process. To provide the necessary reinforcement for a more constructive life style there must be a positive shift in thinking and feeling as well as behavior. Patients who have been so trained learn to develop an independence not only from their therapists, but also from authority figures.

The following new technique, referred to as the Idealized Self-Image (ISI), has been found useful in that area of confidence training in which the goals are the creation of a more positive identity and an enhanced self-esteem. Based upon the concepts of positive reinforcement and the "self-fulfilling prophecy" and accomplished primarily through imagery, the ISI is usually initiated at the onset of therapy after an explanation of the principles involved.

Instructions to the Patient

1. Close your eyes and see yourself as your ISI, i.e., see yourself having all the traits, all the characteristics, and all the qualities you would like to possess.

    a) Select an ISI that you can attain within a relatively short period of time. At this time, do not aspire for one that is beyond your capacity. This should not be interpreted to mean that you cannot set your sights for higher aspirations and long-term planning once these more immediate goals have been successfully achieved. Rather, see this as programmed learning in which you proceed from one level to the next in graduated steps.

    b) Describe your ISI in your own words. Be sure that

your ISI includes those characteristics that you wish to attain, bearing in mind your present problems. (This step is essential. Not only will it reflect the patient's aspirations, it will also reveal whether his goals are realistic. For example, a slightly built, educationally limited young man saw his ISI as President Kennedy. He was made aware that his choice, though admirable, was far beyond him, but that there were some qualities that Kennedy had which he might wish to emulate, such as poise, ability to get along with people, and intellectual curiosity.)

2. Superimpose your ISI on your present self-image and see the enhancement of your self-image as it gradually evolves. The process of evolving from one level to another is an active and viable one. You will not attain your ISI by daydreaming about it or by wishful thinking. This can only be accomplished by actively participating in producing these effects, and by working assiduously towards these goals. This procedure symbolically suggests that you are making a commitment to yourself to achieve your goals.

3. To help you attain your ISI recall an incident or an experience in which you did something quite well and in which you experienced a feeling of accomplishment and a feeling of success.

4. Extend this feeling of accomplishment and success to anything you do in the present and plan to do in the immediate future. In other words, focus on your accomplishments and your successes. This does not mean that you should ignore your mistakes and failures—instead, see them as a "stop" sign, examine them as a process in learning. What am I doing that is wrong? How do I change my tactics? Where do I go from here?

5. Identify with your ISI. As you are walking down the street, as you are working on your job, as you are involved in social situations, begin to act, begin to feel, begin to relate as your ISI. As you see yourself, others will see you. Furthermore, as you see yourself, so you will act, so you will feel, and so you will relate to others.

In my experience this technique has many advantages if used as part of a total behavior therapy program.* It provides the basis for confidence training by focusing on the positive aspects of the personality and capitalizing upon frustrations, mistakes, and failures by showing the patient how to utilize these deficits in a constructive fashion.

It provides the means for self-identification: who he is, where he is going, what he is doing, what he wants to be. In addition, it serves to help maintain the patient's identity within the bounds of reality and his therapeutic goals in focus at all times. For example, the woman who wishes to lose weight sees herself as gradually becoming slim and trim and carries this image with her at all times. It may also provide the patient with an additional technique or crutch for coping with challenging or anxiety-provoking situations. For example, the student who is anxious about speaking up in class includes in his ISI seeing himself speak before the group with ease and confidence. Moreover, the vivid positive self-image enables the patient to cope with the immediacy of a high anxiety experience in the desensitization process, thus eliminating the need for elaborate progressive hierarchies, and provides, in some instances, the opportunity for an accelerated or short-term treatment program.

Exploration of the ISI may facilitate the identification of significant but hitherto unrecognized problems and inconsistencies. For example, a man who requested help for impotency with his wife was asked to include in his ISI seeing himself functioning well sexually with her. He dramatically jumped up from his chair at this suggestion. Exploration of this seemingly curious behavior and attitude brought to light the realization, for the first time, that this was not really what he wanted. Further exploration revealed his partial identification of his wife with his mother, so that having sex with his wife became tantamount to incest. It was then possible to work in behavioral terms with this problem. Sometimes the ISI can serve as the starting-off point for the resolution of quite different problems. For example, the patient who frequently brings about his own rejection, or the patient who

---

* It might be noted that the technique is by no means limited to a patient population. It is equally effective with normal subjects in a variety of settings.

avoids contact with others because he feels inadequate, can be helped by his identification with his ISI to move in the direction of his goals.

It may serve not only as a means for self-control but also as a device whereby the patient becomes aware that he has this ability within himself for control. For example, the patient who is emotionally hyperactive might include in his ISI, in addition to other selected characteristics, seeing himself as a calm, stable person who is in control of a situation. It might be suggested: "You are in the driver's seat—you can be in control."

The ISI may also help in the joint evaluation of therapeutic progress as patient and therapist consider together the extent to which the ISI identification has been achieved and where further reinforcements are needed. In this fashion, it can serve to remind all who use the technique that behavior therapy is a collaborative process. The behavior therapist does not control behavior without the consent of the individual involved. It is the patient who selects his ISI; this is not imposed upon him except to the extent that it is incumbent upon the therapist to ascertain that the ISI is destructive neither to the patient, nor his family, nor his environment; beyond that he is free to choose.

While present rationale and procedure remain tentative and await vertification, the device would seem worthy of further exploration at both theoretical and practical levels.

HYPNOSIS AND THE IDEALIZED SELF-IMAGE

Training in the use of the Idealized Self-Image is often enhanced by the use of hypnosis. Patients who are extremely tense, anxious or depressed, find it difficult to concentrate upon a positive self-image, hence the use of hypnosis in conjunction with this technique is helpful. A most effective approach in the use of self-hypnosis has been the following:

> It is a very, very heavy, hot muggy day in the summer . . . the sun is shining and it is very, very hot . . . it is a heavy, hot, muggy day . . . and as you keep staring at a spot, your eyelids are getting very, very heavy . . . very heavy . . . by the time I count to 5, if you feel like it, you will close your eyes. 1 . . . heavier and heavier 2 . . . very, very heavy . . . 3 . . . heavier and heavier . . . 4 . . . very, very heavy . . . 5 . . . very, very heavy.

In the meantime, your legs are feeling very heavy. It is as if you have weights on your legs, making them feel very, very heavy . . . The heaviness is going from your toes . . . to your feet . . . to the muscles of your calves and your thighs feeling very, very heavy . . . feeling very, very relaxed . . . The heaviness is now going into your hands . . . it is going from your fingertips to your fingers . . . to the muscles of your hands, your forearms and your upper arms . . . feeling very, very heavy, feeling very, very relaxed . . .

The heaviness is going into your chest . . . and now into all the muscles of your stomach . . . the muscles of your back . . . your shoulder-blades . . . the muscles at the nape of your neck feeling very, very heavy . . . feeling very, very relaxed.

The heaviness is now going into all the muscles of your forehead . . . the small muscles around your eyes . . . the muscles around your mouth, the muscles of your cheeks, your chin and your throat . . . feeling very, very heavy—feeling very, very relaxed, very calm, very relaxed, feeling wonderfully well . . .

The heaviness is now going into all the muscles of your forehead . . . the small muscles around your eyes . . . the muscles around your mouth . . . the muscles of your cheeks . . . the muscles around your chin . . . the muscles of your throat . . . feeling very, very heavy . . . feeling very, very relaxed . . . feeling very calm . . . feeling relaxed . . . feeling wonderfully well . . . wonderfully well.

As I count down from 10 to 1, I will ask you to think of a scene that makes you feel calm, relaxed . . . feeling wonderfully well . . . 10 . . . 9 . . . deeply   relaxed . . . 8 . . . 7 . . . very, very deep . . . 6 . . . 5 . . . deep, deeply relaxed . . . 4 . . . 3 . . . very, very deep . . . 2 . . . 1 . . . very calm . . . very relaxed, deep . . . deep . . . deeply relaxed . . . just relax.

ILLUSTRATIVE CASE REPORT

Diane, an extremely obese twenty-year-old single girl, was referred by her dermatologist. He had seen her for several months for treatment of an acne skin condition and hair loss, but she did not respond to treatment. Diagnosing the problem as psychogenic, psychological treatment was recommended.

Initially, she was extremely anxious, tense and very depressed; she reported she hated the way she looked, she "felt very fat, clumsy, ugly and stupid." Her parents, particularly her father, was overindulgent. He made every effort to compensate for her loneliness and depressiveness. Her greatest fear was that her father would die and she would be abandoned. She had been enrolled in an art pro-

gram, but rarely attended classes. Most of her time was spent sleeping during the day, watching TV until the early morning hours, and
eating; she virtually turned night into day, giving her an excuse not
to leave home.

During the first two sessions, we agreed on a program she should
follow rigorously. Her goals (ISI) were to be slim, trim, feel more
feminine (she felt this way when she was slim), feel more confident,
and be more actively involved with people. In subsequent sessions,
training in self-hypnosis and the Idealized Self-Image was given (a
tape recording was made for her) and she was encouraged to practice this regime several times during the day.

The basic principles of learning were explained so that she would
be aware of the contingencies of reinforcement and the antecedent
cues and her consequent behavior. She was also taught how she
could change and control her behavior by cognitive restructuring,
systematic desensitization and the Idealized Self-Image technique.

Within six months, Diane had reached her planned weight loss of
fifty pounds; she was now down to 135 pounds, the slimest she had
ever been. There was marked improvement in her skin and hair; she
became actively involved both in her art work and newly found
social life.

She later said: "In the past I always felt I could not control my
anxieties and depressions—I expected I would have to suffer and
live with them all my life. It feels great to know I can control; that
I know what I can do to avoid those terrible feelings and really feel
good."

THE DEVELOPMENT OF LEARNED RESOURCEFULNESS

The above case illustrates nicely one further therapeutic strategy which is often essential, namely the development of learned
resourcefulness. As Seligman (1973) has made clear, we learn
helplessness in coping with life more often than resourcefulness.
It is, therefore, necessary to develop a new response pattern
based upon the acquisition of resourcefulness rather than a state
of being and feeling helpless. To accomplish this I have developed a procedure which involves weekly monitoring of the
emerging Idealized Self-Image (Fig. 24-2). To facilitate this
process, the patient is introduced to the active principles involved
in diagrammatic form (Fig. 24-3). These principles are discussed
with the patient in detail. Finally, the patient is shown how to
log and monitor his negative behavior (includes thinking, feeling

Figure 24–3. Feedback paradigm for re-education for self-control behavior.

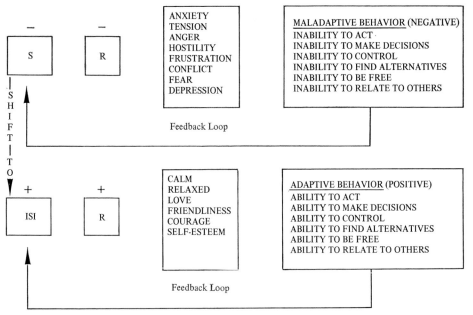

and acting), and how to bring about a more positive life style (Fig. 24–4).

CONCLUSIONS AND SUMMARY

In this paper, I have attempted to make a number of points. First, that behavior therapy is by no means simplistic and mechanistic. Second, that it is possible to expand the horizons of behavior therapy to include such concepts as cognition and awareness without deteriorating into mentalistic or Freudian speculation. Third, I have described a technique, the Idealized Self-Image (ISI) for the enhancement of self-esteem and learned resourcefulness. Fourth, I have shown how this procedure can be used in conjunction with the process of hypnosis to develop the principles of self-control rather than being controlled from without.

Figure 24–4

WEEKLY MONITORING FOR SELF-CONTROL BEHAVIOR *

PURPOSE FOR KEEPING CHART:

1. To make you AWARE of your negative behavior. This IN-CLUDES THINKING, ACTING and FEELING.
2. To help you PREVENT or DETER negative behavior. This INCLUDES THINKING, ACTING, FEELING.
3. To assist you in REARRANGING overwhelming problems into ORGANIZED DISCRETE UNITS.

DATE	− S	− R	+ ISI	+ R	REMARKS

REFERENCES

Franks, C. M.: The practitioner as behavioral scientist-myth, wishful thinking or reality? *New Jersey Psychologist, 19:*4–8, 1969.

Franks, C. M., and Susskind, D. J.: Behavior modification with children: rationale and technique. *Journal of School Psychology, 6:*75–88, 1968.

Franks, C. M., Susskind, D. J., and Franks, V.: Behavior modification and the school psychologist. In M. S. Gottsegen and G. B. Gottsegen (Eds.): *Professional School Psychology, Vol. III.* New York, Grune and Stratton, 1969, pp. 359–396.

Goldfried, M. R., and Merbaum, M.: *Behavior Change Through Self-Control.* New York, Holt, Rinehart and Winston, 1973.

Kanfer, F., and Karoly, R.: Self-Control: A behavioristic excursion into the lion's den. Behavior Therapy, 3:398–416, 1972.

Mahoney, M. J., and Thoresen, C. E.: *Self-Control: Power to the Person.* Monterey (Ca), Brooks-Cole, 1973.

Seligman, E. P.: Fall into helplessness. *Psychology Today,* June, 1973.

Susskind, D. J.: The idealized self-image: a new technique in confidence training. Behavior Therapy, 1:538–541, 1970.

CHAPTER 25

EGO EXHILARATIVE TECH-NIQUES IN HYPNOTHERAPY *

MILTON JABUSH, M.D.

D URING THE ONGOING hypnotherapeutic encounter, instances arise in which certain strategic maneuvers might be pro-ductively employed to assist the patient in achieving a more appropriate and less anxiety provoking level of behavioral adap-tation. Consider, for example, the hypnotherapist confronted with a patient who, despite "insight," is unable to move in the direc-tion of self-assertion. In hypnosis, the patient rehearses the desired behavioral change; desensitization procedures are in-corporated into the hypnotic fantasy experience, leading to self-assertion without anxiety. Hopefully, this change will be trans-ferred to real life experience. Relaxation is the most frequently employed method to inhibit the anxiety component of the self-assertion process. Another approach, usually less successful, con-sists of attempts to strengthen the repressive forces of the ego by hypnotic suggestions directed toward the repression of any anxiety associated with the performance of any sought for be-havioral change.

To the best of my knowledge, no study has attempted to com-pare the therapeutic efficacy of one hypnotherapeutic procedure with another. It has been largely from clinical experience that hypnotherapists have evolved their particular hypnoanalytic and hypnotherapeutic techniques. Here a hypnotherapeutic technique is presented and theoretical considerations offered in an attempt to explain its apparent influence in the therapeutic "cure."

Hypnotic recall and intensification of a previously experienced pleasant affect can easily be accomplished through appropriate

* This is an original manuscript.

suggestions by the hypnotherapist. The hypnotized patient is asked to recall a particular situation, to "see" it vividly with all the details and to experience the pleasing affective component in all its intensity. The patient may or may not divulge the experience to the therapist, though often he will do so. Emphasis is directed to the exaggeration and intensification of the underlying affect of the ego exhilarative experience. It is as if the patient and the therapist are now in possession of a quantity of affect that the patient senses is to be incorporated somehow into the treatment situation for the patient's therapeutic gain. While in hypnosis the patient, who is striving to become more self-assertive, is asked to visualize an image of himself engaging in graduated efforts at self-assertion and to experience, at the same time, the previously intensified affect. It is this intensified affective response that serves as a deterrent to the emergence of anxiety.

Modifications of ego exhilarative recall may be used, depending upon the hypnotherapist's assessment of the ego strength of the patient. If strong ambivalent feelings are present regarding the performance of the sought-for modifications in behavior, resort can be made to the use of the "feeling or experiencing ego and observing ego" (Fromm, 1967). In such cases, the patient is asked, while hypnotized, to visualize himself in a corner as a "watcher" (Klemperer, 1962) observing an image of the self engaging in the particular task. The image will experience the ego-intense affect during the performance, or during participation in the particular activity, without anxiety. The fusion of the "two egos" is permitted to occur, either spontaneously, as is usually the case, or upon direction of the therapist if the patient indicates that this fusion is what he wishes.

Difficulty with exhilarative recall may be encountered with depressed patients. It is as if the recall denigrates their depressive ideation and their morbid preoccupations. Determination and patience are required in such cases to influence the depressed individual's recall of either a childhood or recent situation wherein he experienced an ego exhilarative affect. Another source of difficulty with this approach involves those individuals whose visual imagery is poor. These patients must first develop the ability for imagery through training. Frequently requesting such patients to think of a pleasurable and ego exhilarative experience without necessarily visualizing the data leads to the evocation of the desired affect which can then be intensified.

CASE ILLUSTRATIONS

Case One: A sixty-four-year-old school teacher, spinster, masculine-aggressive, desired to overcome a long standing fear of riding in planes and the rear of automobiles. Although determined to embark on a sabbatical trip to Europe with a group of fellow teachers, she refused any long standing dynamic intervention on the ground that "I don't believe in all that junk!" She appeared to have good ego strength. Hypnotherapy was conducted in six sessions with desensitization and ego exhilarative intensification. Although the recall of an ego pleasing experience was apparently successful, she was unwilling to reveal the nature of this experience; however, marked psychomotor accompaniment consistent with ego exhilarative recall was evident. The therapist permitted the patient to "control" therapeutic sessions; no "probing" into her past experiences was undertaken. The approach was consistent with the patient's needs; within six sessions the patient was able to overcome her phobic reactions. She subsequently toured Europe and wrote to the author on several occasions expressing her delight with her newly developed behavior.

Case Two: A thirty-four-year-old successful businessman suffering with hypertension had developed a number of psychosomatic complaints and was beginning to drink heavily. Following a drinking episode, he would become filled with anxiety and concern with respect to his "heart condition" and blood pressure as well as the concomitant mild precordial discomfort. Numerous electrocardiograms revealed no ischemic change and several cardiologic consultations reported a normal cardiovascular status. He had considerable repressed rage and anger with ensuing guilt, traced to his relationship with his mother-in-law. Ego exhilarative techniques helped to overcome these feelings with good results; he rarely drinks and is no longer preoccupied with his psychosomatic difficulties. Further, his relationships with his mother-in-law and mother are more realistic.

Case Three: A twenty-four-year-old woman, a devout Catholic, presenting an airplane phobia, was seen for nine two-hour sessions. She had previously flown without incident. However, following a broken engagement in which sexual activity had occurred, she suddenly became panic stricken during a stormy return flight from Jamaica. Her family, incidentally, had been instrumental in breaking the engagement and, as if in retaliation, she had undertaken the vacation without her parents' permission; "I didn't ask them. This was the first time I had done this." Her panic feelings were associated with imminent death. She added, "I'm certain that, had I not had sex with him, I'd not have felt so bad." She sought therapy because she wanted to fly to Hawaii to be with her husband (of Jewish faith) who was on leave from Vietnam. She developed considerable insight during her therapeutic sessions. Because of her strong religious inclinations she was referred to a priest to assist in the resolution of her psychoreligious conflict. During the sixth session she voiced fears that her husband might reject her "new image" and guilt feelings concerning her suppressed sexual desires for her employer. Her dreams revealed ambivalent feelings toward her husband and his anticipatory sexual demands. The wide variety of hypnoanalytic techniques used, however, did not produce amelioration of her phobia for flying. Ego exhilarative recall was then introduced, coupled with the previously attempted hypnodesensitization, followed by an actual helicopter flight after the sixth session. These provided a strong forward thrust to therapeutic progress. Her dreams reflected the therapeutic movement when she dreamed of being in Hawaii and noted its resemblance to her home town. During the seventh session the patient was regressed with revivification to a 1960 family flight to Acapulco; an intensification of pleasant affect was produced, coupled with ego exhilarative technique, and the suggestion was given, "You can obtain this feeling whenever you wish." Two days following the visit she reported a dream wherein she again was involved in a pleasant flight but noted further ambivalence regarding her husband. She missed the Honolulu flight in her dream and it was evident that her deeply-rooted guilt feelings toward her husband would determine the success or failure of overcoming her flying phobia. The two days prior to her eighth visit found her quite distraught and beset with doubts. She was regressed once again to the pleasant Acapulco flight and appropriate ego-exhilarative techniques administered. She then stated that she was determined to make the flight. Throughout therapy, the patient utilized self-hypnosis with hypnodesensitization coupled with the ego exhilarative affect. Her flight was successful. Subsequently she became pregnant, her relationship with her husband strengthened, and he told her how proud he was of his "new wife." Her plane phobia did not return, and there was no substitute symptomatology.

DISCUSSION

Therapeutic gain in hypnotherapy is probably related to the regressive aspects of ego functioning inherent in the hypnotic transference. The latter includes simpler levels of ego functioning both in affective and cognitive experiencing. Subtle abreactive experiences probably occur in response to the sensory and imagery correlates of the hypnotic induction or hypnotic involvement (Kline, 1968). Following the "silent" abreaction, there undoubtedly is produced a favorable matrix for spontaneously occurring desensitizations. The hypnotic intensification of an emotion associated with an ego exhilarative event results in an abreactive experience. From a hypnoanalytic viewpoint, one would expect that the abreacted material would be synthesized with insight, appropriate affect, and with waking verbalizations and integrations; that all these ingredients would be necessary in order for meaningful behavioral change to occur. Although this approach is rarely utilized with ego exhilarative techniques, yet therapeutic gain is observed.

SUMMARY

Utilizing the technique of intensification of ego exhilarative affect, catalyzed by the rapidly emerging regressive aspects of the hypnotic transference, evidently encourages multiple and sequential abreactive experiences, both overt and subtle, to occur in a chain-like, autonomous, and self-directed manner. This type of emotional responsivity usually leads to more productive psychotherapy including an increase both in waking verbalizations, and nocturnal dreaming, as well as spontaneous insights with the adoption of new behavior.

REFERENCES

Fromm, Erika: Personal communication, 1967.
Klemperer, Edith: Hypnoanalysis. *J Am Med Wom Assoc, 17*:577, 1962.
Kline, Milton: Personal communication, 1968.

CHAPTER *26*

THE CLINICAL USE OF DIRECT HYPNOTIC SUGGESTION: A TRADITIONAL TECHNIQUE IN THE LIGHT OF CURRENT APPROACHES*

ROBERT G. MEYER, PH.D. AND
HARVEY S. TILKER, PH.D.

Abstract: A psychotherapeutic procedure is described which utilized hypnosis and aspects from the behavior therapies. Direct manipulation of behavior in an efficient, effective, and replicable procedure was the goal. Posthypnotic suggestions for the manifestation of desired behaviors were combined with attempts to induce the patient to reinforce his own behavioral changes. The two cases presented are of male prison inmates diagnosed as having character disorders. Positive and substantiated changes in physiological, behavioral, and attitudinal areas occurred. These continued without decrease over six months (with some indication of healthy adjustment at one year) for one patient, and for fifteen months with some continuous improvements for the second patient. The ease of and need for replication of the procedure is noted.

THE THERAPEUTIC APPROACH employed in the following cases is viewed by the authors as an admixture of hypnotic and behavior modification techniques. The combination is not unique; for example, Wolpe's early work (1958) in behavior modification utilized hypnosis, and hypnosis has been used by other theorists who also view their approach in the context of behavior modifi-

* Reprinted from the April 1969 *International Journal of Clinical and Experimental Hypnosis.* Copyrighted by the Society for Clinical and Experimental Hypnosis, April 1969.

cation (Sipprelle, 1967). It is recognized that the present procedure is not directly comparable to such behavior therapies as systematic desensitization, where the principles are directly based on learning theory. The aspects taken from behavior modification techniques are the attempts to specify clearly a therapeutic procedure and to set up the reinforcement of a desired response.

The efficacy of behavior modification has derived from its rigorous approach to the elicitation, shaping, and control of the responses of the organism. As Greenspoon and Brownstein (1967) state, effective psychotherapeutic change through behavior modification is dependent upon the controlling of stimuli, and verbal stimuli play an extremely important role in this control.

In regard to the elicitation of a response by verbal stimuli, many critics of behavior modification facetiously lament about why one does not simply ask a person to make the desired response, instead of setting up all the verbal gadgetry. This naiveté ignores the environmental context as a whole. Even the most inexperienced therapist knows of the futility and absurdity of such an approach.

The analysis of the interaction process in psychotherapy by Haley (1963) suggests why one can expect such an approach to be futile. Many people develop patterns of eliciting direct suggestions and advice on conflict areas from significant others, only to ignore the proffered advice or fail at abortive attempts to carry it out. This is true in patients to an even more extreme degree. Yet Haley reports that patients do follow direct suggestions if they have been hypnotized. This is, of course, not a unique finding. For example, direct suggestions are followed even when the original context of the hypnotic procedure was to elicit "free associations" concerning conflict areas.

Another question is now relevant: why not simply hypnotize all patients for whom this is feasible and then direct them to make healthy, adaptive responses? This has been ineffective. The primary reason is that the "half-life" of a complex posthypnotic suggestion is rather limited. (This half-life is the last point in time at which a suggestion is responded to in the same form as it was at the first administration of the cue immediately upon the patient's withdrawal from the hypnotic state.) The work of Reyher (1962) and Barber (in press) would suggest, in addition, that many behaviors labeled as the carrying out of posthypnotic suggestions have to be severely reassessed. In any case, there is no strong evidence that any complex posthypnotic suggestion given in one session will persist for a significant period of time.

It should not be surprising that a posthypnotic suggestion has a very short half-life, since it is always treated as an isolated phenomenon. A posthypnotic suggestion can never be expected to become part of a stable response pattern unless an attempt is made to build it into a larger response matrix of the personality. The therapeutic approach in this paper attempts to fit the post-hypnotic responses into that largest of all response matrices, the self-system, as defined by Diggory (1966). This was implemented by first directly suggesting that the desired response be carried out and at the same time directly suggesting that the person reward his own response by strong and immediate self-approval. This aspect of self-reinforcement (Marston, 1965) is an attempt to sustain and amplify the response elicited by hypnotic suggestion.

Case One: While employed at the Psychiatric Clinic of the State Prison of Southern Michigan (SPSM) in Jackson, Michigan, the senior author was confronted with a particularly difficult case. A twenty-six-year-old male (Mr. A.) had been incarcerated for his second narcotics offense. He had an extensive psychiatric history, had been in individual therapy twice outside of prison (for six months and ten months respectively), and had been in group therapy for approximately three months, after which the group had been disbanded. No substantial history or psychological evaluation had ever been completed on him. The working diagnosis had always been that of sociopathic personality, anti-social type.

Mr. A. had received a parole, due to be effective in six weeks. As no progress had ever been made with him, an attempt to implement direct suggestions through the use of hypnosis seemed warranted. He was an excellent hypnotic subject and was able to attain both glove anaesthesia and amnesia for posthypnotic suggestions in the first one-hour session. In the next four weeks he was seen for seven more fifteen-minute sessions and always went into an immediate and "deep" state of hypnosis in response to a rapid induction technique.

During those sessions, only direct suggestions were given for the full fifteen minutes: in this case, that he would stop craving drugs or alcohol. It was emphasized (as a posthypnotic suggestion) that each and every time he was able to resist, or completed any other action that he saw as an indication he was developing a healthier personality, he would think for several moments about how well he had done and how easily he could repeat the event. Blum, Hauenstein, and Graef's (1968) concept of "reverberation" is directly relevant to this aspect of the technique.

He reportedly took no drugs in the next six weeks but drank himself into a stupor three times. He was, however, paroled. Three months later, in a ninety-minute interview, he stated he had not used alcohol or drugs since his discharge, and his conversation indicated that most areas of his life situation had improved. He was holding a good job and he planned marriage. Six months later, by mail, he stated that those trends were continuing. No later contact could be made, but an inmate friend of his stated that Mr. A. had moved to New York to take a different job and was reportedly doing well.

While the improvement was marked, it was premature to assume that the direct hypnotic procedure employed was a factor. In order to provide at least a minimal test situation for this approach, its specific techniques were elaborated and established as an *a priori* procedure for application to another case.

Case Two: The patient selected (Mr. C.), an inmate of SPSM, was markedly different in the majority of respects from Mr. A. Whereas Mr. A. was quite verbal, of bright normal intelligence, aggressive in group situations, self-referred for intrapsychic reasons, and low in subjective and physiological signs of anxiety, Mr. C. was the opposite in all respects. He was a thirty-four-year-old Caucasian serving his third term for larceny. His chief complaint was a chronic weight problem, as well as chronic moderate anxiety. Upon questioning, he admitted to strong feelings of inferiority in situations that he construed as competitive. Mr. C. also expressed resentment toward his two brothers, who had received most of his father's affection, and especially toward his younger brother, who had been quite successful financially.

While in prison, Mr. C. was often in trouble, usually involving passive resistance toward custody officers or the stealing and selling of illegal contraband. He had done nothing to advance himself at any time while in the institution. He had occasionally signed up for courses in order to complete his high school education, but had never remained long in them. He had taken intelligence tests on several occasions and had consistently scored in the 85 to 90 IQ range. On the two prior larceny offenses, Mr. C. had been paroled, but he had violated his parole on both occasions. His first parole had lasted only two months before he was apprehended and returned to prison. He stated he had never interrupted his pattern of stealing at any time from the age of 16 onward. He did not view his problems at this point as intrapsychic, but rather assumed that he would be given pills which would cause him to lose weight and would lower his anxiety.

The first several sessions were directed only toward the patient's rapidly attaining a state of hypnosis marked by both glove anaesthesia (Wolberg, 1948) and amnesia for posthypnotic suggestions. After three twenty-minute sessions, Mr. C. could do so. From that point on, Mr. C. was seen by the senior author in the following sequence (the sequence and procedure set up *a priori*): Week 1—4 times (fifteen minutes each), Week 2—3, Week 3—2, Week 4—1, Week 6—1, Week 9—1, Week 14—1, Week 23—1. This constituted a total of twenty-three weeks and fourteen sessions involving 210 minutes (excluding the three twenty-minute preparatory sessions mentioned above).

In each session, immediately after rapid induction, direct suggestions were repeated and elaborated to the effect that Mr. C. would find himself gradually able to resist eating extra helpings of food (especially bread and potatoes, of which he was particularly fond) and on occasions would even be able to refuse a first serving of various starchy foods. It was emphasized that each and every time this would occur, Mr. C. would feel very proud of himself for having succeeded in spite of his tendencies to do otherwise. He was told that on these occasions he would *immediately* reflect on the fact that he had been able to make some changes by himself and would be justly proud of these changes. It was also directly suggested that he would find himself making changes in other areas that were meaningful to him and at a pace that would be comfortable to him. Areas directly suggested to him were the handling of situations involving competition with other people, and decisions about whether to steal various items and whether he should get into arguments, etc. Again it was emphasized that every time he did anything of a positive nature he would feel good about himself. It was also emphasized that if he failed in particular instances, he would not feel guilty about this but would realize that steps toward improvement are gradual and he would simply wait for a later time at which he would be able to succeed. These direct suggestions were the entire content of all sessions.

Prior to the sessions, Mr. C. weighed 224 pounds. At the end of the sessions, he weighed 189 pounds. He reported he was entirely free of the anxiety that had plagued him most of his life. He spontaneously verbalized that he felt good about himself and optimistic about his life. He once volunteered that he realized there were things about himself that he should be proud of, and that he was not particularly bothered any more about the fact that others might sometimes achieve more than he did.

After the sessions terminated, it was learned that Mr. C. had attained a job promotion within the prison and had also staved off a serious homicidal threat from another inmate without upset or incident. His general prison attitude improved markedly, and his improvement was reported by both his work and recreation supervisors.

Mr. C. was paroled from the prison two months after the termination of therapy. An hour interview a month later by both authors indicated that he was doing well and had maintained a steady job, and there was no suspicion that he was involved in any criminal activities whatsoever. He had stated that he was going to marry the woman with whom he had lived occasionally while on parole, and would attempt to raise her two children as his own. This he had done. Similar checks at both nine and fifteen months from the termination of therapy indicated the same status. At the 15-month mark, Mr. C. reported that he was still free of anxiety, was happy in his marital situation, and had maintained his weight loss. At that time he weighed 186 pounds. As in Case One, a strong effort was made to detect whether any symptom substitution had occurred, and none whatsoever was found.

CONCLUSIONS

The above procedure produced physiological, behavioral, and attitudinal changes in the two cases described. With Mr. C., a very careful attempt was made to employ only the procedures delimited. The patient-therapist interactions were restricted to these, and there was neither supportive chit chat nor discussion of possible improvement during the twenty-three weeks. Also, no conscious communication took place that in any way whatsoever indicated this to be a new, very effective, or experimental procedure, though possible experimenter expectancy effects (Rosenthal, 1966) cannot be excluded. Use of this restricted approach, however, along with the strict adherence to the prior-derived procedure, suggests that the improvements were related to the earlier formulations.

Two points are crucial to the procedure. The first is the use of the context of hypnosis to elicit behaviors, assuming that to request them from a waking patient would have either appeared absurd or proved ineffective. Secondly, all efforts are made to get the patient to reinforce his own positive responses immediately, thereby building them into more stable and permanent patterns while allowing time for the environment to begin acting as a positive reinforcement agent.

The efficiency of the procedure is obvious, and it lends itself to replication. It is also a procedure that could easily be used in conjunction with other psychotherapeutic techniques.

The effects of the therapeutic procedure were stable and substantial in the two cases presented. It should be noted that these two cases were of a type that therapists often hold are not very amenable to any form of psychotherapeutic intervention, especially in regard to any long-term or substantial changes. Further research on larger samples will be required to evaluate the potential benefits of the procedure.

REFERENCES

Barber, T. X.: *A Scientific Approach to "Hypnosis."* Princeton, Van Nostrand, in press.

Blum, G. S., Hauenstein, Louise S., and Graef, J. R.: Studies in cognitive reverberation: Replications and extensions. *Behav Sci, 13:*171–177, 1968.

Diggory, J. C.: *Self-Evaluation: Concepts and Studies.* New York, Wiley, 1966.

Greenspoon, J., and Brownstein, A. J.: Psychotherapy from the standpoint of a behaviorist. *Psychol Rec, 17:*401–416, 1967.

Haley, J.: *Strategies of Psychotherapy.* New York, Grune and Stratton, 1963.

Marston, A. R.: Self reinforcement: The relevance of a concept in analogue research to psychotherapy. *Psychotherapy, 2:*1–5, 1965.

Reyher, J.: A paradigm for determining the clinical relevance of hypnotically induced psychopathology. *Psychol Bull, 59:*344–352, 1969.

Rosenthal, R.: *Experimenter Effects In Behavior Research.* New York, Appleton-Century-Crofts, 1966.

Sipprelle, C. N.: Induced anxiety. *Psychotherapy, 4:*36–40, 1967.

Wolberg, L.: *Medical Hypnosis.* New York, Grune and Stratton, 1948.

Wolpe, J.: *Psychotherapy by Reciprocal Inhibition.* Stanford, Stanford University Press, 1958.

CHAPTER 27

HYPNOTIC AVERSION TO ALCOHOL: THREE-YEAR FOLLOW-UP OF ONE PATIENT*

J. Harry Feamster, Ph.D. and
John E. Brown, M.D.

INTRODUCTION

THE QUESTION OF PERMANENCY of therapeutic changes produced by post-hypnotic suggestion is an important one. According to various experienced therapists, hypnotic suggestions
for symptom removal may need reinforcement. The present report is concerned with hypnotherapy of a patient in which gains
were maintained reasonably well during a three-year period.

CASE REPORT

This white male, whom we shall call Tom Bacchus, is presently
forty-three years of age. He started to work as a messenger when his
father died in 1936, but continued high school and was made a
clerk after his graduation at age fifteen. He continued this employment until 1943, at which time he joined the Navy. He says he
"drank a little" while in the Navy. He was discharged in 1945 because of a subarachnoid hemorrhage and returned to his former position as a clerk, where he continued until 1955. After discharge,
Tom says he drank "to calm me down" six or eight times a year.
He said, "When I did drink, I would take enough to knock myself
out." In 1955 he described himself as being "nervous in mind and
body too." He said, "I get crazy, mixed-up thoughts." He began to

* Originally published in *The American Journal of Clinical Hypnosis,* Vol. VI,
Number 2, October 1963, pages 164–166. Copyright 1963 by the American
Society of Clinical Hypnosis. Follow-up added.

drink heavily, but because of his medical history and his more than fifteen-years service, he was retired from his job at age thirty-three rather than being discharged. His drinking quickly became uncontrollable. After more than two years in another hospital, he was considered a hopeless alcoholic. His wife informed us that she had actually been told by a physician that she should consider divorce because Tom would always require hospital care and close supervision. At almost every opportunity Tom drank steadily until he became unconscious. He received surgery for a right carotid aneurysm in 1957.

His wife arranged a transfer to the Gulfport Veterans Administration Hospital in May 1959. The treatment team rendered the following diagnosis of the then thirty-eight-year-old veteran: (1) Acute brain syndrome associated with alcoholic intoxication and (2) (from history) Chronic brain syndrome with residuals of right carotid aneurysm manifested by poor judgment, lack of response, and indulgence in alcohol.

Psychological tests revealed bright normal intelligence with very little residual effect of the aneurysm which had been operated upon in 1957. He was considered to be an extremely shallow, labile person who attempted to control his intense feelings, especially feelings of rage, by forced passivity and, when this failed, by alcoholic indulgence. The possibility of his turning the rage inward as suicide was considered. He was described in the psychological report as feeling "very vulnerable to attack from an extremely morbid and threatening source," and he manifested a great deal of concern with a phallic reference to sucking and biting animals.

Because it appeared unlikely that Tom would have the depth of feeling necessary for gain from psychotherapy, he was counseled in regard to performing clerical work in the hospital and later going into clerical work outside the hospital.

His hospital adjustment was excellent. However, two brief attempts to adjust outside the hospital resulted in his returning on both occasions with an acute brain syndrome caused by alcoholic intoxication. It was recognized that while the possibility of suicide existed, it would be possible to establish appropriate safeguards; therefore, treatment involving hypnotherapy and hypnotic aversion to alcohol was planned.

In December 1959, a somnambulistic trance state was easily induced. After checking the depth of the trance, the therapist instructed the patient to open his eyes while retaining his depth of trance. He was presented with a glass paper clip container and told, "Smell this whiskey." The expected visual and olfactory hallucinations were noted. He was then told, "From now on, whenever you smell, taste, or even look at alcoholic beverages of any kind, you will begin to relive your worst hangover with all of the headache, nausea, and general discomfort you felt then."

The "whiskey" was presented again, and this time Tom immediately vomited into a container which the therapist had made ready. This procedure was repeated two more times using "wine" and "beer," and the general instructions regarding alcohol were repeated.

Tom was then told, "Whenever you are upset and would ordinarily think of drinking, reliving this hangover will help you to avoid thoughts about drinking. After you have recovered from the hangover feeling you may do three things. (1) You may feel hungry and eat a satisfying meal. This often is a temporary relief of anxiety. (2) If you are still feeling anxious or if no food is available, you can press your left index finger and thumb together. This should help you achieve the desired degree of relaxation appropriate to the situation. (3) If the first two measures are used and intense anxiety or other severe psychological discomfort continues to exist, you will inform your family and return to the Veterans Administration, preferably the hospital at Gulfport." No further hypnotherapy was administered at this time because the patient was given a week-end pass to test the effectiveness of this hypnotic treatment.

Through repeated extensions of his pass to ninety days trial visit, Tom remained at home until June 1960 (about six months). At that time a Social Service visit to the Bacchus home was reported as follows: "On May 31, I visited Mr. Bacchus and his wife at her place of employment and was very much pleased to receive the report that he is doing exceptionally well since his return home. He continues to have moody, depressed spells when in the past he has sought drink as a relief, but so far states that he has not even been tempted in that direction. Mrs. Bacchus can hardly believe it and is most anxious to know how long she can depend on the suggestion remaining with him. Is it possible to answer this question? The Bacchuses have become interested in square dancing, have joined a class, and are having a really good time in that field. It is an entirely new group of associates, who know nothing of the veteran's past history, and he is much more at ease with them. He is very optimistic about the future, as is Mrs. Bacchus, and the only question they seem to have at this point is how long they can expect the present situation to hold. Mr. Bacchus is able to talk about his situation freely and frankly and is amazed at himself for his loss of interest in drinking."

Two weeks after this report was received, Tom was admitted to the hospital in a state of acute intoxication. The hypnotic aversion to alcohol was no longer effective. Further hypnotherapy, including reinforcement of his aversion to alcohol, was administered. At each session he was instructed to "have a three-minute dream which may help us to understand your problems better, which may help you to feel better, and which may eventually aid in your making a better adjustment over a long period of time." The first of these dreams revealed more clearly the symbolic morbid fear of biting animals first noted in the Rorschach. This dream about "snapping turtles biting me" was re-dreamed with instructions that "this time it will be a pleasant dream." The patient complied, described the second dream and said, obviously with very marked relief, while still under hypnosis, "I feel good—best I ever felt in my whole life. I want to keep feeling this good always." Other dreams revealed poor communications with family members and the day-to-day building up of stress due to minor annoyances. He was instructed to re-dream these dreams with the suggestion that "this time you'll handle the situation better." This hypnotic dream repetition stimulated some ingenious creative thinking on Tom's part. Some of the solutions developed during the repeated dream were extremely well thought out and were promptly verbally reinforced by the therapist. Little or no therapy was conducted in the waking state.

After receiving intensive hypnotherapy for two weeks, Tom returned home in June 1960. His wife had been counseled at this hospital and by a Veterans Administration Regional Office social worker for several months beginning in January 1960. In March 1961, the following Social Service report was received: "The wife stated that the opportunity to take over the management of a small store and post office came quite suddenly. It was formerly managed by a relative who had to give it up because of a death in the family. Veteran and the wife were somewhat hesitant about accepting the responsibility. Thus far, they are very much pleased with the venture. On March 1st the veteran and the wife were interviewed at their grocery store. Veteran was serving customers at the time of my visit and the wife was working in the post office, which is a small room with the one door opening into the grocery store. Veteran immediately explained that he had just returned from another trip to the hospital and was very pleased with the treatment he received. The wife stated that going to the hospital is 'like a miracle' for the veteran. He was extremely despondent before he went and has returned in an entirely different frame of mind. Veteran stated that he had worried too much about not being able to collect from the customers. He thinks now that he probably did exaggerate his problem and thinks that after discussing it with his doctor he will be able to manage his affairs differently and will be able to take a different attitude toward his business. He and the wife simultaneously remark that the veteran is able to control his drinking and has been able to control it successfully for several months. Both are extremely well pleased at this improvement."

Recent follow-up contacts at this hospital reveal that Tom relies on self-hypnosis and eating to relieve anxiety from day to day. While he has gained some weight, he is not obese; and the minor gain in weight is not considered to be a problem. Tom has started to drink, become ill with the posthypnotic "hangover," and returned to the hospital briefly on a number of occasions to "get away from it all" for a few days at a time. The hospital authorities continue the arrangement whereby he is free to come in at any time, day or night.

Both Tom and his wife have profited from counseling and from hypnotherapy and psychotherapy respectively. The plan for Tom to leave the hospital, which was initiated during his first week here, has been fulfilled. However, we offer him hospitalization as a ready defense against temporary crises. Thus, in keeping with our treatment philosophy, his brief periods of rehospitalization are considered by Tom and his family, as well as by our treatment team, to be a therapeutic source of maintaining his improvement rather than an indication of failure.

SUMMARY

A three-year follow-up of a patient successfully treated for alcoholism by hypnotic aversion to alcohol and hypnotherapy is described. Although no hypnotic treatment has been administered for more than a year, his brief attempts to drink have resulted in a strong aversion to alcohol and his return to the hospital as a form of "safety-valve."

CONCLUDING REMARKS

According to Rachman and Teasdale (1969) "the surprising thing about aversion therapy is not that its effects are uncertain, but rather that it works at all. . . . Why should the patient refrain from carrying out the deviant behavior after he has left the clinic? . . . . Even so, for long periods after the termination of treatment, many patients do not carry out their deviant acts." The use of hypnosis in applying aversion therapy offers interesting advantages when its use is feasible. The phenomenon of generalization is well known. Use of hypnosis appears to maximize response generalization. Hypnosis affords the ability to apply the aversive stimulus during all of the patient's waking hours rather than only in the clinic situation. The factors of safety (no electric current), convenience, immediacy of presenting and withdrawing the aversive stimulus in relation to the target experience, are all important advantages. Fewer treatment sessions are needed. Hypno-aversion is versatile. For example, I have used hypnotically induced electric shocks as an aversive and "emotion-stopping" technique. It can be combined with other treatment methods. I have come to call this "hypno-shock."

In one instance a young woman who had a violent temper which was set off by being teased was being treated using a transactional analysis model. A hypnotically induced shock became the aversive stimulus applied "when family members 'hook your child.'" The instructions were, "Whenever you feel that your husband or children are about to 'hook your child,' and you feel yourself losing control, you will receive a painful, but momentary electric shock on your hand except when driving the car, or when it would be otherwise dangerous. This shock will help you to focus on the insight you have achieved into how you were originally 'programmed' to respond to teasing and will help you to stop the developing emotional reaction and keep your adult in control." Although the hypnotically induced shock needed weekly reinforcement, the patient reported no more difficulty after three weekly sessions. This patient was followed for three months after treatment and continued to report 100 percent success.

Some major disadvantages have prevented my using hypno-aversion more widely. All potential candidates for hypno-aversion cannot be successfully hypnotized. Of those who do achieve adequate trance depth, some fail to report back for reinforcement of the original hypnotic suggestions. Mr. Bacchus was intensely motivated for improvement, and therefore was more faithful than most of our other hypno-aversion patients. However, a more recent follow-up disclosed that even he eventually failed to avail himself of aversion therapy.

In September, 1973, a ten-year follow-up Social Service report indicated that the improvement reported in 1963 was maintained

until 1967 and the patient was gainfully employed at least periodically until that time. During the period of time from 1967 to
present, Mr. Bacchus has experienced eleven VA hospital admis-
sions, six for the treatment of various medical diagnoses and five
for psychiatric reasons. Primary diagnoses on psychiatric admis-
sions have included acute brain syndrome secondary to alcoholism and chronic organic brain syndrome secondary to subarachnoid hemorrhage with paranoid reaction. In recent years he has
avoided reinforcement of hypno-aversive suggestions. However,
he is able to remain at home most of the time. This adjustment is
still an improvement over his need for continuous hospitalization
for approximately four years prior to hypno-aversive treatment.
The contrast between the four years prior to treatment and eight
years of employment after treatment have led us to conclude that,
for this individual, hypno-aversion combined with other hypnotherapy methods and family counseling was the best possible
treatment method.

REFERENCES

Rachman, Stanley J., and Teasdale, John: Aversion Therapy: An Appraisal.
     In Franks, Cyril M. (Ed.): *Behavior Therapy: Appraisal and Status.*
     New York, McGraw-Hill, 1969, pp. 279–320.

CHAPTER 28

HYPNOTHERAPY IN A CASE OF CLAUSTROPHOBIA AND ITS IMPLICATIONS FOR PSYCHOTHERAPY IN GENERAL *

JEROME M. SCHNECK, M.D.

INTRODUCTION

THE PURPOSE OF THIS PAPER is to report on hypnotherapy for a patient with claustrophobia. The precipitating events in symptom formation possess points of interest. Certain aspects of treatment warrant elaboration. The account presented here deals with one phase of a longer and more involved therapeutic procedure for this patient who had a number of additional problems.

CASE DATA

This thirty-four-year-old patient revealed that he was troubled by a closed-in feeling. His discomfort would appear when he entered any building. He would notice it when sitting in a room, especially a small room. He experienced it in subways. He was badly frightened by the roar of subway trains. At times he would leave the subway before arriving at his destination and smoke a cigarette in the street before continuing. When in the street he would feel comfortable. He claimed that he began to experience the claustrophobia following his Army service, but as will be shown later this recollection was incorrect.

On inquiry as to whether he could link his symptom with any past occurrence, the patient told about a nightmare he had experienced a few days before. He saw an Army tank coming at him, was

* Reprinted from the October 1954 *Journal of Clinical and Experimental Hypnosis*. Copyrighted by The Society for Clinical and Experimental Hypnosis, October 1954.

frightened, and awoke from his sleep. He added that this night-mare was a repetition of what had occurred on maneuvers when a tank came at him while he and another soldier became trapped in a trench. The sides of the trench collapsed and they had to be ex-tricated.

The patient was placed in a deep hypnotic state and instructions were given him for revivification of the tank episode at which time the patient and his buddy were in the trench. As he was being prepared by instruction for this revivification, he appeared to be developing anxiety. His breathing became rapid and irregular. Then he inhaled deeply but did not exhale freely. He began to shake. He started to whine, "Get us out of here! Get us out of here! Dirt's piling in on us! How'll we get out? Can't get out of here! Stuck! Holla for the guys! Quick! Tell 'em to get us out! Here they come!" The patient's hands waved and his head shook. "It feels good to be free. What's the matter with my legs? Can't move my legs! Give me some water! Take it off! Take 'em off! Go ahead! Pour it over my head! Leave me alone!" The patient started to cry. He was asked why he was crying. "I don't know." The patient apparently experi-enced altered time-place orientation because on questioning he could reply that he felt better, but when asked whether he knew the therapist he said he did not. When asked where he was, he said "Lying down in the field." He was asked what he was thinking about when the tank passed over him and he replied, "Couldn't get out." On inquiry he claimed this did not remind him of anything else. The patient was then reoriented to the present with the tank episode to remain as a memory.

With the patient still in hypnosis, he was asked whether he re-called anything about the tank episode which he had been unable to recall in the waking state. "The captain called it a big joke when I started to cry. He laughed. Thought it was funny. I couldn't help crying."

In order to explore further and link up what might otherwise be apparently unconnected data, the patient was instructed to visualize a crystal ball and in it he was to see a scene involving something emotionally connected with the tank incident. The patient related, "I see that slit trench, three feet deep. Just perfect in case we had to jump out. I insisted on making it deeper. That's why we couldn't get out. We even had that step cut out so that we could get out. He made us dig out that step. The captain made us dig it deeper than theirs (the other soldiers)."

The patient was instructed to visualize a scene for the same purpose mentioned above. "There's the captain talking to the in-structor. The captain is going away now. The instructor told us the only way (the patient) and Whitey will get out of camp is in a box."

On inquiry, the patient revealed that this scene occurred before the tank incident. On further questioning he claimed having had the feeling that the captain may have arranged for the tank to stop over the trench. He believed this might have been done to scare him or perhaps even to hurt him. He said that ordinarily the tank would have continued over the trench without stopping.

The same imagery technique was used again to elicit a scene which, according to the instructions, would appear if it was in fact valid and that if it were fantasy or a dream it would be known as such to the patient. He was told this would occur in order to link it with the claustrophobia. The patient revivified the episode again. "There comes that tank again." He struggled and breathed rapidly. "It's right over our trench! Tell him to move! Dirt's coming down! Getting us out now." Then the patient said, "Cole, get me some water." To evaluate the nature of the patient's time-person orientation he was asked whether he knew who the therapist was but he did not respond. He tugged at his tie, pulling it open. He was again reoriented and asked to fill in gaps which had been present. He told how the soldier in front of him had just managed to duck under the tank as it came along and how the tank had squashed this man's canteen.

When an attempt was made to have the patient retrieve an episode preceding the tank event but which would be linked with the claustrophobia, he pictured a particular person who in a subsequent scene turned out to be the instructor during a gas mask drill which did not appear to be especially traumatic, but following which the patient commented, "It's good to be out in the fresh air." The purpose of the treatment effort was to elicit predisposing material on which the precipitating tank trauma might have been superimposed. As these efforts continued, the patient described a variety of scenes in different parts of the country, none of which seemed to be highly charged emotionally. Afterwards when verbalizing spontaneously about these scenes, he said, "Everything is going underneath the tank. The tank is on top. All these scenes are going underneath the tank. The tank is coming down on them now, making a pancake of them. The tank seems to be in front of it all the time—in front of everything." Then, later, "It's moving all the time. The treads keep moving. It keeps coming and coming and coming."

An attempt was made to investigate past occurrences involving one or more persons who might be dynamically related in some way to the closed-in aspect of the patient's feelings and to the Army incident, but nothing of note was uncovered. When the claustrophobia theme was centered upon, the patient reverted to the tank issue. "There's a tank coming up the road. Coming into our area. He stopped for a little while. We're digging away at the trench.

It's hot. Me and Whitey. It's so dry and thirsty, yet we can't touch our water. Have to dig under that hot sun." This preceded the traumatic event previously revivified and the current description of the trench digging was offered in a relatively matter of fact way. Again the patient was asked to fill in details of the tank episode which he had not revealed previously in the waking state. "My legs felt numb. Whitey and I cried and lay down for a couple of hours. Then they checked us at the hospital. The Colonel said we were a couple of brave boys. A lot of good that did. They let us out of the review parade, but our Captain didn't give us any passes."

The session had to be terminated at this time and the patient was brought out of the hypnosis with instructions for posthypnotic recall of the material elicited. The patient then mentioned spontaneously that he had not remembered during his nightmare or in his waking recollections all of the elements involved in the traumatic occurrence. The additional details were retrieved during the hypnosis. More important was his assertion that the significant point was his having relived the episode completely. He stated that the feeling of real reliving had not been experienced even during his nightmare. He said that during the hypnosis he was "scared stiff." Interestingly, and this will be commented on later, he was perplexed about the link between the symptom and the tank experience. He felt strongly the emotional tie between the two but on an intellectual level he was puzzled that such a connection between emotional trauma and symptom formation could exist. The patient was not told in any way that symptom disappearance would follow. One important reason for this was the uncertainty that all pertinent elements had been uncovered. He wondered whether he would experience relief at this time and was told that we would observe him further.

The patient revealed further that he had hesitated telling about the closed-in feeling he would experience even in the consultation room. It would occur each time he was there, and as he sat in his chair he would feel that the closed door would move close to him. The walls too would move in toward him. On emerging from the hypnosis he observed that this did not happen. He felt surprised and pleased and mentioned this of his own accord. He felt after this hypnosis, but while still in the office, that a burden had been lifted from him. There was a discussion of certain aspects of his life situation wherein he felt closed in, stifled, unable to do the things he wished. When the link was made with the tank episode, the patient reacted suddenly as with a burst of insight. Despite this emotional reaction, as mentioned previously he was perplexed on intellectual grounds that such a relationship could exist.

The therapist mentioned the subway anxiety and asked whether the patient was frightened by the noise of the trains. When this was confirmed he was asked whether they sounded like the tank he described. Again the patient appeared startled, said that he experienced the noise as being the same and claimed that he had not connected the two before. When a train would noisily approach him, the closed-in feeling came on immediately. An attempt at reevaluation of earlier years in relation to this material was not fruitful.

The patient felt well for the remainder of that day, but the following morning he experienced an intensification of the claustrophobia and attempted to open a window when riding in the subway. He was uncomfortable for a number of days.

At his next visit a hypnotic state was induced again. He was asked to visualize a blackboard. With this as background he was to visualize the words "yes" and "no" whirling through the air and finally one of the words was to appear on the board in chalk. This would indicate whether other issues were to be learned about his symptom. The word "yes" appeared. The technique was repeated using numbers and the number appearing on the board would indicate his age at which time something pertinent had happened in connection with the claustrophobia. The number "30" was seen. An attempt was made to regress the patient to that age level for the purpose of inducing significant revivifications but this approach proved to be unproductive despite successes on other occasions. It was believed that the patient might be warding off anxiety and a more indirect approach was then made. He was instructed to have an hypnotic dream which would entail an event of importance in connection with his symptom. "We were on a camping trip—me and Whitey slept in a pup tent and during the night we were closing the flap and something seemed to grab Whitey's hand. He pulled it away. It scared the daylights out of us!" The patient revealed that he was thirty years old when this event occurred. It happened after the tank incident previously described. He told about their fear that a bear might be outside the tent and they were unable to sleep. A storm came up and the tent collapsed on them. They were afraid to get out to fix it. The next morning they saw a skunk nearby but were not sure what had grasped Whitey's hand. The hand was badly scratched. This remained an unsolved puzzle.

An additional dream induction was attempted with similar instructions. His defenses may have been reenforced because he was unable to follow through until the hypnotic state was deepened further and the patient related the following material. "Seems to be four of us sleeping in a lean-to. I woke them up early in the morning." He went on to relate that he had the feeling someone had been stealing the food. He woke up. A lot of snow fell from the roof of the shelter and it seemed to him that the roof was caving in. He was very frightened. They ran out and noticed that sunlight was streaming in through cracks in the roof, giving the impression of a searchlight beam and apparently resulting, according to the patient, in his feeling that theft of the food was being attempted. When the snow fell from the roof there was a roaring noise. Asked what kind, he replied, "Like the rumbling of a tank." This was linked then with the subway noise. Again he revealed he was thirty years old when this event occurred and that it followed the tank incident.

Following through with the patient's tendency to respond with actual events to the dream induction approach, the latter was employed again with instructions that the material would deal with a closed-in and frightened feeling, and with roaring noise. "We were just coming off maneuvers." He went on to relate that they were marching in column, there was a thunderstorm, and a tree fell about five feet in front of him. He was quite frightened. "It seems to me one of the fellows was caught under the tree. Yes, because we did lift the tree and move it over." Again his age was thirty and the occurrence was subsequent to the tank episode.

The hypnotic state was then deepened and the patient was reoriented to the subway setting the day after his preceding visit. A revivification was attempted with instructions to retrieve his very thoughts at the time. He began to breathe heavily. "The tank seems to be rolling over my head. It seems like it's closer and closer all the time. It went away now." When asked where he was he replied, "On the platform." Then, "Isn't it funny—the subway looks just like a tank!" Asked what he was doing, he replied, "I'm getting out of the way. Instead of wheels it looks like treads." His thoughts then were, "I'm a little scared to go in. I don't see why it should be all closed up that way. Why can't they keep the windows open!" Then again, "The treads of the tank look so menacing!"

Regressions were then effected for the indefinite past in order to elicit data which might have predisposed the patient to develop the claustrophobia following the precipitating experiences. Nothing crucial was obtained and his productions as a matter of fact possessed pleasant attributes in general for him. He appeared to be counterbalancing some of the anxiety he had been experiencing.

Before the hypnosis session was terminated the blackboard and chalk technique was used. The patient was asked whether any other elements were involved in his phobia and whether he felt that anything had been omitted. The word "no" appeared in response each time. It reappeared when he was asked whether he felt anything else should be taken up. The hypnosis was terminated following suggestions for posthypnotic recall. This was effected satisfactorily. On emerging from the hypnosis the patient looked content and pleased, stretched and commented that he felt as if he had come out of a long sleep. He said he felt rested. The tank episode and subway discomfort were discussed. He reaffirmed what were evidently marked perceptual distortions as he described how he would see tank treads instead of subway wheels coming toward him. This was of special interest to him because most of the time he would see the treads when he could not even have seen wheels as the train pulled into the station.

Prior to the hypnotic induction the patient had been asked what he noticed and he described again how the door and walls were closing in on him. Following the session this feeling was no longer with him. The patient at this time gave the impression of intense personal satisfaction.

After this session the patient experienced some apprehension about the symptom returning. This apprehension is a common finding in such problems. It then disappeared. In the meantime the symptom itself had disappeared too under all settings as described. It had been with the patient almost four years and had dated from the tank incident. Its resolution constituted a partial success in total treatment because there were other problems with which he had to deal. At a subsequent visit the patient mentioned his interest in the fact that the tank episode on retrospect seemed so very frightening, although at the time it occurred he did not experience the frightening feeling to such degree.

DISCUSSION

In routine practice involving a large number of patients it has become increasingly clear to psychotherapists that the summation and dynamic interplay of a variety of life experiences are involved usually in symptom formation. In keeping with professional group affiliations stress is placed often on one or another life periods as being the more fundamental for investigation. The two extremes are, of course, the years of childhood and the years of adulthood. In fact it would appear that there is a tremendous variation in periods for emphasis when evaluating symptom formation in a large variety of patients. Furthermore, when evaluating problems and the frequently encountered range of specific symptoms in any one patient, the life periods most significant for each will vary considerably with each symptom. In the patient described, for example, one phobic reaction was strongly linked with recent adult trauma, yet an investigation of early family involvements proved crucial to an understanding of the problem and in effecting relief. With the claustrophobia, it appeared from this study

that events of relatively recent occurrence were crucial in symptom formation even though the psychological connotations of the
phobic reaction could be linked with oppressive, closing-in feelings clearly relating to the patient's early family ties and later
environmental and family pressures. All of this has bearing on the
issue of how far into the past one must reach, how much time
must be consumed, and how much one can depend on results
which may be obtained. Conclusive answers are most certainly
not available despite a variety of claims. Symptom removal as a
result of direct attempts, hypnotic or otherwise, may be transient
or permanent. Symptom removal concurrent with the fathoming
by the patient of related dynamic issues is believed generally
more likely to be lasting. Even so, there is considerable variation
from patient to patient. There are claims that in the course of
analytic work, as underlying problems are worked through, symptoms will disappear without specific investigation. It is probably
accurate to say that such relief can be shown often to be as
permanent or evanescent as relief through the aforementioned
approaches. Even relief through prolonged and intensive treatment with dynamic evaluation of symptoms does not insure in
many instances against the recurrence which various therapies
strive to obviate. The complexity of personalities confounds the
complexity of techniques. Need it be said again that the field
remains fertile for exploration.

With the present patient, the tank episode was devastatingly
traumatic and the threat with which he had to cope was that
against his life. There can be no doubt, however, that the patient,
as a result of previous experience, had developed a low threshold
for anxiety. Perhaps it may be unwarranted to state this in so
positive a fashion. It was at least the impression of the therapist.
Within the setting of time limited but very pointed attempts to
explore predisposing elements from earlier years for the development of the claustrophobia, no specific factors were uncovered,
although the pressures of certain difficult family interpersonal relations and other environmental pressures were known at the time.
It seems that the threat to life as exemplified in the closing in and
crushing experience set the pace for symptom formation and
utilization of the specific symbol theme. Subsequent events in-

volving the tent collapse and lean-to fright apparently reenforced the traumatic impact of the tank episode. The latter may have predisposed to the development of more marked reactions to the additional occurrences by which the patient might not otherwise have been as greatly affected. It is not possible now but it would have been of interest to know whether the patient's buddy sustained any lasting emotional problem stemming from the tank episode or the other events. The relief experienced by the patient as a result of dealing only with the data as described in this report suggests greater optimism for offering some assistance to patients with similar traumatic experiences and without assuming that for symptom relief a time-consuming therapeutic approach would be essential. This issue is to be differentiated from that of dealing with acute problems as emergencies wherein time-limited therapy is a necessity rather than a choice. The point just made does not deny that patients of this type may well have involved problems calling for long-term-intensive treatment. The patient reported here does in fact fit into this category.

The exploratory approach in this case allowed for the patient's unconscious awareness of certain issues touching on his problem. The search described with the blackboard technique was predicated on this possibility. It is unwarranted, with the little that is known about personality functioning, to assume that this type of exploration if pressed strongly enough would produce results invariably. Clinical experience has demonstrated that it has definite limitations but when effective it would appear that hypnotic methods may be of special assistance.

There is widespread belief that the type of dream revealed by this patient constitutes an attempt to master the anxiety relating to a traumatic experience. Combat dreams have received special attention in regard to this. It was of interest to hear that the hypnotic revivification far surpassed in emotional impact not only simple recall but the nightmare recollection of the tank episode. The powerful emotional hold on the patient by this experience was undoubtedly reflected in his tendency during hypnosis to reproduce the event, although the anxiety apparently felt by the patient in the revivification seemed to decrease on repetition.

Of special note is the reaction of the patient to the link between the tank trauma and the claustrophobia. His immediate reaction was one of experiencing the connection on an emotional level, but he was puzzled by it as an intellectual concept. A favorite theme in literature dealing with such material is the separation between emotional and intellectual insight with reiteration of patient's acquiring intellectual insight but failing to improve owing to lack of emotional insight. In relation to this there is the issue of having an emotional experience in therapy stemming from transference involvements. Experiencing an integration of material on an emotional level prior to absorption of concepts as intellectual issues as illustrated in this case is, it would seem to this therapist, far more frequent than generally recognized. A number of patients have been encountered in whom this type of reaction has been decisively exhibited. There may well be a variety of reasons for this. One example would be the patient whose intellectual level of functioning might preclude early or eventually adequate intellectual integration, although the emotional experience is conclusive for him. Then there is the patient who may repress acknowledgment of the intellectual integration while permitting admission of the emotional connections in the same way that the alleged schism may occur with patients who freely acknowledge viewing connections in terms of ideas but deny a concurrent reaction in terms of feeling. It would appear important then to recognize the diversity of responses under such circumstances.

The use of the dream induction stimulus to elicit recall of life experience when the patient's pattern of response had been observed previously deserves comment. Similar occurrences have been noted elsewhere. The issue involved is to contend with the patient's anxiety and defenses, to further progress, and to permit the patient's active participation in the advance. A patient, for example, may supply a hypnotic dream on instruction to do so. If he sets up a barrier to this but offers a description of a current emotion or a past experience, his very response may be integrated into therapy and similar responses elicited with further integration even though the nature of the response is to all appearances inconsistent with the nature of the stimulus. Some patients will produce automatic writing under certain circumstances. Others when so instructed will produce no writing but will offer meaningful verbal associations to the instructions. Such responses may prove to be consistent and the data may prove to be of dynamic significance. The responses then are pseudo-failures in appearance but constitute successes for their role in treatment. In a nontherapeutic, or more specifically a non-scientific setting where dynamic issues are not the goal, the reactions of such subjects would be viewed as failures. Similar patterns of response are found also in non-hypnotic therapeutic settings. If the pattern is discerned by the therapist, he may capitalize on the data elicited. In treatment it is necessary to deal at times with the patient's feeling that his divergent response constitutes a failure.

The relationship between the tank experience and the subway phobia is of some interest. The patient experienced what probably should be called an illusion rather than a hallucination in which the oncoming train would appear to have tank treads. The quality of this perception, however, was almost hallucinatory. Despite this, the connection between his anxiety and fears and the Army episode was not assimilated satisfactorily as a grouping of ideas so that he demonstrated his puzzled reaction even after the revivification despite what appeared to be his emotional realization of the link between the two. Such functioning is an additional demonstration of the manifold aspects of levels of awareness in personality operation. In line with this was the patient's initial claim that he became aware of his claustrophobia after leaving military service. His final awareness of its development was effected after the specific repression had been eliminated.

The use of the crystal ball imagery is not an essential for the type of recall described in one part of this report, but it has advantages with some patients and has been discussed more thoroughly elsewhere (Schneck, 1954).

The attitude of the patient toward his officer seemed to have a paranoid quality. This was not investigated in detail and the impression may well have been valid, although the basic elements involved in symptom formation as elicited here would have remained crucial. Contact with varieties of military settings and with soldiers undergoing diverse Army experiences tends to diminish skepticism about what would otherwise seem to be situations and relationships hardly likely to occur.

The data involved in this case suggest that therapeutic approaches of this type might well be considered in highly traumatic and comparable occurrences within a civilian rather than a military setting. A number of the comments already made would apply likewise in such instances.

Care was taken to avoid implying during any phase of this study that the patient would not reexperience his symptoms. It was felt that transference or other issues might influence a positive result of this type with subsequent relapse if inadequate work had been done on this problem. On the other hand, failure to improve might well have discouraged the patient and jeopardized further progress. An attitude of watchful waiting allowing for further investigation was therefore adopted and when this step was shown to be correct, it was evident that further probing could be attempted.

The work on the major trauma evidently permitted the patient to experience a brief respite. Reactivation of the symptom on the following day might be explained in various ways. First, there were other issues touching on the problem which had to be dealt with. Second, the patient had to contend with alteration of inner psychological processes which would permit obliteration of the symptoms as means of coping with and compartmentalizing over-all anxiety. The total defense structure in personality functioning had to undergo revision. Third, and as part of the preceding issue, any secondary gain issues which were not investigated had to undergo realignment and revision or elimination. The holding on to symptoms for a variety of reasons is well known, and threat to their elimination is combatted, often with temporary exacerbation. At this phase of treatment, patients with weak ego structures or for other secondary considerations, are prone to leave treatment so that the investigation remains incomplete. This occurs too in therapy on a non-insight level and it is, of course, not limited to hypnotic therapy.

Data elicited revealed that the tank episode was apparently the major element in the development of the claustrophobia, although subsequent events served as reinforcement. The tremendous impact of the tank episode is demonstrated by the perceptual distortions in subway settings. It is illustrated also in the hypnosis when a variety of visual images appeared to the patient to be inundated by the shadow of the tank event.

The last comment by the patient as described in this report regarding the fright element during the tank trauma and on recall of the trauma is in keeping with what has often been observed and recorded. The sudden, overwhelming threat to life did not allow, it seems, for sufficient time for the patient to experience and master his emotions. Their free expression and management was prevented by the precipitous occurrences. The emotions were blocked and sealed and the impact of the experience could not be appreciated fully on a conscious level and mastered as such. The fright in connection with the tank trauma was consciously experienced to a significant degree as a result of subsequent evaluation and elaboration. It appears that the revivification was required for significant therapeutic effect in contrast to unsuccessful spontaneous efforts through nightmare, fantasy and conscious recall. This may account in part for the emotional acknowledgment of the link between the tank trauma and the claustrophobia with a delay in the assimilation of its implications on an intellectual level following the crucial revivification.

SUMMARY

This report presents the hypnotherapy of a patient with claustrophobia. The crucial event responsible for symptom formation occurred in military service when the patient was trapped in a trench by a tank which stopped over the patient before proceeding, and at which time the sides of the trench began to cave in. Subsequent traumatic events served as reenforcement. It is likely that a low threshold for the development of anxiety predisposed this patient to the development of the claustrophobia, although the major trauma sustained was undoubtedly of tremendous impact and a distinct threat to life. Emotional experiences were sealed and free expression was permitted through hypnotic revivification. The dynamics, further elaborated in the report, suggest that similar occurrences not necessarily in military settings may be approached therapeutically in this way. Aside from the re-living technique, recall stimulation through a dream induction approach was employed. Other hypnotic methods were described and further implications for psychotherapy in general were elaborated. Hypnotherapeutic and hypnoanalytic approaches to phobic reactions have been described at length elsewhere (Schneck, 1954).

REFERENCES

Schneck, J. M.(Ed.): *Hypnosis in Modern Medicine.* Springfield, Thomas, 1953.

Schneck, J. M.: *Studies in Scientific Hypnosis.* New York, Nervous and Mental Disease Monographs, and Baltimore, Williams and Wilkins, 1954.

CHAPTER *29*

PREVENTING CRYING THROUGH DESENSITIZATION *

PETER B. FIELD, PH.D.

INTRODUCTION

SYSTEMATIC DESENSITIZATION has been widely applied in the treatment of anxiety, phobias, and related avoidance responses, but its applicability to other problems needs greater definition. This paper reports the use of systematic desensitization and hypnotherapy in an unusual problem, the prevention of crying during a wedding ceremony. Although compulsive crying has been treated by assertive training, it has rarely been treated by desensitization or reciprocal inhibition. Rimm (1967) reported a case in which crying spells were eliminated by replacing them with assertive behavior. In that case, anger-induced crying was successfully treated by pairing termination of electric shock with the emission of assertive responses.

CASE REPORT

The present case report describes desensitization treatment of a bride for stress-induced crying, which she feared would take place during her wedding. Eight days before the wedding, the patient consulted the author and requested hypnotherapy to enable her to get through the ceremony without crying. When I protested that some crying was natural in a bride, she explained with occasional tears that she had a serious problem. She was certain that she would cry a great deal throughout the wedding in an inappropriate way, and that she would be unable to pay attention to the ceremony. The emotional impact of the wedding was exacerbated since this was her first marriage after many years as a spinster.

* Originally published in *The American Journal of Clinical Hypnosis,* Vol. 13, No. 2, October 1970, pp. 134–136. Copyright 1970 by the American Society of Clinical Hypnosis.

The patient had a history of crying out of proportion to the provocation in a variety of emotional and innocuous situations. When scolded as a child she would not try to suppress her feelings, but would go to her room, put on a recording of an old waltz that she associated with tears, and feel sad and sorry for herself. She would weep over fairy tales as a child, and still wept as an adult when reading sentimental material. Tears would well up at the lines of verse in a birthday card, or at the National Anthem. If a motion picture had a sad theme, she would never go with anyone else, so that she would be free to "tear all over the place." She responded with tears not only to sadness and sentimentality, but also to anger, happiness, and almost any kind of feeling. Although she cried at funerals and weddings, she did not cry at her father's funeral, and cried at her mother's funeral only because others were doing so. Three years of psychotherapy elsewhere had not changed her crying, although she felt they had been helpful in other ways.

Her usual defense against inappropriate crying was to avoid thinking about the provocation. For example, she would count objects in a room to keep her mind off the emotion. At times she would conceal her feelings by pausing in a conversation, catching her breath for a moment, and pretending she could not remember what she wanted to say next. She expected that she would have to work hard to keep her mind off her wedding ceremony, which would destroy much of the value of the ceremony to her, and would be unsuccessful to boot. The wedding ceremony is pervaded by symbols and images designed to provoke sentiment, and the problem was to help the patient keep her responses to them within normal limits.

TREATMENT

Treatment possibilities were limited by the brief time available. A simple direct suggestion approach was immediately discarded as unlikely to be effective. Chertok (1966, p. 79) reports the unsuccessful hypnotic treatment of a bride for stress incontinence, which finally forced her to absent herself in the middle of the church ceremony. Therefore, the treatment chosen was a variation on systematic desensitization, in which the patient was instructed not only to relax during successive presentations of the items in a hierarchy, but was repeatedly told to be "calm, objective, and detached" as she imagined them. This approach was selected because the psychological opposite of exaggerated sentimentality is an objective, dispassionate, hard-headed "scientific" response. The responses of inappropriate emotion were to be replaced by detachment, control, and studied calm.

A seven-item hierarchy was constructed as described by Wolpe (1958). The items were drawn from aspects of the Unitarian ceremony, and comprised the following:

1. The wedding vows, looking at each other, the ring. (Most disturbing.)
2. Readings from *The Prophet*—e.g. "Make not a bond of love."
3. Apache benediction—"no more loneliness."
4. The opening—"For as much as we are gathered together," and the "I do's."
5. Coming out to the altar from the minister's study.
6. Busy work in the minister's study.
7. Greetings and walking up the aisle at the end. (Least disturbing.)

Three desensitization sessions were conducted, on the fifth, fourth, and second days before the wedding. Hypnosis was induced at all sessions. The patient showed spontaneous fixation of her gaze and spontaneous eye closure, tilting her body to the side as she went deeper into hypnosis. She reported that she had tried to lift her arm and to pull herself up during hypnosis and had been unable to do so, although the therapist did not suggest these phenomena. A total of fifty-four item-presentations were made over the three sessions, and the patient showed disturbance by raising a finger on thirteen (24%) of these. The median difficulty of the items presented was six on the first day, three on the second, and two on the third, indicating steady progress in imagining more and more difficult items. When a tear appeared during the desensitization, the therapist deepened the hypnosis. The latter procedure terminated incipient crying.

OUTCOME

The patient did not cry at all during her wedding. Her testimony was confirmed by the bridegroom and by candid photographs. At one point her voice was almost inaudible and her hands trembled enough to shake petals from the bouquet onto the floor, but she was happy and aware of the entire ceremony.

She was very pleased by the outcome, and reported no substitute symptom on five-month follow-up.

The procedure, although successful, did not produce a generalized change in her emotional response in other situations. She wept lightly during a follow-up interview. She attended another wedding several months later, and cried. It was not important for her to be in control at that time.

REFERENCES

Chertok, L.: *Hypnosis.* New York, Pergamon Press, 1966.

Rimm, D. C.: Assertive training used in treatment of chronic crying spells. *Behav Res Ther,* 5:373–374, 1967.

Wolpe, J.: *Psychotherapy by Reciprocal Inhibition.* Stanford, Stanford University Press, 1958.

CHAPTER 30

THE MODIFICATION OF HYPNOTIC BEHAVIOR OR EXTENDING THE VERBAL CONTROL OF COMPLEX HUMAN BEHAVIOR *

Ian Wickramasekera, Ph.D.

U NTIL RECENTLY hypnotizability has been regarded as relatively unmodifiable behavior (Hilgard, 1965; Shor, Orne and O'Connel, 1966; London, 1969; Gill and Brenman, 1959). Several psychotherapist-hypnotists have implied that hypnotizability can be significantly altered (Bernheim, 1884; Erickson, 1952; Moll, 1958). It appears likely that the early interpersonal techniques (Gill and Brenman, 1959; As, Hilgard and Weitzenhoffer, 1963) used to modify hypnotizability were relatively ineffective because the specific experiential behavioral targets of change were poorly defined and the interventions unsystematic. Recently the following procedures have been found to be promising approaches to disinhibiting or shaping up expanded hypnotic repertoires: 1) Verbally and behaviorally (modeling) presented instructions and training directed at private events, e.g. attention, imagery, misconception, critical thinking, sensory focus and comfort under conditions of fading reality orientation; 2) Training in interpersonal risk taking, closeness, self disclosure and arranging the conditions for "trust"; 3) Special procedures intended to alter perception (sensory deprivation and psychedelic drugs); 4) Biofeedback training procedures (EEG and EMG).

* This is an original manuscript.

Shor, Orne and O'Connel (1966) have stated that it is important to distinguish between variations in hypnotic performance and the modification of hypnotizability per se. But it is important to note that all statements about changes in hypnotizability are necessarily inferences from performance because hypnotizability per se, like learning, is an unobservable construct. From a practical standpoint it is important to know 1) if the four general types of pre-hypnotic procedures identified above will reliably expand hypnotic behavior (response to test suggestions) above baseline levels; 2) if the expanded hypnotic repertoire will generalize to a standard induction procedure minus the special pre-hypnotic procedures; 3) if changes induced in hypnotic performance in the laboratory will generalize to the clinical situation; 4) if pre-hypnotic procedures that are reliably effective in the laboratory will also be reliably effective in the clinic.

It is also important to know if these four general types of hypnosis increasing interventions have most impact on initially (baseline measurement) low or moderately hypnotizable subjects. It would also be useful to know which technique to use with which type of subject and which experimental procedures are most suitable for shaping up or disinhibiting which hypnotic phenomena. Unfortunately, secure answers to all the above questions are not yet in.

The procedures to be outlined below appear to significantly increase the probability of boosting hypnotic performances above baseline levels by facilitating the subject's skill in manipulating internal events or by educating him subjectively. Through subjective education or the development of effective and reliable skills in controlling private events (thoughts and their physiological consequences) the range of personal self management and control may be expanded, beyond the limits that are environmentally imposed. It is probable that if subjective education is made part of the regular elementary and secondary school curriculum there will be a less sharp drop off in longitudinal curves of hypnotizability and related phenomena from childhood to adulthood. It is also possible that the average adult who comes to the psychotherapist will bring with him more subjective skills and a higher baseline of subjective education, which, of course, may improve the prognosis for therapy. Hypnotic training, biofeedback, transcendental meditation and related procedures may contribute to a technology of subjective education.

The following techniques appear to increase the probability of hypnotic experience:

1.) *Verbally and behaviorally (modeling) presented systematic instructions and training directed at private events.*

It has been shown that modifying a subject's expectations regarding hypnosis either in the direction of inculcating positive attitudes or correcting misconceptions can increase hypnotizability. Positive attitudes may be induced by defining the situations as easy to respond to, a pleasant and interesting experience, or a consent situation. (Barber and Calverley, 1964, 1966; Diamond, 1972). Positive expectations may also be experimentally induced by manipulating a subject's estimates of his own ability to respond (Wilson, 1967; Gandolfo, 1971; Gregory and Diamond, 1973). For example, Wilson (1967) used unobtrusive types of "prompts" (e.g. hidden lights) to increase the probability that the subject would experience hypnotic suggestions. Gregory and Diamond, (1973) used false personality test results to alter in a positive direction a subject's expectation of hypnotic experience.

Positive attitudes towards hypnosis may also be elicited by exposing hypnotic subjects to a very susceptible hypnotic model who verbalizes his subjective experiences, sensations and responses to discrete hypnotic suggestions. Inviting the subjects whose hypnotizability is to be increased to question the highly susceptible hypnotic model raises the probability of increasing hypnotizability. A model who has high status in a context that is relevant to the hypnotic subject appears to contribute to the enhancement of hypnotizability (De Voge and Sachs, 1973). In general, exposing hypnotic subjects to a highly susceptible hypnotic model, who openly verbalizes his subjective reactions to hypnosis and who responds freely to questions will increase the probability of hypnotic responses in participating observers (Zimbardo, Rapaport and Baron, 1969; Marshall and Diamond, 1969; Diamond, 1972; De Voge and Sachs, 1973; De Stefano, 1971).

The alteration of misconceptions regarding hypnosis and provision of counter information will also raise the probability of hypnotic response (Cronin, Spanos and Barber, 1971; Diamond, 1972; Gregory and Diamond, 1973; Diamond and Harada, 1973). Exposure of misconceptions and provision of counter information may be provided by written instructions on paper, by the observation and questioning of a highly susceptible hypnotic model or by looking at a responsive hypnotic model on video tape. Extinguishing anxieties which stem from misconceptions like loss of consciousness, loss of personal self control, inability to wake from hypnosis, are also powerful cognitive procedures to increase hypnotizability.

The systematic provision of information and training (self-paced successive approximations) on what to do internally (privately and experientially) provided by a responsive hypnotic model or through verbal instructions will also increase hypnotizability (Pascal and Salzberg, 1959; Sachs and Anderson, 1967; Zimbardo, Rapaport and Baron, 1969; Diamond, 1972; Gregory and Diamond, 1973; Diamond and Harada, 1973; Sachs, 1970). The following are effective procedures: 1) Provision of a clear verbal concept of the desired sensory experience; 2) The use of "prompts" to shape up vivid sensory experiences (e.g. to acquaint subject with immediate sensations of heaviness, place a heavy weight on hands); 3) Self-paced successive approximations using just noticeable-difference (JND) steps; 4) Structuring the procedure to place the subject in a double bind situation where he has to validate his subjective report with increased objective performance. In essence, this is a cognitive dissonance procedure; 5) Inviting the subject to imagine vividly, to suspend reality orientation and critical judgment and to permit himself to become totally absorbed (e.g. like at an exciting movie); 6) Verbal reinforcement of hypnotic responsivity; 7) Eliciting the subject's active responsible participation by the use of task relevant motivational instructions presented either verbally or in the form of a programmed text (Havens, 1973).

2.) *Training intra- and interpersonal risk taking.*

We hypothesize that systematically increasing a subject's personal risk taking behavior will increase hypnotizability. This increase in risk taking behavior may be induced by increasing his confidence in the outcome and/or by lifting his intrapersonal inhibitions (defensiveness) to risk taking. Confidence in outcome may be shaped with first a continuous reinforcement schedule and eventually a variable reinforcement schedule. The resulting positive expectancy and the conditions for "trust" are prompts and props which may be faded after risk taking behaviors are internalized and have become high probability events under appropriate conditions. Specifically it is predicted that any manipulations that increase confidence and trust in the Self or confidence and trust in a specific person in the social environment will increase hypnotizability.

In terms of increasing hypnotizability by arranging conditions for "trust" (Wickramasekera, 1973) and confidence in an individual in the social environment, it has been shown that a hypnotist who speaks in a forceful voice (Barber and Calverley, 1964b), behaves warmly (Greenberg and Land, 1971) and who is perceived by the subject (through instructional and situational manipulations) to be an experienced expert (Balaschak, Blocker, Rossiter and Perin, 1972; Wuraftic, 1971; Small and Kramer, 1969; Coe, Bailey, Hall, Howard, Janda, Kobayashi and Parker, 1970) elicits greater hypnotizability. It is hypothesized that systematic provision of the "core conditions" at high levels plus increasing patient "self exploration" (Truax and Carkhuff, 1965) will also increase hypnotizability in that interpersonal context by reducing defensiveness and resistance.

Hypnotizability may also be increased by increasing confidence in the self (mature self confidence). Tart (1970a) found that a nine month training program that stressed interpersonal risk taking (encounter groups and Gestalt therapy) and subjective experiential experimentation (directed imagery and sensory awareness) at Esalen Institute increased hypnotizability as measured by the Stanford Scales. If high interpersonal and intrapersonal trust are an important aspect of both positive mental health and hypnotizability, then the generally poorer hypnotizability of psychiatric patients is partially explained (Gill and Brenman, 1959; Barber, Karacan and Calverley, 1964; Webb and Nesmith, 1964). The clinical-empirical observation (Hilgard, 1965) that adventurous behavior is correlated with hypnotizability may be explained by postulating a risk taking construct that may facilitate both behaviors (mental health behaviors and hypnotizability). It is hypothesized that a systematic program of subjectively oriented personal and social risk taking which incorporates the elements of successive approximation, reinforcement and corrective feedback will increase the probability of hypnotic behavior.

3.) *Special procedures to alter perception.*

It is probable that impairing reality testing with psychedelic drugs and/or sensory deprivation will increase hypnotizability by inhibiting left cerebral hemisphere functions like sequential, analytic and critical-judgmental verbal operations (Sperry, 1964; Milner, 1971; Galin and Ornstein, 1972; Gassaniea, 1967). In terms of the effects of psychedelic drugs, it has been shown that both hypnotic phenomena and hypnotizability may be enhanced by LSD-25 (Fogel and Hoffer, 1962; Levine, Ludwig and Lyle, 1963; Levine and Ludwig, 1965; Sjoberg and Hollister, 1965; Netz, Morten and Sundwall, 1968; Negz and Engstrom, 1968; Middefell, 1967; Ulett,

Akpinar and Itil, 1972) and mescaline (Sjoberg and Hollister, 1965). Two recent studies report a high degree of association between self reported use of marijuana, LSD, mescaline and psilocybin and hypnotizability scores on the Harvard Group Scale (Shor and Orne, 1962; Van Nuys, 1972; Franzini and McDonald, 1973). It is possible that prior use of marijuana and/or psychedelic drugs creates a sense of familiarity and comfort with right hemispheric mental functions and inhibits chronic vigilance and analytic thinking. The disinhibition of these mental functions creates an intrapersonal condition that increases the probability of entry into the hypnotic experience.

Sensory deprivation and restriction procedures appear to be a promising technique of increasing hypnotizability (Pena, 1963; Wickramasekera, 1969, 1970; Sanders and Rehyer, 1969) at least temporarily. Pena (1963) found that three hours of sensory restriction increased hypnotizability in a prison population. Wickramasekera (1969) found that thirty minutes of sensory restriction was sufficient to increase hypnotizability in a college female population, and later Wickramasekera (1970) found that one hour of sensory restriction increased hypnotizability in a group of male prisoners who were generally younger than Pena's (1963) subjects. Sanders and Rehyer (1969) reported that four to six hours of sensory restriction significantly increased the hypnotizability of previously resistant subjects. In the above studies sensory restriction or perceptual deprivation (Zubek, 1973) was imposed on the visual, auditory and tactual-kinesthetic sensory systems to varying extents and with varied instrumentation (sensory deprivation chamber, wearing goggles constructed to decompose visual patterns or listening to "white" noise through headphones). Under the above conditions many subjects spontaneously reported hallucinatory experiences. The above sensory restriction studies used control groups, but there were no tests for transfer of the increased hypnotizability outside the laboratory or to later points in time.

4.) *Biofeedback training procedures (EEG and EMG)*.
Some studies appear to show a relationship between the duration of EEG alpha and hypnotic susceptibility (Galbraith, London, Leibovitz, Cooper and Hart, 1970; London, Hart and Leibovitz, 1968). The biofeedback training procedure (Barber et al., 1971) was used by Engstrom, London and Hart (1970) to demonstrate that six sessions of contingent alpha feedback training was productive of greater increases in hypnotic susceptibility than six sessions of non-contingent alpha feedback training. It appeared from verbal reports that the alpha-on state and hypnosis were subjectively similar. In a single blind study, Wickramasekera (1971) showed that six sessions of contingent EMG feedback training increased hypnotizability more significantly than an equal number of sessions of non-contingent EMG feedback training. In a double blind study Wickramasekera (1973) replicated the above results with another sample of college students of identical age and sex. Ten sessions of shorter (thirty minutes) EMG feedback training were used in the replication study. Currently we are collecting data on pre and post measures of hypnotizability in patients who are learning temperature control with feedback for the management of migraine. These data appear to confirm the hypothesis that any procedures that increases comfort and skill in the self control of internal responses increases the probability of hypnotic behavior.

In summary, then it appears that certain procedures and environmental arrangements increase the probability of hypnotic experience. These arrangements appear to externally alter perception or to increase comfort and skill in subjective functioning. The technology of experimental hypnosis is only one of the streams converging to improve the general technology of subjective education. The availability of reliable and effective procedures to elicit or shape subjective responses (private events) may contribute saliently to a precise and powerful future technology for the control of complex human behavior.

REFERENCES

As, A., Hilgard, E. R., and Weitzenhoffer, A. M.: An attempt at experimental modification of hypnotizability through repeated individualized hypnotic experience. *Scand J Psychol*, 4:81–89, 1963.

Balaschak, B., Blocker, K., Rossiter, T., and Perin, C. T.: The influence of race and expressed experience of the hypnotist on hypnotic susceptibility. *Int J Clin Exp Hypn*, 20:38–45, 1972.

Barber, T. X., and Calverley, D. S.: Comparative effects on "hypnotic-like" suggestibility of recorded and spoken suggestions. *J Consult Psychol*, 28:384, 1968a.

Barber, T. X., and Calverley, D. S.: Effect of E's tone of voice on "hypnotic-like" suggestibility. *Psychol Rep*, 15:139–144, 1964b.

Barber, T. X., Karacan, I., and Calverley, D. S. Hypnotizability and suggestibility in chronic schizophrenics. *Arch Gen Psychiat, 11:439–451*, 1964.

Barber, T. X., Ascher, L. M., and Mavroides, M.: Effects of practice on hypnotic suggestibility: A re-evaluation of Hull's postulates. *Am J Clin Hypn*, 14:48–53, 1971.

Bernheim, H. M.: *De la suggestion dans l'etat hypnotique et dans l'etat de veille*. Paris, Librairie Scientifique et Philosophique, 1884.

Coe, W. C., Bailey, J. R., Hall, J. C., Howard, M. L., Janda, R. L., Kobayashi, K., and Parker, M. D.: Hypnosis as role enactment: The role-location variable. *Proceedings*, APA, 5:839–840, 1970.

Cronin, D. M., Spanos, N. P., and Barber, T. X.: Augmenting hypnotic suggestibility by providing favorable information about hypnosis. *Am J Clin Hypn*, 13:259–264, 1971.

De Stefano, M. G.: The modeling of hypnotic behavior. Paper presented at the Annual Meeting of the Society for Clinical and Experimental Hypnosis, University of Chicago, October, 1971.

De Voge, J. T., and Sachs, L. B.: The modification of hypnotic susceptibility through imitative behavior. *Int J Clin Exp Psychol*, 21:70–77, 1973.

Diamond, M. J.: The use of observationally presented information to modify hypnotic susceptibility. *J. Abnorm Psychol*, 79:174–180, 1972.

Diamond, M. J., and Harada, D.: The use of direct instructions to modify hypnotic susceptibility. Unpublished manuscript, University of Hawaii, 1973.

Engstrom, D. R., London, P., and Hart, J. T.: EEG Alpha feedback training and hypnotic susceptibility. *Proceedings*, APA, 5:837–838, 1970.

Erickson, M. H.: Deep Hypnosis and its induction. In Cron, L. M. (Ed.): *Experimental Hypnosis*. New York, Macmillan, 1952, pp. 70–112.

Franzini, L. R., and McDonald, R. D.: Marijuana Usage and Hypnotic Susceptibility. *J. Consult Clin Psychol, 40*:176–180, 1973.

Fogel, S., and Hoffer, A.: The use of hypnosis to interrupt and to reproduce an LSD-25 experience. *J. Clin Exp Psychopathol, 23*:11–16, 1962.

Galbraith, G., London, P., Leibovitz, M., Cooper, L., and Hart, J.: An electroencephalographic study of hypnotic susceptibility. *J. Comp Physiol Psychol,* 72:125–131, 1970.

Gandolfo, R. L.: Role of expectancy, amnesia, and hypnotic induction in the performance of posthypnotic behavior. *J Abnorm Psychol* 77:324–328, 1971.

Galin, D. and Ornstein, R. E.: Lateral specialization of cognitive mode: An EEG study. *Psychophysiology, 9:*412–418, 1972.

Gazzaniga, M. S.: The split brain in man. *Sci Am, 217*:24–29, 1967.

Gill, M. M., and Brenman, M.: *Hypnosis and Related States.* New York, International Universities Press, 1959.

Greenberg, R. P., and Land, J. M.: Influence of some hypnotist and subject variables on hypnotic susceptibility. *J Consult Clin Psychol, 37*:111–115, 1971.

Gregory, J., and Diamond, M. J.: Increasing hypnotic susceptibility by means of positive expectancies and written instructions. *J. Abnorm Psychol,* 1973, in press.

Havens, R.: Using modeling and information to modify hypnotizability, Unpublished Ph.D. thesis. West Virginia University, 1973.

Hilgard, E. R.: *Hypnotic Susceptibility.* New York, Harcourt, Brace and World, 1965.

Levine, J., and Ludwig, A. M.: Alterations in consciousness produced by combinations of LSD, hypnosis and psychotherapy. *Psychopharmocologia, 7*:123–137, 1965.

Levine, J., Ludwig, A. M., and Lyle, W. H.: The controlled psychedelic state. *Am J Clin Hypn, 6*:163–164, 1963.

London, P.: *Behavior Control.* New York, Harper and Row, 1969.

London, P., Hart, J. and Leibovitz, M.: Alpha rhythms and hypnotic susceptibility. *Nature, 219*:71–72, 1968.

Marshall, G. D., and Diamond, M. J.: Increasing hypnotic susceptibility through modeling. Unpublished manuscript, Stanford University, 1969.

Middlefell, R.: The effects of LSD on body sway suggestibility in a group of hospital patients. *Brit J of Psychiat, 113*:277–280, 1967.

Milner, B.: Interhemispheric Differences in the Localization of Psychological Processes in Man. *Brit Med Bull,* 27, 3:272–277, 1971.

Moll, A.: *The Study of Hypnosis.* New York: Julian Press, 1958.

Netz, B., Morten, S., and Sundwall, A.: Lysergic Acid diethylamide (LSD-25) and intellectual functions, hypnotic susceptibility and sypatho adrenmedullary activity. A pilot study. MPI B-rapport nr 19, 1968, Stocholm, Militurpsykologiska Institutet.

Orne, M. T.: The nature of hypnosis: Artifact and essence. *J Abnorm Soc Psychol, 58*:277–299, 1959.

Pascal, G. R., and Salzberg, H. C.: A systematic approach to inducing hypnotic behavior. *Int J Clin Exp Hypn, 7:*161–167, 1959.

Pena, F.: Perceptual isolation and hypnotic susceptibility. Unpublished doctoral dissertation. Washington State University, 1963.

Sachs, L. B.: Comparison of hypnotic analgesia and hypnotic relaxation during stimulation by a continuous pain source. *J Abnorm Psychol 76:* 206–210, 1970.

Sachs, L. B.: Construing hypnosis as modifiable behavior. In A. Jacobs and L. Sachs (Eds.): *Psychology of Private Events.* New York, Academic Press, 1971, pp. 61–75.

Sanders, R. S., and Reyher, J.: Sensory deprivation and the enhancement of hypnotic susceptibility. *J Abnorm Psychol, 74:*375–381, 1969.

Shor, R. E., and Orne, E. C.: *The Harvard Group Scale of Hypnotic Susceptibility, Form A.* Palo Alto, California, Consulting Psychologists Press, 1962.

Shor, R. E., Orne, M. T., and O'Connell, D. N.: Psychological correlates of plateau hypnotizability in a special volunteer sample. *J personal Soc Psychol, 3:*80–95, 1966.

Sjoberg, B. M., and Hollister, L. E.: The effects of psychotomimetric drugs on primary suggestibility. *Psychopharmacologia, 8:*251–262, 1965.

Small, M. M., and Kramer, E.: Hypnotic susceptibility as a function of the prestige of the hypnotist. *Int J Clin Exp Hypn, 17:*251–256, 1969.

Sperry, R. W.: The Great Cerebral Commissure. Sci Am, 1964, *210, #1,* 42–52.

Tart, C. T. Increases in hypnotizability resulting from a prolonged program for enhancing personal growth. *J Abnorm Psychol, 75:*260–266, 1970a.

Truax, C. B. and Carkhuff, R. R.: Experimental manipulation of therapeutic conditions. *J Consult Psychol, 29:*119–124, 1967.

Ulett, G. A., Akpinar, S., and Itil, T. M.: Hypnosis: Physiological, pharmacological reality. *Am J Psychiat, 128:*33–39, 1972.

Van Nuys, D.: Meditation, attention, and hypnotic susceptibility: A correlational study. *Int J Exp Hypn,* 1972.

Webb, R. A. and Nesmith, C. C.: A normative study of suggestibility in a mental patient population. *Int J Clin Exp Hypn, 12:*181–183, 1964.

Wickramasekera, I.: The effects of sensory restriction of susceptibility to hypnosis: A hypothesis, some preliminary data, and theoretical speculation. *Int J Clin Exp Hypn, 17:*217–224, 1969.

Wickramasekera, I.: Effects of sensory restriction on susceptibility to hypnosis: A hypothesis and more preliminary data. *J Abnorm Psychol, 76:* 69–75, 1970.

Wickramasekera, I.: Effects of EMG feedback training in susceptibility to hypnosis: Preliminary observations. Proc. 79th annual convention of Amer Psychol Assoc, 1971, 6, 783–784 (Summary).

Wickramasekera, I.: Effects of "hypnosis" and task motivational instructions in attempting to influence the "voluntary" self-deprivation of money. *J Personal Soc Psychol, 19:*311–314, 1971.

Wickramasekera, I.: The effects of EMG feedback on hypnotic susceptibility: More preliminary data. *J Abnorm Psychol,* 1973, in press.

Wilson, D. L.: The role of confirmation of expectancies in hypnotic induction. Unpublished doctoral dissertation, University of North Carolina,
1967.

Wuraftic, R. D.: Effects of experimenter status on hypnosis and suggestibility. Unpublished doctoral dissertation, University of Tennessee, 1971.

Zimbardo, P. G., Rapaport, C., and Baron, J.: Pain control by hypnotic
induction of motivational states. In Zimbardo's, P. G. (Ed.): *The Cognitive Control of Motivation.* Glenview, Illinois, Scott, Foresman, and
Company, 1969, pp. 136–152.

Zubek, J. P.: Behavioral and physiological effects of prolonged sensory and
perceptual deprivation: A review. In Rasmussen (Ed.): Man in Isolation and Confinement. Aldine, 1973.

CHAPTER 31

BEHAVIOR MODIFICATION AND HYPNOTIC CONDITIONING IN PSYCHOTHERAPY *

WILLIAM S. KROGER, M.D.

INTRODUCTION

BEHAVIOR MODIFICATION THERAPY is receiving increasing recognition in clinical psychology and psychiatry. The basis for classical conditioning therapy was established by Pavlov and Thorndike. Watson and later Mowrer experimented with behavior modification. In 1950 Wolpe used counterconditioning or systemic desensitization, often with hypnosis, for eliminating the anxieties of certain neuroses. About the same time, disciples of Skinner demonstrated that they could modify behavior, especially in psychotics, by operant conditioning and reinforcement learning. These principles now are successfully applied to such clinical conditions as mental retardates, autistic children and even chronically hospitalized patients. The rationale is that whenever a particular behavior is "reinforced" or rewarded, there is a greater chance that it will be repeated.

I have taken these methodologies and combined them with the wisdom and lore of even older healing modalities such as Yoga, Zen and hypnosis. The *raison d'etre* for the adjunctive use of hypnosis, applicable for most models of psychotherapy, enables patients to "tap forgotten assets and hidden potentials." If this assumption is valid, then hypnotic conditioning should potentiate behavioral modification.

* This is an original manuscript.

I have obtained best results in chronic psychosomatic disorders, phobias, compulsions, sexual neuroses and such habit patterns as obesity and smoking. Poorest response was in psychotics, deep-seated characterologic disorders, chronic alcoholics and drug addicts. I am aware that a subtle placebo effect is present in all forms of psychotherapy including hypnotherapy per se. More than 60 percent of the "garden variety" types of disturbed persons recover irrespective of the treatment procedures employed. Many of the patients referred to the hypnotist-psychiatrist are the miserable peripatetic "medical shoppers," the "port of last call patient." Nearly all are looking for magic, and most have been refractory to conventional psychotherapy.

PROGRAM PHASES

(1) *Historo-diagnosis:* Taking a careful history, making a diagnosis and establishing good rapport.

(2) *Hypnotic Induction:* I try for some degree of hypnotic depth, even though a formal induction procedure often is not necessary. However, I use the standard progressive relaxation method, familiar to all of you, because the structured nuances of this induction builds in a *control system* to be used later for desired behavioral changes. For instance, I suggest that development of eye-lid and leg heaviness, lightness of the arm during levitation, rigidity of the limbs demonstrated by catalepsy, and relaxation of the entire body—any or all determine how well greater control of autonomic system functioning (A.N.S.) as well as the desired changes are to be attained. Thus behavior modification is instituted early. Some of the imagined somatic activities can be detected even electromyographically.

Thus, words, self-generated thoughts and covert feelings act as conditioned stimuli for specific autonomic responses even though the original stimulus has been forgotten. As Pavlov stated "Suggestion is the simplest form of a conditioned reflex."

About two sessions are required to produce a suitable depth of hypnosis. The next one or two sessions are used to deepen it by the "elevator" technic described elsewhere (Kroger, 1963).

(3) *Training in Autohypnosis:* During autohypnosis full use of mnemonic material (reviving past experiences similar to those

desired) via the imagination is employed for inducing the typical sensory alterations of the eyelids, toes, feet, chest, trunk, and head. Doubling back over each of these areas acts as reinforcement; the reward is the associated relaxation and increased control over these autonomic processes. It is axiomatic that whenever the imagination (the experiential background) and the so-called "will" come into conflict, the imagination always "beats the will to the draw." Therefore, "the battle to establish a beachhead on the periphery of the patient's neurosis" is going to be won or lost on the field of imagination. If full control of simple feedback subsystems (the "how am I doing" error correcting information transmission mechanisms) producing relaxation are learned, then more complex and resistant processes become amenable to at least semi-volitional regulation. This is similar to autogenic training.

After sufficient practice, autohypnosis is attained by a triggering cue as closing the eyelids or as in Zen and Yoga—a mantra. This by-passes the need for the progressive-relaxation technic. The purpose of this meditative and self-reflective state, somewhat like communion or prayer, is to repeat the indicated autosuggestions or affirmations taught in phase 4, *long enough, strong enough,* and *often enough* to reinforce positive conditioned responses. The negative ones responsible for the symptom-complex are inhibited. This is direct symptom removal, but yet permissive and patient-centered. The patient is now taught dehypnotization.

I tell patients they should learn autohypnosis for the following reasons: (a) "you will have a feeling of pride and self-esteem that you removed the symptom"; (b) "you will not be dependent upon any other physician"; (c) "if the original symptom returns, you will use the same affirmations that once removed it"; (d) "should a substitute symptom replace the removed one (and this is highly equivocal), you can readily remove it as you did the original symptom." A new symptom does not replace a removed symptom, especially if the patient himself eliminated the original symptom. Eysenck (1967) states, "Behavior therapists consider it a trifle odd that they should be criticized for only curing 'symptoms.'"

(4) *Affirmations:* If the four premises mentioned above are

understood, I then suggest the affirmations required for dissolution of the symptom. I prefer to have these repeated by interoceptive conditioning, as we all have "bells in our brain that we can ring." From now on I shall use obesity for my model to show how behavioral modification is employed. The aversive and other goal directed affirmations utilized for weight loss are described in detail elsewhere (Kroger, 1970).

"Inner speech" based on "scene visualization" of past experiences (sensory imagery conditioning), or in the language of the behaviorists, "visual voyages," "imagery conditioning" and "self-feeling talk," enhance (ANS) control. As mentioned, this is relatively easy if control of the *non-learned, nonconditioned* or *involuntary* reflexes such as heaviness and lightness are first taught. These ideosensory activities are functions of the "instinctual" or primary signaling system described by Pavlov. They are mobilized readily since they are necessary to preserve the integrity of the organism. Because they are on or off they have been compared to "digital" notions in central nervous system functioning.

Patients are also trained to develop "heat" by imagining their foot being placed in a tub of hot water and "cold" by their hand being put in a glass of ice water. After these ideosensory mechanisms are perceived as real, more complex ones as aversive tastes for specific foods are readily developed by recalling the representations of disgusting thoughts and feelings. Such symbolic activities are *learned, conditioned* and *voluntary.* They are part of the secondary signaling system of higher nervous elaboration. They act slowly by analogy and have therefore been referred to as analogic notions—the latter controls the former. This method is not new but differs from classical-type Pavlovian conditioning initially produced by external stimuli—*exteroceptive conditioning.*

My approach is similar to the extraordinary "mind-body" responses provided by Yoga, Zen, and other Eastern therapies. These indicate that the ANS is not as autonomic as believed and that some portions of it can by appropriate training come under volitional control. If Yoga and Zen conditioning are examined objectively within our own culture their similarities with behavior modification and hypnotic conditioning is self-evident. All rely on relaxation, concentration, exquisite receptivity and greater objectivity for acceptance and facilitation of the affirmations.

In other words, autogenous biofeedback cues can trigger and reinforce pleasant states in a similar manner to the alpha "beeps" of biofeedback training (B.F.T.). Well trained Yogians and Zennists do not need biofeedback training to alter pulse, blood pressure and other autonomically established conditioned reflexes.

Recent data (Platonov, 1955; Paterson, 1967) indicate that conditioned reflexes established under hypnosis are more durable and less likely to go into extinction. I have taken this type of conditioning one step further by employing sophisticated hypnotic technics with reinforcement learning to establish corrective behavioral changes. The punishment and reward alternatives implicit in behavioral and operant conditioning can be incorporated, particularly if the affirmations and posthypnotic suggestions (PHS) are oriented around the patient's emotional needs. It is recommended that the affirmations be used at least four to five times a day during autohypnosis. As reinforcement learning increases, weight loss becomes a reward and the weight gain acts as punishment. Thus far, my treatment has been directed toward the symptomatic level. A noncondemnatory attitude when failure occurs combined with encouragement, facilitates acceptance of the affirmations. I have successfully used a similar approach for treatment of the tobaccomaniac.

(5) *Symptom-Manipulation:* Most of these technics have been described by Erickson (1954). The first is *symptom-substitution.* Through PHS, one can "trade down" to other eating behaviors such as chewing gum, or get patients interested in organic or dietetic foods. In *symptom-transformation* the overeating can be transferred by an appropriate PHS to other behaviors such as physical exercise, shopping, child raising, P.T.A. meetings and interest in community affairs. Although seemingly similar to symptom-substitution, reduction of excessive eating occurs by transformation of the symptom into a less noxious one without directly attacking the character of the symptom itself. In *symptom-amelioration* the overeating is reduced. First, it is deliberately increased by PHS; if this is done volitionally it eventu-

ally can be decreased. *Symptom-utilization* consists of encouraging, accepting and redefining cooperative activity of an aversive nature toward the faulty patterns. This differs from symptom removal by direct suggestion. Any one or all can be used in various combinations.

(6) *Holistic Approach:* The final phase is directed to the holistic approach. The dictum is treating the personality who has the obesity rather than the symptom per se. Otherwise, "we will have a fat personality crying to get out of a thin body." The significance of the overeating in the *here* and *now* is more important than its relationship as to how the symptom developed. I concur with Rado (1953), "Fishing into the past only yields diminishing returns."

Briefly, the therapeutic design is structured around the following: (a) "how much of the overeating do you really need to keep?"; (b) "Perhaps you could overeat just enough to lose one and one half pounds a week?"; (c) "What are you trying to prove by overeating?"; (d) "How rapidly can you divest yourself of the emotional needs for the overeating?"

To expedite therapy, most of the patients are given an interview-in-depth and a complete psychometric evaluation by my clinical psychologist. This is time-saving and brings many hidden facets of the personality into focus. Behavioral modification and conditioning under hypnosis always requires treatment of the associated anxieties. Desensitization (exposure to small amounts of anxiety-laden material at each hypnotherapeutic session) is effective for some but worthless for others.

As Conn (Kroger, 1963) has described in detail there are needs inherent in all anxiety ridden persons, i.e. the need to talk, the need to be told what to do, the need to be accepted, the need to be one's real self, and the need to emancipate oneself from any undue dependency on the therapist.

Briefly, and this applies to nearly all kinds of psychiatric cases, there are only three therapeutic avenues open to the anxiety-ridden patient; (a) He can "develop a thicker skin" and learn to live with his problems; (b) he can walk away or retreat from his life situations to fight another day when stronger; (c) he can come to grips with his difficulties, provided, and if, the therapist gives him the necessary coping mechanisms.

Patients sense the physician's interest and warmth. Who can deny that the strength of the interpersonal relationship is the important vector in any therapy, and it is the therapist who motivates the patient to achieve self-mastery over his behavior? This best can be achieved by the best co-pilot any healer can have— faith in the therapist's methods. Successful behavioral conditioning is therefore a collaborative and reciprocal effort between therapist and patient—each learning from the other. Though I have no statistical data to support my contention that behavioral modification and hypnotic conditioning are more effective than conventional psychotherapy, empirically they appear to be.

Behavioral conditioning and hypnosis are both derivatives of ancient therapies. That they have survived as meaningful therapeutic adjuncts indicates these will not be hailed as the "treatments of the year." There are drawbacks—not all patients are amenable to hypnotic conditioning, it is a time-consuming process for the therapist, and by no means are the methods described above a panacea. I have had dramatic successes as well as dramatic failures.

REFERENCES

Eysenck, H. J.: Behavior therapy and techniques: evaluation. *Medical Opinion and Review,* February, 3:61, 1967.

Kroger, W. S.: *Clinical and Experimental Hypnosis.* Philadelphia, Lippincott, 1963.

Kroger, W. S.: Comprehensive management of obesity. *Am J Clin Hypn,* 12:165, 1970.

Paterson, A. S.: Acquisition of cortical control over autonomic malfunction in psychosomatic medicine through hypnosis. Presented at the International Congress of Hypnosis and Psychosomatic Medicine, Koyto, Japan, July 13, 1967.

Platonov, K. I.: *The Word as a Physiological and Psychological Factor.* Moscow, Foreign Language Publishing House, 1955.

CHAPTER 32

CONCLUDING REMARKS

THIS BOOK IS DIRECTED primarily towards behavior therapists and hypnotherapists with the aim of acquainting practitioners of one school with the techniques and concepts of the other. A marriage of convenience is thereby established, for hypnosis adds leverage to behavior therapy and shortens treatment time, while behavioral techniques harmonize with hypnotherapy like a hand into a well-fitting glove.

Behavior therapists tend to neglect hypnosis, feeling that there is no need for it in their particular approach to treatment, while hypnotherapists, who have—albeit unwittingly—used behavioral techniques for ages past, have done so neither in an organized manner nor with full knowledge of their potential.

A basic approach in behavior therapy involves contact with the feared object, situation or feeling, a graduated approach to this contact (except in flooding), motivating the patient to make this contact on a regular basis, and assisting him to reduce his fears by whatever means the therapist finds successful. However, exposure to the basic phobic unit (the lowest common denominator in many neurotic disorders) is not always possible. As Susskind points out, the evolution of behavior therapy brings with it the recognition that modern day behavioral practices are by no means simplistic.

Hypnosis can produce experiences most like real life and thus add another dimension to therapy. It makes treatment easier by relaxing the patient, easing the path to visual imagery, and providing techniques which aid in the management of more difficult subjects.

There are numerous overlapping techniques mutually available to the behavior therapist trained in hypnosis, and to the hypnotherapist trained in behavioral techniques, for the accomplishment of these tasks. Hypnotic vivification can intensify the visual image to a point where fantasy and reality blend and the patient lives through the exposure as if it were an *in vivo* experience. A statement given in the hypnotic state, such as "When I touch your shoulder, you will visualize it with ease and comfort," will often gently nudge the patient along.

Time distortion techniques can project a patient into the future and have him live through an anxious situation as if it was happening in the present. The patient comes out of the trance state with the feeling that he has been through all of this before and has progressed adequately. The induction of dreams by hypnosis, particularly if they are repetitive, is a useful desensitiza- tion device with graduated responses. Patients are given tasks to perform in the "dream state" and suggestions are paced to the progress of the patient, or the patient may be told to set the pace for himself.

By associating new and pleasant stimuli with the old response, it is possible to diminish general anxiety. At the conclusion of a session, posthypnotic suggestions to the effect that the patient will continue to feel relaxed and will carry out that which he per- formed in the sessions can be most helpful.

The hypnotherapist has much to gain by adding behavioral procedures to his armamentarium of therapeutic modalities, and will find no difficulty in adapting to this different orientation in order to use these techniques successfully. Much is to be gained by this sharing of knowledge, to the betterment of the patient and the satisfaction of the therapist.

SUBJECT INDEX

A

Abreaction, 114, 123, 229, 233, 288, 333, 334
Acceleration, 84, 96, 99, 103c
Acrophobia, 281
Age regression, 58, 63, 65, 133, 137, 150, 228–30, 232, 333, 353, 354
Aggression, 246, 332, 338
Agoraphobia, 22, 194
Air blast, 202
Air swallowing, 21
Alcoholism, xxi, 10, 11, 32, 33, 103, 165, 188, 191, 202, 203, 262, 286, 292, 332, 338, 342–48, 380
Alpha rhythm, 83, 86, 87, 374, 383
American Society of Clinical Hypnosis, 243
Amnesia, 26, 41, 47, 52, 53, 133, 150, 151, 153–55, 228, 298, 337, 339
  selective, 294
Amobarbital, 247
Amphetamine, 247
Analgesia, 150, 151
Anesthesia, 47, 51, 87, 88, 89, 103b, 153, 232, 275, 279
  glove, 279, 337, 339
Aneurysm, carotid, 343
Anger, 9, 13, 17, 54
Anguish, 97
Animal magnetism, xiv
Antianxiety drug, 22, 23
Antidepressant drug, 13, 15
Antipsychotic drug, 15
Anxiety, 5–10, 12, 14–17, 19–22, 31, 32, 113–20, 123–28, 136, 140, 166, 181, 183, 185, 196, 206, 208–17, 228, 234, 245, 247, 248, 250, 255–59, 272, 286, 293, 296, 307, 309, 312–15, 323–27, 330–32, 338–40, 344, 346, 350, 352–54,

Anxiety (*Continued*)
  356–58, 360, 361, 363, 370, 379, 384, 387
  free-floating, 31
  test, 146, 193, 236, 238–40, 272
Apomorphine, 202
Arm levitation, 30, 153, 164, 169, 170, 247, 380
Assertive training, 5, 9, 146, 185, 224, 251, 252, 257, 258, 285, 286, 307, 317, 330, 337, 363
Association, 16, 27, 42, 43, 51–55, 86, 100, 101, 124, 126, 139, 202, 272, 274, 292, 295–97, 303, 332, 359, 373, 381, 387
  covert, 249
  free, 6, 13, 275, 336
  letter, 6
Asthma, 103
Attention conditioning, 145
Attitude,
  subject, xv, 5, 72, 74, 148, 155, 156, 158–64, 172, 182, 193, 239, 240, 242, 244, 286, 300, 302, 232, 335, 340, 345, 359, 369
  therapist's, 186, 311, 383
Audiotape recording, 139–41
Audiogram, 87, 89
Autistic children, 379
Autogenic training, 381
Autohypnosis, 31, 106, 229, 232, 380, 381, 383
  (*See also* Self-hypnosis)
Automatic writing, 278–80, 359
Autonomic nervous system (ANS), 18, 43, 47, 87, 99, 100, 380, 382
Autosuggestion, 29, 31
Average evoked response, 91
Aversive conditioning, xx, 11, 33, 145, 150, 249, 255, 268, 269, 286, 299, 301, 303, 342–48, 382, 384

AUTHOR INDEX

A

Aaronson, B. S., 112, 236, 243
Abraham, H. A., 195, 199
Abramovitz, A., 17, 24
Abramovitz, C. M., 23
Abrams, S., 33, 69, 80, 198, 199, 292, 304
Agras, C., 252
Agras, W. S., 12, 18, 23, 24, 25, 29, 35, 157, 161, 163, 172, 176, 177, 191, 199
Akpinar, S., 373, 377
Alexander, L., vii, xix, 37, 39–44, 69, 80, 83, 103, 285, 286
American Academy of Psychotherapists Tape Library, 251
Anderson, W. L., 72, 82, 167, 178, 370
Appley, M. H., 284
Arnold, W. J., 177
As, A., 375
Ashem, B., 191, 199
Ascher, L. M., 194–6, 199, 375
Astrup, C., 252
Ayllon, T., 12, 23

B

Bailey, J. R., 371, 375
Balaschak, B., 371, 375
Ban, T., 252
Bandura, A., 12, 14, 23, 115, 128, 217
Barber, T. X., vii, xv, xx, 30, 32, 34, 64–6, 69–72, 74, 79, 80, 105, 112, 145, 148, 151–5, 157, 159, 160, 166, 167, 169, 170, 172–5, 178, 179, 181, 186, 337, 341, 369–72, 374, 375
Barlow, D. H., 157, 161, 172, 176, 191, 199
Baron, J., 370, 378
Barrett, C. L., 170, 173

Barrios, A. A., vii, xix, 37, 68, 69, 72, 74, 75, 78, 80, 81, 209, 217
Bass, M. J., 52, 56
Baumann, F., 295, 296, 305
Baxter, J. C., 125, 128
Baykushev, S. V., 72, 81
Beahrs, J. O., 286
Beecher, H. K., 18, 23
Bell, G. K., vii, xx, 146, 271
Bellak, L., 280, 283
Bendig, A. W., 117, 129
Bergin, A. E., 180, 187
Bernheim, H. M., 292, 305, 367, 375
Bertrand, A., xiv
Biddle, W. E., 69, 81
Bilz, R., 142
Birbaumer, N., 174
Black, S., xix, 83, 87, 88, 89, 90, 103
Blocker, K., 371, 375
Blum, G. S., 154, 173, 216, 338, 341
Borkovec, T. D., 29, 34, 161, 162, 173
Bower, G. H., 289, 291, 299, 303, 304, 305
Bowers, 216
Bracchi, F., xix, 83, 97, 103
Braid, J., xiv
Brenman, M., 127, 128, 280, 284, 367, 372, 376
Bridger, W. H., 217
Brock, L., 162, 163, 176
Brown, B. M., 160, 170, 174, 273, 276, 286, 292
Brown, H. A., 157, 174
Brown, J. E., vii, xxi, 33, 191, 200, 305, 342
Brown, W., 56
Brown, W. F., 243
Brownstein, A. J., 336, 341
Budzynski, T. H., 157, 174

H4